CASH'S TEXTBOOK OF ORTHOPAEDICS AND RHEUMATOLOGY FOR PHYSIOTHERAPISTS

Second Edition

First Edition edited by
Patricia A. Downie

SECOND EDITION EDITOR

MARIAN E. TIDSWELL

MA, BA, MCSP, DipTP, ONC

Oswestry and North Staffordshire
School of Physiotherapy
Oswestry
Shropshire
England

Mosby—Year Book Europe Limited

Copyright © 1992 Mosby–Year Book Europe Ltd
First edition published in 1984, reprinted 1988 and 1990,
by Faber and Faber Ltd
Printed by BPCC Hazells Ltd, Aylesbury, England.
ISBN 0 7234 1843 8

A CIP catalogue record for this book is available from the British
Library.

For full details of all Mosby–Year Book and Wolfe titles please write to
Mosby–Year Book Europe Ltd, Brook House, 2–16 Torrington Place,
London WC1E 7LT, England.

Contents

Foreword

This second edition has been completely revised in its present format, and is the work of the physiotherapy and medical staff of the Robert Jones and Agnes Hunt Orthopaedic Hospital, Oswestry and its associated Unit at the North Staffordshire Group of Hospitals. Authors from two University Departments, that of Birmingham and that of Keele, have also been involved.

These authors are national and international experts in this field and most of them have been welcomed as new authors to this edition.

The information contained covers the vast field of disorders and injuries of the neuro-muscular-skeletal system, and provides information of value not only to physiotherapists, but also to nurses and doctors involved in caring for people with such disorders and injuries.

Brian T. O'Connor
MS, MChOrth, FRCS, FRACS
Robert Jones Professor of Orthopaedics
in
The University of Birmingham
at
The Robert Jones and Agnes Hunt
Orthopaedic and District Hospital
Oswestry

Editor's Preface — First Edition

More than 30 years have passed since Joan Cash wrote *Physiotherapy in Medical Conditions* and *Physiotherapy in Some Surgical Conditions*. At first she wrote them herself seeking advice from medical and physiotherapy colleagues. As medicine and surgery became more specialised, as well as technical, she invited additional contributors to share their expertise in these two books.

Joan Cash recognised the growth of specialisation and from chapters in the original titles she developed first, *Neurology for Physiotherapists* and, then, *Chest, Heart and Vascular Disorders for Physiotherapists*. Now I, too, have felt the need to rationalise the present medical and surgical textbooks. They have both continued to grow haphazardly, with overlap and idiosyncratic division. It seemed logical that the orthopaedic, fracture and rheumatology chapters could come together, and so this title is born.

This has not been an easy volume to assemble and I am conscious of omissions and failures! Some of the chapters are technical and academic, others reflect the absolute practical approach by physiotherapists to their patients. Some are heavily referenced, others are not. Different approaches to the same problems are clearly evident, indicating the importance for the physiotherapist to understand the rationale of different treatments and then to apply what she considers is best for the individual patient, after consultation with the doctor.

What I hope I have done is to provide a solid background to that area of medicine which has, in the past, been described as 'carpentry on the human body'. While nuts, bolts and plates may indeed be used, and saws, files and levers are stock in trade instruments, the patient on whom these are used is a human being who requires an understanding approach. Some orthopaedic patients require little or no physiotherapy, but others require it over many months and, in some cases, years. This applies to the rheumatology patient also, and orthopaedic surgery is inextricably bound up with many of them: it is for this reason that a large section of the book is devoted to the clinical and physiotherapeutic management of those with a rheumatological disorder.

Readers will note that many of the contributors are from the Robert Jones and Agnes Hunt Orthopaedic Hospital, Oswestry.

Why so? First, when I devised this volume I wanted the contributors to be fully aware of the needs of students as well as trained therapists. Oswestry has a School of Physiotherapy, an Institute of Orthopaedics and a Department of Rheumatology — it seemed the perfect answer. Secondly, I admit it was a personal choice. I have long admired the pioneering role of Dame Agnes Hunt who started the cripples' home at Baschurch in 1900, and then interested Robert Jones, a Liverpool orthopaedic surgeon, to become the honorary surgeon to it. I have recently reread the *Heritage of Oswestry*, a private publication which describes the development of the hospital from its inception as the cripples' home to the world renowned centre it is today. There is an interesting mention of the beginning of the School of Physiotherapy:

> It is interesting to record that in 1918 Dame Agnes Hunt started what was then a Massage School with one Swedish Masseuse and three young ladies who were to combine this work, if they so desired, with a Housekeeping course, to take six months to complete. This School was taken over by Miss Dalton, who remained with the Hospital until 1945, and increased the course to one of 15 months.

In the early days, orthopaedics revolved round bone tuberculosis, osteomyelitis, rickets, bone-setting, etc.; later it was poliomyelitis and the devastations of war injuries; today it is joint replacement, bone transplants, biomechanical assessments, etc. In all this Oswestry has been in the forefront of teaching generations of surgeons, nurses and allied professionals.

It is invidious to select individuals for acknowledgement, but on this occasion I must. Professor Brian O'Connor, the present Robert Jones Professor of Orthopaedics at Oswestry, has been enthusiastic, helpful and persuasive as the needs demanded and I am most grateful. Mr Gordon Rose OBE, FRCS has been a respected adviser to physiotherapists for many years and I count it an honour that he has provided four chapters for this book as well as advising on others. From myself as editor, and for all the prospective readers, I extend to him our sincere thanks. Miss Winifred Cannell was Principal of the School of Physiotherapy based at Oswestry when this book was devised; she organised the Oswestry contributors, discussing content and timing, and in her well-earned retirement she has acted as the local co-ordinator. I am most grateful to her.

As in a previous title I accept full responsibility for including two chapters from Miss Sandy McLaren. They will be controversial to some purists, but they do show so clearly how enjoyment can be used to conquer the fear which so often hinders final restoration to activity.

I cannot forget the artists and photographers who have provided the many contributors with illustrative matter — I thank them all, but particularly the Photographic Department at Oswestry for many superlative pictures. Audrey Besterman, as ever, has laboured diligently on new drawings as well as providing a most helpful 'touching-up' service; for all of which I am indeed appreciative.

Without the great pioneers we should not, today, be able to provide so much skilled help to the physically disabled (the cripples of a past era), and in such a book as this it is right that we honour the memory of them: Hugh Owen Thomas, Robert Jones, Agnes Hunt, Gathorne Girdlestone, Rowley Bristow, George Perkins, Reginald Watson-Jones to name but a few. In my edition (the fourth) of *Fractures and Bone Injuries* by Reginald Watson-Jones there is a dedicatory quotation which sums up the gratitude we owe them and which we must never forget:

They, whose work cannot die, whose influence lives after them, whose disciples perpetuate and multiply their gifts to humanity, are truly immortal.

Patricia A. Downie, 1984
London

Editor's Preface — Second Edition

Editors of an original textbook have the unenviable task of selection from an extensive range of knowledge and skills, which are available and appropriate to the subject areas of relevance to the chosen title. The choice is made as to which areas will be included in the book, which will be emphasised, and inevitably, which shall be omitted.

Editors of later editions evaluate the choices made for the first edition and repeat the selection process. Some chapters will then be updated, new areas of knowledge will be commissioned and, with regret, some areas covered in previous editions will have to be omitted. So has it been with this second edition of *Orthopaedics and Rheumatology for Physiotherapists*. The first edition, edited by Patricia A. Downie, was published in 1984 and, in the intervening eight years between publications, orthopaedic practice has altered significantly in some areas, while other aspects of care that were appropriately included in the first edition have, with regret, been excluded from this text.

This edition, as with the first, has been written by members of staff currently practising in the National Health Service, the majority of the contributors, as before, being employees in departments or units based at the Robert Jones and Agnes Hunt Orthopaedic and District Hospital. The text reflects current practice at this world-renowned hospital. It will guide student physiotherapists towards appropriate management strategies for the range of situations encompassed by the text, and for qualified therapists, will provide indications as to when and how they should intervene to effect maximal therapeutic benefit for their patients. Several chapters have been submitted by consultant medical staff who provide the surgical, pathological and medical information about patients necessary for appropriate physiotherapeutic practice and we are grateful to the contributors.

A major omission from the first edition was detailed reference to the upper limb. By the inclusion of a chapter on Biomechanics of the Shoulder and another on Surgery and Associated Physiotherapeutic Management of Conditions Affecting Joints of the Upper Limb, this omission has been rectified, but the cost has been high. The Editor has, with regret, omitted from this text the chapter on Footwear as, with practice development, this area of responsibility is now seldom devolved to physiotherapists. The chapter on Traction has similarly been omitted as, with the development of sophisticated modern surgical immobilisation strategies, the need for extensive traction in routine trauma and orthopaedic patient management has been largely superseded. Traction has now been integrated in specific chapter texts as part of the relevant patient management strategy. The final area that has been excluded is that of Sports Injury as it is considered there are many comprehensive texts now available covering this aspect of physiotherapy.

The National Health Service is in the throes of significant reorganisation and the emphasis of practice is changing. With the increase in care in the community, physiotherapists must be confident in the knowledge they possess in order to treat a greater number of patients individually, outwith the facilities of a well-equipped department or gymnasium. In addition, physiotherapists need to be effective in final rehabilitation of patients who are to return to heavy manual work or vigorous sporting activities and this is tending to be lost from individual physiotherapist's repertoires. For these reasons, the two chapters by Miss Sandy McLaren have been included in this edition. As rehabilitation centres are closed, responsibility for these areas of practice are resumed by physiotherapy staff.

Management of chronic pain is now occupying a greater proportion of the physiotherapist's time, particularly in management of patients with disorders of the spine. A recent development, emerging from pain clinics, has been the School for Bravery approach to the management of chronic pain and it is appropriate that this area should be included in the book. Miss Ellingworth is a pioneer in this field and we are grateful for her contribution to the text.

I would like to thank the Institute of Orthopaedics at the Robert Jones and Agnes Hunt Orthopaedic and District Hospital for their continued support of this second edition: Professor Brian T. O'Connor, the present Robert Jones Professor of Orthopaedics at Oswestry, for his encouragement and enthusiasm, and all contributors for their text, photographs, artwork and tolerance over the years of gestation of this book.

Finally, I thank the staff at Mosby—Year Book Europe who have enabled completion and publication of this new edition.

Marian E. Tidswell, MA, BA, MCSP, DipTP, ONC, 1992
Oswestry and North Staffordshire School of Physiotherapy

List of Contributors

Mrs C.E. Apperley, MCSP
Formerly Senior Physiotherapist
Robert Jones and Agnes Hunt Orthopaedic and District Hospital
Oswestry SY10 7AG
England

Mrs A. Biggs, MCSP
Physiotherapist
Robert Jones and Agnes Hunt Orthopaedic and District Hospital
Oswestry SY10 7AG
England

Mrs P.B. Butler, MSc, MCSP
Research Physiotherapist
Institute of Orthopaedics
Robert Jones and Agnes Hunt Orthopaedic and District Hospital
Oswestry SY10 7AG
England

Dr R.C. Butler, MD, FRCP
Consultant Rheumatologist
Robert Jones and Agnes Hunt Orthopaedic and District Hospital
Oswestry SY10 7AG
England

Dr A.J. Darby, MB, BS, FRCPath
Consultant Histopathologist
Robert Jones and Agnes Hunt Orthopaedic and District Hospital
Oswestry SY10 7AG
England

Dr J.J. Dixey, MD, MRCP
Consultant Rheumatologist
Robert Jones and Agnes Hunt Orthopaedic and District Hospital
Oswestry SY10 7AG
England

Mrs V. Draycott, MCSP, ONC
Senior Physiotherapist
Robert Jones and Agnes Hunt Orthopaedic and District Hospital
Oswestry SY10 7AG
England

Mr S. Eisenstein, MB, BCh, PhD, FRCS(Ed)
Director
Department for Spinal Disorders
Institute of Orthopaedics
Robert Jones and Agnes Hunt Orthopaedic and District Hospital
Oswestry SY10 7AG
England

Miss C.M. Ellingworth, BSc, Grad.Dip.Phys., MCSP
Superintendent Physiotherapist
Doncaster Royal Infirmary
Doncaster DN2 5LT
England

Mr G.A. Evans, MB, BS, FRCS, FRCS(Ortho)
Consultant Orthopaedic Surgeon
Children's Orthopaedic Unit
Robert Jones and Agnes Hunt Orthopaedic and District Hospital
Oswestry SY10 7AG
England

Mrs E. Goss, MCSP
Senior Physiotherapist
Robert Jones and Agnes Hunt Orthopaedic and District Hospital
Oswestry SY10 7AG
England

Mr D. Jaffray, MB, ChB, FRCS(Ed)
Consultant Orthopaedic Surgeon
Robert Jones and Agnes Hunt Orthopaedic and District Hospital
Oswestry SY10 7AG
England

Mr A.M. Jamieson, MB, ChB, FRCS
Consultant Orthopaedic Surgeon
Robert Jones and Agnes Hunt Orthopaedic and District Hospital
Oswestry SY10 7AG
England

Mrs R. Jones, MCSP, ONC
Senior Physiotherapist
Robert Jones and Agnes Hunt Orthopaedic and District Hospital
Oswestry SY10 7AG
England

Mrs M. Kerr, MCSP
Senior Physiotherapist
Robert Jones and Agnes Hunt Orthopaedic and District Hospital
Oswestry SY10 7AG
England

Mrs K. Major, MCSP
Senior Physiotherapist
North Staffordshire Royal Infirmary
Princes Road
Hartshill
Stoke on Trent ST4 7LN
England

Miss S.H. McLaren, MCSP, DipPE
Formerly Superintendent Physiotherapist
The Hermitage Rehabilitation Centre
Chester-le-Street
County Durham DH2 3RF
England

Mr M.D. Northmore-Ball, MA, MB, BChir, FRCS
Consultant Orthopaedic Surgeon
Robert Jones and Agnes Hunt Orthopaedic and District Hospital
Oswestry SY10 7AG
England

Mr J.H. Patrick, MB, BS, FRCS
Director
Orthotic Research and Locomotor Assessment Unit
Robert Jones and Agnes Hunt Orthopaedic and District Hospital
Oswestry SY10 7AG
England

Mr E.R.S. Ross, FRCS, FRACS
Consultant Orthopaedic Surgeon
Wythenshawe Hospital
University of Manchester School of Medicine
Southmore Road
Manchester M23 9LT
England

Mr Rutter, BA, Dip Visual Communication
One Ash
West Lane
Chester-le-Street
County Durham DH3 3HZ
England

Mr J. Stallard, BTech, CENG, FIMECH, IMBES
Technical Director
Orthotic Research and Locomotor Assessment Unit
Robert Jones and Agnes Hunt Orthopaedic and District Hospital
Oswestry SY10 7AG
England

Mr P.B.M. Thomas, MB, BS, FRCS(Eng), FRCS(Ed)
Senior Lecturer in Traumatic Orthopaedic Surgery
University of Keele School of Post-Graduate Medicine and
Biological Sciences
Department of Traumatic Orthopaedic Surgery
North Staffordshire Hospital Centre
Hartshill
Stoke on Trent ST4 7QB
England

Dr D.J. Ward, MB, FRCP
Formerly Consultant Rheumatologist
Robert Jones and Agnes Hunt Orthopaedic and District Hospital
Oswestry SY10 7AG
England

1 The Mechanics of Lower Limb Orthoses

J. Stallard

Introduction

It is well known that mechanics are based on Newton's three Laws of Motion (Williams and Lissner, 1977a). Contrary to popular opinion, engineers do not constantly recite these to themselves and it is not suggested that therapists should either! However, Newton's Third Law is not only easy to remember, it is also self-evident and of great benefit to those who wish to have an elementary understanding of the subject. 'To every action there is an equal and opposite reaction.' What this means is that unless there is *resistance*, there cannot be *force*. If you pull with a force of 10 Newtons, then something must oppose that pull with the same force in order to maintain equilibrium.

Force

Force is the physical action which tends to change the position of a body in space. Some confusion exists about the units in which force can be expressed. Many different units have been used over the years, but the one which has been adopted as an International Standard is the Newton (N). An appropriate way of remembering the magnitude of 1N is to think of it as approximately the force which one apple (from which Newton developed his ideas!) exerts at rest under the influence of gravity. Thus a lightweight man would weigh between 600–800N.

In orthotics, force derives from two main sources: muscles and gravity. These can combine with other mechanical systems to produce force from stored energy (springs, etc.) or from inertial reaction, which will be discussed in more detail later.

Since force always acts along a straight line it may be represented graphically by a line, the length of which is proportional to the *magnitude* of force, the *direction* of which corresponds to that of the force, the start of which represents the *point of application* of force. Drawing this line (a vector) is a convenient way of indicating the effect of a force applied to a mechanical system. The application of force by a therapist on the lower limb of a patient (*Figure 1.1(a)*) can be represented vectorally (*Figure 1.1(b)*), as can the reaction (the equal and opposite force of the leg on the hand (*Figure 1.1(c)*).

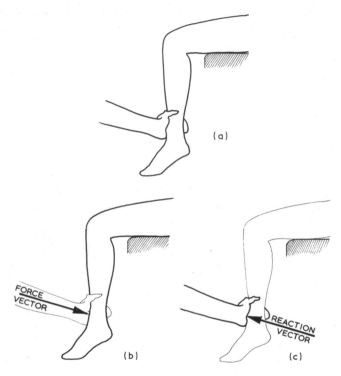

Figure 1.1. Representation of force by a vector.

The weight of the body acts vertically downwards. There is necessarily an equal and opposite force and this is known as the *ground reaction force*, which can be represented vectorally (*Figure 1.2*).

Centre of gravity, or *centre of mass*, is defined as the point in a RIGID BODY at which the mass may be considered to act. While it may be appropriate to use this concept for individual body segments, it can be misleading when applied to the whole body, which is multisegmental with freely articulated interconnections.

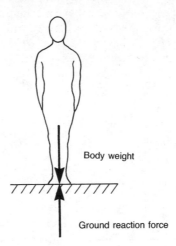

Body weight

Ground reaction force

Figure 1.2. Body weight and ground reaction force.

Moments

A force system is rarely simple since it is frequently a combination of forces, and because secondary effects (most commonly moments) also occur. In order to gain some understanding of the problems that result, it is convenient to examine the problem of an unstable knee caused by extensor paralysis. Every therapist knows that with the knee fully extended the lower limb can support the weight of the body even when it is muscularly deficient (*Figure 1.3(a)*). They further know that when this same knee is put into a small degree of flexion (*Figure 1.3(b)*), it collapses under the weight which it is carrying. The reason this happens is that the weight of the body acting vertically downwards produces a *moment* about the knee — the direction of which changes when the knee moves from full extension into flexion.

A *moment* is the action of a force which tends to cause rotation of a body about a point (known as the fulcrum or moment centre). When giving passive movements to the elbow (*Figure 1.4*) the therapist applies a force some way from the fulcrum (the elbow joint) in order to cause the forearm to rotate about the elbow. The farther away from the fulcrum the force is applied, the easier it is to produce the turning effect. A *moment* is *force* (F) multiplied by the perpendicular *distance* (L) from the line of force to the fulcrum or moment centre (*Figure 1.4*).

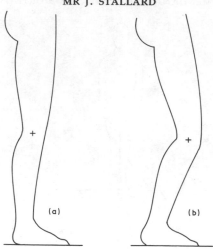

Figure 1.3. Knee in (a) extension; (b) flexion.

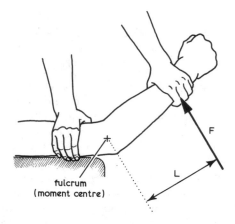

fulcrum
(moment centre)

Figure 1.4. Turning moment about the elbow joint. Applying passive
movements to the elbow. Moment = F × L.

In (*Figure 1.5(a)*) the moment produced about the knee from
the shoe (the weight which acts vertically downwards) is 10N ×
40cm = 400Ncm. However, this ignores the weight of the shank
of the lower limb, which is itself heavy and very significant. In
order to understand the turning effect of the shank it is necessary
to know where its centre of mass is located. *Centre of mass* is the
point at which the mass of a body is considered to be concentrated
and is the point of perfect balance (Williams and Lissner, 1977b).
Figure 1.5(b) shows the same leg without the boot, with the centre

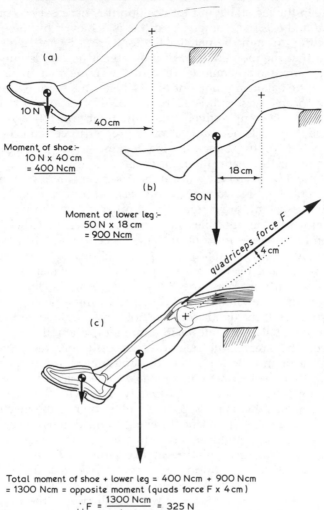

Figure 1.5. Balancing a moment about the knee with the quadriceps muscle. The circles indicate the centre of gravity for (a) shoes; (b) shank and foot, and (c) these combined.

of mass marked at 18cm horizontal distance from the knee centre and the weight of the shank indicated as 50N. In the position shown the shank produces a moment of 900Ncm (i.e. 50N × 18cm). Thus the overall effect when the shoe is worn is shown in *Figure 1.5(c)* and the total moment about the knee is the summation of the two effects, which gives a moment of 1300Ncm.

To keep the leg stable in that position it is necessary to provide an *equal* and *opposite* moment, and this is achieved by the quadriceps acting through the patellar tendon. From *Figure 1.5(c)* it can be seen that the moment arm of the patellar tendon is only 4cm, and by simple mathematics we can determine that in order to produce the balancing moment of 1300Ncm, the force with which the quadriceps must pull is 325N (i.e. 325N × 4cm = 1300Ncm). Notice that the comparatively small moment arm through which the quadriceps acts demands a much greater force than the combined action of the boot and leg weight acting through their respective much greater moment arms.

Care must be exercised with units when considering moments. *Force* units, e.g. Newton (N) and *moment* units, e.g. Newton centimetres (Ncm), are different and must *not* be confused.

To return to the unstable knee: it can be seen that the ground reaction force passes in front of the knee centre when the knee is fully extended (*Figure 1.6(a)*). This produces an extending moment which is resisted by the posterior capsule thus maintaining the knee in extension. With the knee in flexion, the line of force passes behind the knee centre, thus producing a flexing moment (*Figure 1.6(b)*). If the quadriceps are not active, or are insufficiently powerful to balance that flexing moment, then the knee will collapse. The greater the degree of knee flexion, the larger the moment arm and the less likely the quadriceps are to cope.

The orthotic solution to an unstable knee is almost axiomatic, and a long-leg caliper is universally fitted to the flail knee (*Figure 1.6(c)*). What is perhaps less well known is the mechanical effect of this device. The cliché 'three-point fixation' is oft repeated, and is true enough, but it obscures to many people the real effect. Newton's Third Law will reveal everything. 'To every action there is an equal and opposite reaction.' When a fixed flexion deformity occurs it is inevitable that a knee-flexing moment will be produced, the magnitude of which will rise as the degree of flexion deformity increases. Without a caliper, a flail knee with flexion deformity has an unbalanced flexing moment applied to it which is equal to body weight (W) multiplied by the perpendicular distance (L) from the knee (*Figure 1.6(b)*). When the orthosis is applied it resists this unbalanced moment by producing an *equal* and *opposite* moment through *three-point fixation* (*Figure 1.6(c)*). Anyone who has ever broken a stick over his knee will understand how this is effective in producing a 'bending' effect (*Figure 1.7*).

If it can be arranged that the line of force acting at the knee passes directly through its centre, then clearly no moment would be applied. When a long-leg caliper is fitted to an unstable knee with a full range of movement, it is set so that negligible moments are produced about the knee. In this situation the orthosis is

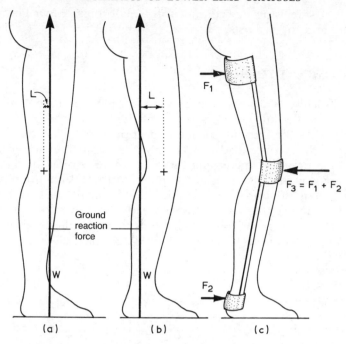

Figure 1.6. *Balancing a moment about the knee with a caliper.*

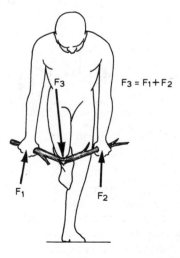

Figure 1.7. *The bending effect of three-point fixation.*

merely a stabilising device and only small forces occur between the leg and the orthosis.

Interface pressure

One difficulty which can occur with a caliper is high interface pressure at the knee or, less often, at the thigh band.

Pressure is the intensity of loading applied to a particular area (*Figure 1.8*). A large load concentrated on a small area will give very high pressure. Increasing the area, or decreasing the load, is the only way in which pressure can be reduced. With any type of bracing it is advisable to minimise the applied loads as far as possible, and at the same time spread them over the greatest possible area. It is for this reason that, for example, thigh bands on calipers should be made as broad as is practical.

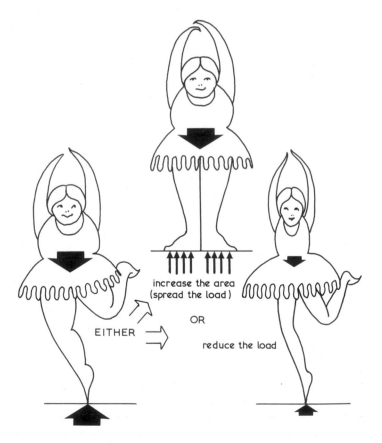

Figure 1.8. Pressure: the distribution of load.

To reduce pressure further, the forces F_1, F_2 and F_3, required to achieve stabilisation of the knee, can be minimised by increasing to a maximum the moment arm through which F_1 and F_2 act (*Figure 1.6(c)*). Moments are a product of both force and moment arm, and increasing or decreasing one has the opposite effect on the magnitude of the other to maintain the same moment. Thus it is in the interest of the patient to locate the thigh band as high as possible since this will decrease not only F_1 but also F_3, because (as indicated by Newton's Third Law) $F_3 = F_1 + F_2$. *Figure 1.9* gives a comparison of forces for different application points on a long-leg brace.

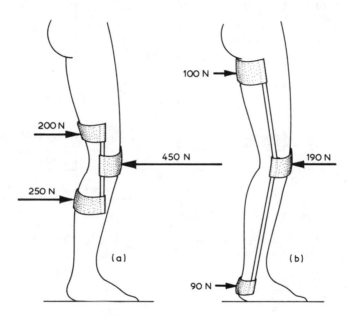

Figure 1.9. The beneficial effect of long lever arms.

Another well-known fact is that 'the higher the degree of knee flexion deformity, the larger the forces required to suport the leg'. Once it is understood how the unbalanced moment about the knee centre is developed, then the reason becomes obvious. As was stated earlier, the line of ground reaction force passes behind the flexed knee centre (*Figure 1.10(a)*). With larger flexion deformities the moment arm from knee centre to line of action of force increases (*Figures 1.10(b) and 1.10(c)*). Even though nothing else changes (body weight must stay the same) this increases the flexing moment about the knee in proportion with the increased moment arm, and a consequent increase in stabilising forces occurs.

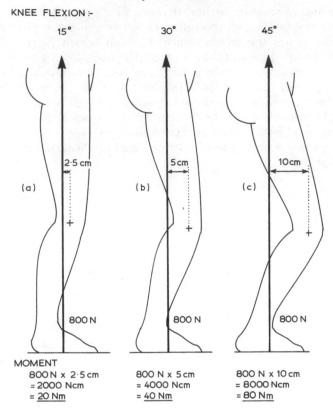

KNEE FLEXION :-

15°   30°   45°

(a)   2·5 cm   (b)   5 cm   (c)   10 cm

800 N   800 N   800 N

MOMENT

800 N x 2·5 cm	800 N x 5 cm	800 N x 10 cm
= 2000 Ncm	= 4000 Ncm	= 8000 Ncm
= 20 Nm	= 40 Nm	= 80 Nm

Figure 1.10. The increase in bending moment with increasing knee flexion (the vertical arrows represent the ground reaction force).

Resolution of forces

Patients who use calipers frequently need also to use crutches. These have two primary functions:

- To improve stability by increasing support area.
- To provide a means of propulsion through ground reaction forces.

In both of these functions it is necessary for the crutch to apply forces to the ground, and this is generally done through the handle along the axis of the crutch. During ambulation the crutches are always sloping, which means that the applied forces are never perpendicular relative to the ground. The implication of this is that there must be a proportion of the overall force which acts *vertically* and a further proportion which acts *horizontally* with the ground (*Figure 1.11*). Provided that the magnitude and direction of the force along the crutch axis is known, it is possible to determine these two 'components' of that force by simple manipulation of its vector representation. This is done by dropping a perpendicular line from the 'top' end of the vector and drawing a horizontal line from the other end (*Figure 1.11*). The point of intersection of these two lines will show their magnitude − the direction of force being indicated by following the 'component' vectors around from the top to meet the other end of the overall force vector.

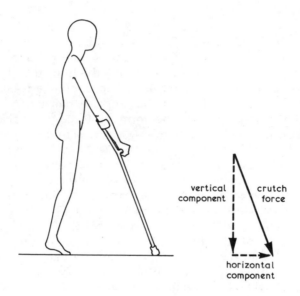

Figure 1.11. The resolution of crutch force.

Friction

From Newton's Third Law it can be seen that for a horizontal component of crutch force to exist, there must be an *equal* and *opposite* force. This comes from the friction between the crutch tip and the floor surface. Without this frictional opposing force the crutch would slide on the floor surface and fail to fulfil its function. *Coefficient of friction* describes the frictional properties which exist between two surfaces (*Figure 1.12*). Clearly it is in the

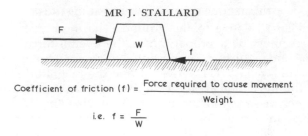

Coefficient of friction (f) = $\dfrac{\text{Force required to cause movement}}{\text{Weight}}$

i.e. $f = \dfrac{F}{W}$

Figure 1.12. Coefficient of friction.

patient's interest that crutches should resist slipping, and so the tips are made from a high friction material such as rubber.

Stability

Stability, which crutches can help to provide, is vital for any form of ambulation, an activity which requires both intrinsic and extrinsic stability. *Intrinsic stability* prevents the human body (which is a multi-segmental structure) from collapsing under itself. Where muscular deficiency exists — for example a flail hip or knee — then orthotic assistance in the form of three-point fixation is required. In the static situation, *extrinsic stability* ensures that an intrinsically stable body does not topple over. This means that the centre of mass, when projected vertically downwards, must be contained within the support area of the body.

An illustration of three forms of extrinsic stability can usefully be gained from the study of a cone (*Figure 1.13*). On its point a cone will require only tiny movements sideways to take the centre of mass outside the support area. This is known as *unstable equilibrium*. When lying on its side, the cone may be rolled and the centre of mass then follows the support area so that it takes up a new position of equilibrium: this is known as *neutral equilibrium*. However, when a cone which is standing on its base is tilted it will drop back to its original position, as long as the centre of mass does not pass outside the support area. This is known as *stable equilibrium*. Once the centre of mass goes beyond the outside edge of the cone it loses its stable equilibrium and falls on to its side. More interesting is the concept of degrees of stability within the category of stable equilibrium. This can be considered with a funnel standing on its large and small ends (*Figure 1.14(a)*). Standing on the small end requires a much smaller angular movement before stability is lost (*Figure 1.14(b)*) than when the funnel is standing on the large end (*Figure 1.14(c)*). The more stable situation is better able to resist external disturbances.

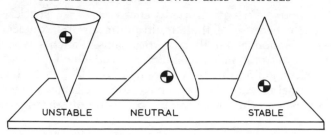

Figure 1.13. Stability: conditions of equilibrium.

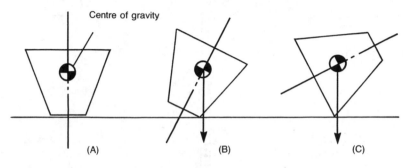

Figure 1.14.

Walking aids

Walking aids fall into three categories and can perform a number of functions. The categories are:

- Sticks.
- Crutches.
- Frames.

The functions include:

- Provision of increased extrinsic stability.
- A means of exerting propulsive forces.
- Part of the intrinsic stabilisation system.

Sticks
Sticks give the lowest level of assistance and in most cases provide a degree of increased *extrinsic stability* by enlarging the support area. They also enable some injection of *propulsive force* by reacting against the ground through the arm (or arms).

The tripod and quadropod sticks are a special case (*Figure 1.15*): because of their multi-point ground contact, they can resist rotation about their vertical axis. Patients who have difficulty with rotational instability around the hips find that these particular aids can be of great assistance. In addition to their rotational reaction they also have some resistance to forward or side thrust and this enhances the provision of *extrinsic stability*.

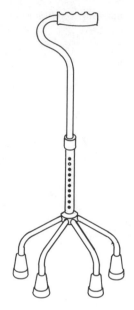

Figure 1.15. A quadropod stick.

Crutches

Crutches provide support across at least one joint in the arm. There are three main types: axillary, Canadian and elbow crutches (*Figure 1.16*). Axillary and Canadian crutches cross both the wrist and elbow joints, and give patients a greater level of stability. In contrast elbow crutches cross only the wrist joint, and as such they, of the three main types, least enhance patient stability.

Crutches are usually grounded at points farther from the body than are sticks, and because of this give larger support areas. This, coupled with better arm stabilisation, means that they provide a higher level of *extrinsic stability* (*Figure 1.17*).

For patients who use long-leg calipers and have no hip control (e.g. paraplegics with lesions at lumbar-1 level and above) crutches

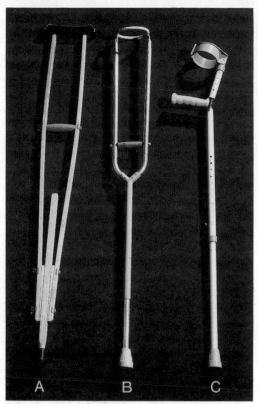

Figure 1.16. Crutch types: A, axillary; B, Canadian; C, elbow.

form an important part of the *intrinsic stabilisation* system. By leaning forward to support themselves on the crutches they ensure that the applied forces produce an extending moment about the hips (*Figure 1.18*). This condition must be satisfied at all times for such patients. It is a difficult feat and explains why so few paraplegics are able to ambulate with long-leg calipers.

In addition to providing stability, crutches enable patients to exert *propulsive forces*. The most common means of achieving this is for the arms to pull against the crutches – the equal and opposite reactive forces being the crutch tip/ground interface friction. It is essential for patients to have intact latissimus dorsi muscles if they are to generate these forces, for it is the arms pulling towards the body under their influence which causes the crutch to react against the ground.

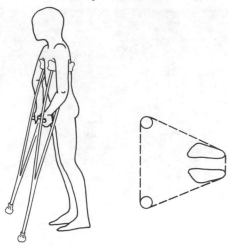

Figure 1.17. The support area provided by crutches. The extrinsic stabilisation is improved with crutches because of the increased support area.

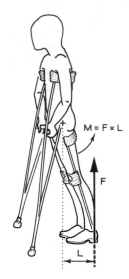

Figure 1.18. Stabilising flail hips with crutches. M = moment; F = force; L = length.

Frames

The third category, namely frames, comes in a variety of forms (pulpit frames, Rollators, etc.). They all provide a large support area for improved *extrinsic stability*. Since many of these enable patients also partially to 'suspend' themselves in the frame using their arms, they can additionally improve *intrinsic stabilisation*. All types of frame have good contact points, which make it possible to inject *propulsive forces*. Some (e.g. the Rollator) also incorporate wheels so that frictional resistance is greatly reduced when support points are lifted from the ground, thus making it easier to push the device forward to begin the next phase of the gait cycle.

Stabilisation of the foot

The weight-bearing foot has a condition of stable equilibrium. As it supinates (*Figure 1.19*) the point of application of ground reaction force moves towards the outer border of the calcaneus (3) and fifth toe (2). Stability will be retained until the point of application reaches the border of the support area. At this point stability becomes uncertain and collapse may occur because the moment from the forces acting on the body can change from being corrective into one which increases supination.

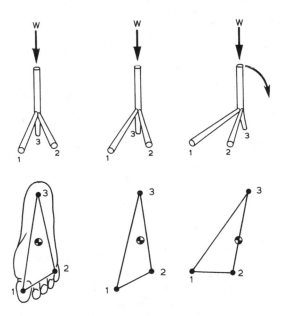

Figure 1.19. Stability of the foot in supination. 1 = great toe; 2 = fifth toe; 3 = calcaneus; W = body-weight (the quartered circles show the point of application of the ground reaction force).

Limited range in the subtalar joint means that this does not normally occur in pronation. However, in the rheumatoid foot the centre of mass can move outside the line 3–1 (*Figure 1.19*) if the disease is in an advanced stage. When this happens an orthosis of the type shown in *Figure 1.20* is necessary if the patient is to walk. As can be seen from the diagrammatic representation (*Figure 1.20(a)*), the resolution of forces tends to pull the strap down the outside iron and pull the foot (represented by the cone) towards the iron. Thus in order to make the orthosis work effectively it is necessary to put a loop on the outside iron (*Figure 1.20(b)*) to provide the *equal* and *opposite* force to the vertical component and a wedge in the shoe to oppose the horizontal component of the strap force.

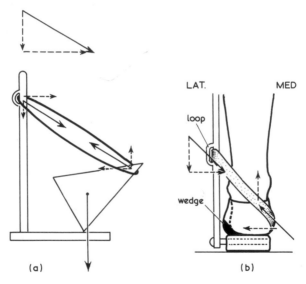

Figure 1.20. Stabilising the pronated foot.

Dynamic forces

One of the aims of a lower limb orthosis is to enable patients to walk. This is, in mechanical terms, a dynamic activity in that forces over and above those required to maintain the status quo (i.e., the 'static' situation) are involved. When a change of state occurs, such as starting to walk from standing still or changing speed and direction when walking, extra force is required to bring that about. While it is possible to determine the magnitude of these increased forces, given the various parameters, the mathematics can be complex and it is really only necessary for therapists to understand the effect of dynamic situations.

During walking, the centre of mass rises and falls and also sways from side to side. This implies that the body is accelerated upwards and downwards and from side to side. The force required to raise the body upwards is over and above that of body weight, and in order to permit the body to fall back again the force of the body on the ground must be less than body weight. Swaying of the body sideways is brought about by small side-thrust forces on the ground.

Thus it can be seen that the ground forces involved in walking are quite complex. The forces are monitored by a force platform (force plate). This is flat rigid plate, set flush into a walkway, which registers components of force applied to the top surface. The use of force platforms over more than 40 years has established the levels and patterns of the various components of ground reaction force for normal walking. For convenience, ground reaction force is split into three components:

- The vertical (Fz).
- Horizontal in line of walking (Fy).
- Horizontal at right angles to line of walking (Fx).

Typical patterns for normal steady pace walking are shown in *Figure 1.21.*

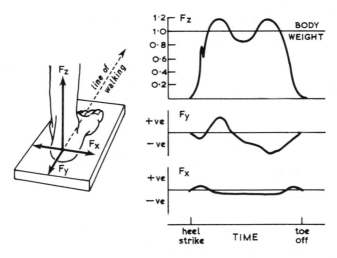

Figure 1.21. Ground reaction forces in walking. Fz = vertical; Fy = horizontal in line of walking; Fx = horizontal at right angles to line of walking.

Notice that Fz (the vertical component) rises to approximately 1.2 body weight just after heel strike, drops to around 0.8 body weight at mid-stance and rises again at the end of single stance phase – once again to approximately 1.2 body weight. For running, a different pattern of Fz emerges and the force on the lower limb can rise to almost 3 × body weight (*Figure 1.22*).

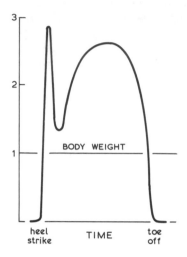

Figure 1.22. Vertical ground reaction force in running.

In the normal leg, these dynamic forces put greater demands on the bones, tendons and muscles. However, with a braced lower limb, the orthosis also has to bear the increased burden. Many patients perform swing-through gait when wearing calipers and this introduces forces greater than those experienced in reciprocal ambulation (Stallard *et al.*, 1978a; 1980). The design of orthotic devices must reflect the need to withstand the extra forces involved in the dynamic activities which are undertaken by patients.

Work done and energy

One of the reasons for treating patients by physical therapy or orthotics is to enable them to get some work done. In mechanics the term 'work done' has a very specific meaning and it involves moving bodies. *Work done* is the *force* applied to a body multiplied by the *distance* through which the body moves under the influence of and in the direction of that *force* (*Figure 1.23*). An object can be

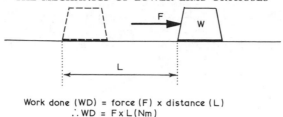

Work done (WD) = force (F) x distance (L)
∴ WD = F x L (Nm)

Figure 1.23. The definition of work done.

pushed extremely hard, but unless it moves no 'work' will be 'done'.

On the other hand *energy* is the ability to do *'work'* and has the same unit (Nm) as *work done*. There are many forms of energy:

- Biochemical energy (muscles).
- Stored energy (stretched springs).
- Kinetic energy (motion − momentum).
- Heat.
- Potential energy (gravity), etc.

Clearly the act of walking involves doing *work* and expending the various forms of *energy* available to the body (biochemical, kinetic and potential energy in particular), and it is the interchange of *energy* to *work done* which is at the heart of mechanical *dynamic* systems. The *efficiency* with which we move is the *ratio of work done to energy expended.*

Inertial forces

Any object tends to retain the mechanical state in which it finds itself. This *resistance to change* is known as *inertia*, and dynamic forces are required to overcome this effect. When running to catch a bus, it takes an effort to slow down and stop. That is because of the momentum of the running body and its inertia. To every action, Newton states, there is an equal and opposite reaction, and the reactive effect to forces applied to overcome inertia is known as *inertial reaction*. This effect is an integral and important part of walking. At the end of swing phase for example, the hip extensors apply a decelerative force on the swing leg, and this in turn produces an inertial reaction on the trunk which pulls it forward in space.

Any orthosis applied to the lower limb will alter the dynamics of walking. The increase in weight of the 'lower limb system' will obviously increase its inertia and so affect the inertial reaction. Long-leg braces prevent knee flexion, and this limits the ability of the patient to 'smooth out' the rise and fall of the centre of mass during walking. Thus the amount of energy required to walk will be increased and the overall efficiency of ambulation decreased.

Conclusion

Much research is being done to establish more efficient forms of walking for the heavily handicapped. Orthotics can play a major part in this, and a number of devices have been developed within the Robert Jones and Agnes Hunt Orthopaedic Hospital, Oswestry, to enable the paralysed to walk more effectively (Davies and Lucas, 1977; Rose, 1979; Rose et al., 1981; Stallard et al., 1978b; Stallard et al., 1986a; Stallard et al., 1986b; Butler and Major, 1987; Beckman, 1987; Summers et al., 1988.

Attention to detail by therapists can improve the efficiency of their patients. Careful consideration should be given to orthotic devices and walking aids. Even the type of crutch used to perform swing-through gait can affect the efficiency of the patient. Dounis et al. (1980) and Sankarankutty et al. (1979) showed that Canadian crutches are the most efficient for swing-through gait. The need to quantify performance is increasingly a requirement and new techniques of monitoring ambulation for various levels of ability are becoming available. Functional performance can be established, even in high levels of handicap, using the concept of physiological cost index (PCI; Butler et al., 1984) and the effect of ground reaction forces on the joints of the lower limb can be easily monitored using a video vector generator (Stallard, 1987).

References

Beckmann, J. (1987). The Louisiana State University reciprocating gait orthosis. Physiotherapy, 73(8), 393—397.

Butler, P.B., Englebrecht, M., Major, R.E., Tait, J.H., Stallard, J., and Patrick, J.H. (1984). Physiological Cost Index of walking for normal children and its use as an indicator of physical handicap. Developmental Medicine and Child Neurology, 26, 607—612.

Butler, P.B. and Major, R.E. (1987). The ParaWalker: A rational approach to the provision of reciprocal ambulation for paraplegic patients. Physiotherapy, 73(8), 393—397.

Davies, J.B. and Lucas, D. (1977). The Salop Skate. *Physiotherapy*, **63**(4), 112–115.

Dounis, E., Stevenson, R.D., and Wilson, R.S.E. (1980). The use of a portable oxygen consumption meter (Oxylog) for assessing the efficiency of crutch walking. *Journal of Medical Engineering and Technology*, **4**(6), 296–298.

Rose, G.K. (1979). The principles and practice of hip guidance articulations. *Prosthetics and Orthotics International*, **3**, 37–43.

Rose, G.K., Stallard, J., and Sankarankutty, M. (1981). Clinical evaluation of spinal bifida patients using hip guidance orthosis. *Developmental Medicine and Child Neurology*, **23**, 30–40.

Sankarankutty, M., Stallard, J. and Rose, G.K. (1979). The relative efficiency of 'swing through' gait on axillary, elbow and Canadian crutches compared to normal walking. *Journal of Biomedical Engineering*, **1**, 55–57.

Stallard, J. (1987). Assessment of the mechanical function of orthoses by force vector visualisation. *Physiotherapy*, **73**(8), 398–402.

Stallard, J., Sankarankutty, M., and Rose, G.K. (1978a). Lower-limb vertical ground reaction forces during crutch walking. *Journal of Medical Engineering and Technology*, **2**(4), 201–202.

Stallard, J., Rose, G.K., and Farmer, I.R. (1978b). The ORLAU Swivel Walker. *Prosthetics and Orthotics International*, **2**, 35–42.

Stallard, J., Dounis, E., Major, R.E., and Rose, G.K. (1980). One leg swing through gait using two crutches. *Acta Orthopaedica Scandinavica*, **51**, 71–77.

Stallard, J., Farmer, I.R., Poiner, R., Major, R.E., and Rose, G.K. (1986a). Engineering design considerations of the ORLAU Swivel Walker. *Engineering in Medicine*, **15**(1), 3–8.

Stallard, J., Major, R.E., Poiner, R., Farmer, I.R., and Jones, N. (1986b). Engineering design considerations of the ORLAU ParaWalker and FES hybrid system. *Engineering in Medicine*, **15**(3), 123–129.

Summers, B.N., McClelland, M.R., El Masri, W.S. (1988). A clinical review of the adult hip guidance orthosis (ParaWalker) in traumatic paraplegics. *Paraplegia*, **26**, 19–26.

Williams, N. and Lissner, H.R. (1977a). *Biomechanics of Human Movement*, ch 2, p 10. W.B. Saunders Co, Philadelphia.

Williams, N. and Lissner, H.R. (1977b). *Biomechanics of Human Movement*, ch 2, p 8. W.B. Saunders Co, Philadelphia.

Bibliography

American Academy of Orthopaedic Surgeons (1975). *Atlas of Orthotics: Biomechanical Principles and Applications.* C.V. Mosby Co, St Louis.

Brunnstrom, S. and Dickinson, R. (1977). *Clinical Kinesiology*, 3rd edition. F.A. Davis Co, Philadelphia.

Carlsoo, S. (1972). *How Man Moves.* William Heinemann Limited, London.

D'Astrous, J.D. (ed) (1981). *Orthotics and Prosthetics Digest.* Edahl Productions, Ottawa.

Day, B.H. (1972) *Orthopaedic Appliances.* Faber and Faber, London. (Out of print; available in libraries.)

Department of Health and Social Security (1980). *Classification of Orthoses.* HMSO, London.

Frankel, V.H. and Burstein, A.H. (1970). *Orthopaedic Biomechanics.* Lea and Febiger, Philadelphia.

Freeman, M.A.R. (1973). *Adult Articular Cartilage.* Pitman Medical, London.

Frost, H.M. (1973). *Orthopaedic Biomechanics.* Chas Thomas, Springfield, Illinois.

Kennedy, J.M. (1974). *Orthopaedic Splints and Appliances.* Baillière Tindall, London.

McCollough, N.C. (1978). Orthotic management in adult hemiplegia. *Clinical Orthopaedics,* (131), 38.

Murdoch, Geo. (ed) (1976). *The Advance in Orthotics.* Edward Arnold (Publishers) Limited, London.

Rehabilitation Engineering Centre, Moss Rehabilitation Hospital. *Lower Limb Orthotics — A Manual.* Temple University, Drexel University, Philadelphia.

Rose, G.K. (1980). Orthoses for the severely handicapped — rational or empirical choice? *Physiotherapy,* **66**(3), 76—81.

Stewart, J.D.M. (1975). *Traction and Orthopaedic Appliances.* Churchill Livingstone, Edinburgh.

Tohen, Z.A. (1973). *Manual of Mechanical Orthopaedics (Prosthetics and Orthotics).* Chas Thomas, Springfield, Illinois.

Williams, N. and Lissner, H.R. (1977). *Biomechanics of Human Movement.* W.B. Saunders Co, Philadelphia.

2 Biomechanics of Gait

J.H. Patrick

Introduction

The *Oxford English Dictionary* definition of gait is 'the manner of walking, bearing or carriage as one walks'. Locomotion is commonly used as a synonymous term — literally 'the power of motion from place to place', but is obviously a term with a wider application since it would include inanimate motion. The term gait implies mobility using limbs, and our interest is in bipedal gait, rather than that of a four-legged animal. The erect human form has given man great evolutionary advantage — the development of his special senses helped by massive brain convolution and growth, together with the freeing of the arms and the use of the hands and thumb to produce dexterity in manipulation of his surroundings. To be safe in ancient society, primitive man had to move over a varied terrain, both flat and mountainous, slowly to gather food, and often quickly to avoid capture or danger. The co-ordination of the special senses with the ordering of limb muscle (and trunk) movement, and with the necessary cardio-pulmonary support, can be traced by any parent watching the process of learning to walk in a baby about one year old.

It is worth pointing out at this stage that the immense nervous feedback to allow control of our walking is highly 'redundant'. One can explain the concept best by thinking of a stroke victim who learns to walk again. No longer does he have a normal gait, but he can move. Maybe he now has to recruit trunk musculature to circumduct the hip for progression, or use a stick to assist a weakened hip abductor, but retains mobility. By suitable compensations he can walk, but is less liable to succeed if furthur difficulties or disability occur. In Duchenne dystrophy, the lordotic lumbar posture and equinus walk are compensations for increasing weakness in the hip and knee extensors. If the knee or hip should flex, for any reason, stability of the trunk over the foot is lost and collapse occurs. Tendo achilles lengthening can have serious effects on the knee by leaving it flexed; walking is then lost. The manner of our walking can be divided into sections for study and understanding. Clearly all parts interrelate.

Lower limb functions

Functions of the lower limbs include:

- Obviously to support the trunk, head and upper limbs.
- By movement, the legs produce a propulsive force to get us around.
- To conserve energy during movement.

    Inman (1981) showed that energy conservation was of major importance. Even the smallest adult will raise and lower his body centre of gravity as little as possible. We know that climbing up several flights of stairs is tiring. Similarly during a stride (defined as one full cycle of left heel strike through (R) foot strike and on to (L) heel strike again), the body centre of gravity rises and falls. In *Figure 2.1* to move forwards from pelvic position at X requires the opposite swinging leg and the remainder of the body to be raised to Y. Instinctively we choose the most energy-efficient method of doing this, and the rise of the centre of gravity is at most 2cm; but in disease states it is often more, shown most dramatically in the paraplegic three-point, or swing-through, gait with crutches. We prevent too much sideways movement also, again to conserve this precious energy. Our preferred walking speed and cadence (number of steps per minute) remain remarkably the same, because of this conservation policy.

- The legs are used as shock-absorbers. This may seem obvious since they hit the ground alternately, but several protective

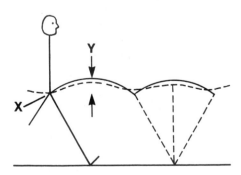

Figure 2.1. Vaulting action of stance leg considered as a non-articulated limb. Note the large rise and fall and jerky acceleration/deceleration produced compared with the normal relatively smooth sinusoidal curve with much less amplitude. This makes clear the 'uphill' phase which requires the injection of energy, largely returned in the downhill, and spilling over to the next uphill as an inertial contribution.

mechanisms exist to lower the force imparted to the skeleton. For example, during jumping this force rises to over eight times the body weight. The heel pad of fatty skin is very 'elastic' and compresses under load, then expands. Eccentric contraction of the ankle extensors and quadriceps muscles helps to dissipate the shock of sudden deceleration at the beginning of the stance phase (loading response).

Essential requirements of gait

Three mandatory aspects of locomotion need to be present:

1. The multisegmented structure we call the skeleton needs to be stabilised. *Intrinsic stabilisation* confers to the 'bag of bones' of the

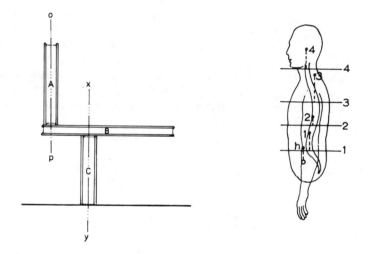

Figure 2.2. (left) Three books in a balanced stable position. The general centre of mass line x−y is irrelevant when considering the stability of the 'joint' between books A and B. The centre of mass of A lies in line O−P; it is within the support area of A which is therefore stable on B.

Figure 2.3. (right) Considering balance stability about any joint, it will be clear from Figure 2.2 that the only relevant centre of mass is that of all the portion of the body above that joint. Lines h1, 2, 3 and 4 correspond to hip, lumbo-sacral, thoraco-lumbar, mid-thoracic and mid-cervical articulations, and it will be seen that the centre of mass of the relevant portion of the body is above their respective articulations. Therefore, although the human spine is curved, each segment is in fact balanced on the one below it, and requires no muscular effort to support this. It does require muscle activity to maintain the balance.

lower limb a connection through joints, one with another. To conserve muscle energy the limb bones 'stand' one on top of another by balance in the same manner as the three books in Figure 2.2. The books do not fall over since the centre of mass of book A lies in the line O−P and is within the support area of A which is therefore stable on book B. As the books balance on one another by virtue of the relationship of their own centre of mass over their own support area, so do individual segments of the body. In *Figure 2.3* we see that the only relevant centre of mass is that of the part above the articulation. It balances nicely on the second book (or spinal segment) below. No muscular activity is required to maintain this balance. Reference to the caber diagram (*Figure 2.4*) shows how little muscle contraction is necessary to achieve balance, although clearly if the pole becomes unstable then the children will have difficulty in holding it still. *Figure 2.5* shows the situation when the posture is changed, here the centre of mass lies outside the body. There is no balance, and muscle activity is required to retain posture. Clearly this activity 'costs energy'. As the centre of mass is moved to lie over the support area (the feet) we can appreciate that *extrinsic stability* has been achieved. This is an important concept in normal as well as abnormal gait (*Figure 2.6*). Provided that the centre of mass is not displaced outside the one foot support when the displacing force is removed, the whole body 'falls back' and is stable again (like an upturned cone on a motorway).

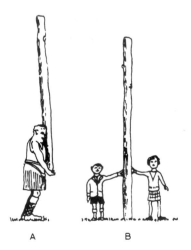

A   B

Figure 2.4. The energy saving of muscle used to balance as opposed to support. The energy required to hold the caber in A is clearly much greater than in B, particularly if the children have a controlled feedback to act quickly and promptly before the caber has tilted more than very slightly.

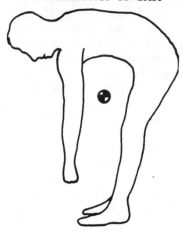

Figure 2.5. The location of the centre of mass outside the body in this position. It is possible in modern techniques of high jumping that the body goes over the bar and the centre of mass below it. To keep extrinsic stability by moving the centre of mass over the feet the buttocks go backwards. Hence the impossibility of bending forward like this and remaining stable with heels against the wall.

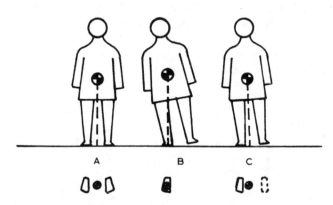

Figure 2.6. A. A static stable standing position with centre of mass within the support area of the two feet. B. Static stable position with one-foot support area; clearly not as assured as (A). C. Dynamic stable position — not in itself stable, but will fall back to stable position (A).

2. The generated power is from muscle activity. There has to be transmission and modification of this muscle energy through the limb to a point of external reaction with the surface walked upon. The body segments are all involved in muscle activity, producing

a 'flux' from one part to another – again a helpful concept since as little of it as possible is squandered. During the first part of stance phase ('loading response', see below) the body centre of mass is elevated by up to 5cm, producing a potential energy storage which is released as kinetic energy as the body enters the downhill phase (*Figure 2.1*) during opposite leg swing. At the end of this phase the energy is translated into a momentum which assists in the next uphill phase. Thus any patient who has to take each step as a separate event, because of disease, will squander 'saved' energy, and will not be energy efficient. The swing leg has a stored potential energy at initial swing, and this becomes kinetic. During the sudden deceleration after initial contact, inertial energy assists in moving the body forward, a useful contribution to propulsion. We have already mentioned stability as a mandatory requirement of gait and for walking this must be present in both stance and swing phases. The trunk requires active hip abductors and extensors to restrain any tendency to flexion abduction at the hip in standing still; and to counter the necessary hip flexion during swing phase. Similarly stance-phase stability in the limb requires co-ordinated action of the hip extensors, quadriceps and soleus to restrain passive flexion forces at the lower limb joints.

3. Walking requires movement of the body and the limbs forward. To avoid frictional loss of energy between the foot and the ground, we must also 'clear' the limb (i.e. lift the foot clear of the ground). Adequate hip and knee flexion plus ankle dorsiflexion is required for this, and muscle action from psoas, hamstrings, triceps surae and ankle extensors is seen.

Components of gait

Pendulum motion

Consideration of the action of a swinging leg makes us think of pendulum motion. If we construct a compound pendulum model of thigh, shank and foot, the swinging model moves similarly to a walking human limb. As clock-watchers will know, a pendulum clock requires very little energy to keep moving, and the human animal walks at a surprisingly uniform cadence which corresponds to the experimental harmonic of a disarticulated cadaveric lower limb. Such basic details of our motion have been unchanging over centuries – the Roman legions had regular camps or resting points along their highways corresponding to 20-mile distances covered in 5 hours of marching with a regular step.

The vaulting action of the stance leg

Consider *Figure 2.1*: At point X the hip and body have to move 'uphill' as the head and trunk weight is transferred forwards at the flexing (stance) hip. Work is done by applying forces to the skeleton to move the body in this way, but at point Y when the centre of mass is some 2cm higher, the body has acquired potential energy which is expended freely in the 'downhill' phase. To prevent jerky individual phases which 'waste' energy by reason of staccato stops and starts, the brain brings into play learned consecutive muscle actions to damp-down the excesses of movement and smooth the path of the moving body. Physiotherapists will instantly be aware of the awkward high-energy expenditure of the stiff-kneed cerebro-vascular accident patient, or the spastic child, who has to circumduct the hip to swing the leg forward. Often the step is a single unco-ordinated event and great transfers of energy are required to lift the affected leg upward and forward. It is known that a 25% increase in energy consumption occurs with a stiff-kneed gait. In normal walking, the smoothing of the rise and fall (and latent displacement) of the centre of mass is of paramount importance to prevent tiredness or waste of muscle work. Normal level walking is about 50% efficient in energy conversion for each gait cycle, but some energy, as metabolic cost, must be injected during each step at the toe-off to ensure that the uphill phase is achieved.

Pelvic rotation

This is difficult to visualise, but consider for a moment the left hip in stance with the right left swinging forward: you are looking from above with the trunk amputated above hip level. As the right leg swings, the right hemipelvis must move forwards, and the fulcrum of movement is at the left hip socket. Relatively, the left hip internally rotates since the right hemipelvis is moving forward; if the external rotators of the right hip are paralysed, then the right femur will also be internally rotated, but normally they act to rotate the swinging leg, so keeping the foot pointing forward in the line of progression. Clearly, disorders of the hip joint(s) will alter this rotation, and gait is affected, particularly by reduction of the step length. As normal rotation occurs at the hip, so the upper limbs alternately swing − importantly to counter the above-mentioned rotatory movement, thus acting as a damping device to 'smooth' these abrupt changes in trunk or pelvic rotation.

Foot clearance and advance

We have already mentioned the vaulting action of the stance leg and pelvic movement, which we now must consider together, since shortening of the swing-leg to get it off the ground is the objective. The knee bends at the initial swing, the hip also flexes to overcome its extended position. In Figure 2.1, the opposite ankle plantar flexes – resulting in shortening of the swing leg.

Abduction of the swing leg hip at the initial swing must also occur if the leg leaving the ground is not to 'bang into' the stance leg. Similarly, the stance hip *adducts* slightly. This must be so, as the *stance side* hip abductor (gluteus medius) contracts to raise the opposite hemipelvis (thereby opposite leg elevation). Because this adduction would produce a great deal of sideways movement (and this requires energy expenditure) there is stance-leg subtalar joint movement resulting in less pelvic motion laterally. The centre of body mass thus moves towards the stance leg (*Figure 2.7*), but never over it in normal walking, again reducing the energy cost.

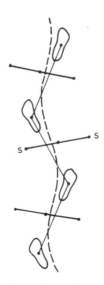

Figure 2.7. The dotted line is the path of the centre of mass. Note that it does not go over each foot as this assumes support. S–S is the shoulder line and moves in the opposite direction to the pelvis.

Spinal movement

Spinal movement has been stated to be the generator of leg movement (Gracovektsky and Lacano, 1986). Although maintenance of the body segments one over the other has already been mentioned as a conserver of energy, its application to the moving subject is rather obstruse. However, as spinal surgery and biomechanics have become more successfully understood, we can now appreciate how the energy cost of walking rises if spinal segments are fused. Fine adjustments of the position of the centre of mass occurs in the spine as the walk continues.

Scientific study of gait is now possible with the advent of gait laboratories, and gait can be considered kinematically, kinetically, and by looking at the all-important energy cost.

Kinematics

The study of the pattern of movement of locomotion is called kinematics.

Scientific study to assist treatment by physiotherapist or doctor may include study of joint-angle movement in the lower limbs. From the side, the familiar stick-diagram (*Figure 2.8*) must be studied. The moving limb is described in 'swing-phase'; the stance phase has a simple 'rule-of-three' — three joints which have rotations in their sagittal plane. These are: one flexion/ extension range for the hip; two flexions for the knee (one as a shock-absorber after initial contact; the second, to allow limb clearance in swing phase); the third movement at the ankle—foot complex has three rockers of movement, the heel, ankle and toe rockers. The ankle rocker is the most important since as the tibio-talar joint dorsiflexes, small angular changes at shank to floor produce a large movement forwards of the body. The heel rocker

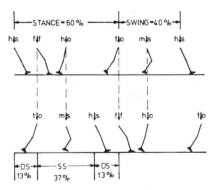

Figure 2.8. hs = heel strike; ff = foot flat; ho = heel off; to = toe off; ms = mid-swing; DS = double stance; SS = single stance. Sub-divisions of the phases of walking commonly used to describe the events which occur.
Note *the relationship of events in one leg with the other, and that twice in each phase of walking double stance occurs when both touch the ground, and share the load in varying degrees.*

is, however, important also, since at *initial contact* the specially adapted skin and subcutaneous tissues of the heel pad 'squash' down, dissipating shock energy. The third rocker, at toe-off (used to be called 'push-off'), occurs in the pre-swing phase with the forefoot dorsi-flexing at the metatarsophalangeal (MP) joints, leaving only these MP joints and toes on the ground.

From *Figure 2.9*, we can see three parts of swing phase — where the limb is advanced through space providing forward reach for the next step while maintaining toe clearance. During *initial swing* (IS; *Figure 2.9(f)*) the limb lifts from the floor, the hip flexes to 20°, while the knee bends to 70°; the ankle dorsiflexors keep the toes clear. Hip flexors and abductors advance and control the limb, the hamstrings are silent since inertial forces and gravity make the knee bend (provided that there is no genicular disease). *Mid-swing* (MSW; *Figure 2.9(g)*) occurs at the opposite leg mid-stance. The swinging limb advances until the tibia is vertical, causing passive knee extension, hip flexion increases slightly (to 30°) and the ankle and foot become horizontal. Muscle activity is almost entirely in the ankle dorsiflexors.

Terminal swing (TSW) is at terminal stance phase (*Figure 2.9(h)*) of the opposite leg, and allows the tibia to swing forward a little more to create maximum step length. This depends upon the knee assuming full extension itself. Clearly, any limitation of movement will cause limitation of step length. During TSW the hip reaches 30° of flexion, and the ankle dorsiflexes to neutral to get ready to 'land' under the influence of the ankle extensor muscles. The leg travels forward too fast, and at this stage the hip extensors fire to brake the forward swing and both knee flexors and extensors are active to produce a synergistic stabilisation of the joint. TSW ends as the heel hits the ground — the initial event of the next cycle — *initial contact* (IC; *Figure 2.9(a)*). It will be appreciated that at this moment *both* feet are on the ground, thus a *double support* phase occurs (this becomes a definition of walking where in every stride one foot has just contacted the ground, before the other leaves it).

The foot has reached the ground (IC; *Figure 2.9(a)*) at 0% of the gait cycle. The hip is flexed to 30° and is neutral in both rotation and ab/adduction. The knee is almost fully extended, and the ankle is in neutral, so unsurprisingly muscle activity is as mentioned above in TSW.

We now have to support body weight with this new leg, and facilitate body advancement over the stance foot. The next stage is *loading response* (LR; *Figure 2.9(b)*), 0–10% of the gait cycle. As its name suggests, the limb accepts body weight, and body weight is moving towards this new stance foot. Because of the shock of landing, the limb joints are all flexing to minimise the

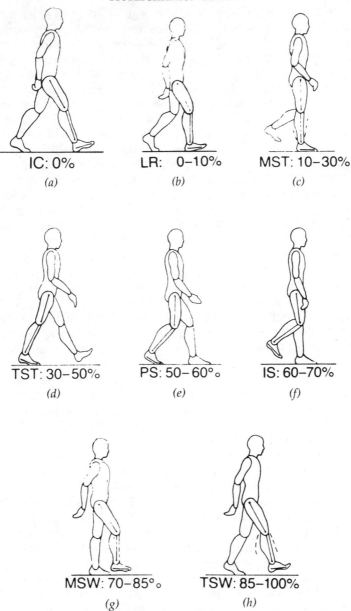

IC: 0%

(a)

LR: 0–10%

(b)

MST: 10–30%

(c)

TST: 30–50%

(d)

PS: 50–60°○

(e)

IS: 60–70%

(f)

MSW: 70–85°○

(g)

TSW: 85–100%

(h)

Figure 2.9. (a) IC: 0%, touchdown; (b) LR: 0–10%, limb accepts weight; (c) MST: 10–30%, limb supports weight; and body advances over foot; (d) TST: 30–50%, body advances ahead of foot; (e) PS: 50–60%, limb unloaded and prepared for swing; (f) IS: 60–70%, limb lifts and thigh advances; (g) MSW: 70–85%, limb advances until tibia vertical; (h) TSW: 85–100%, limb advances to create step length.

upward movement of the pelvis, which also is stopping its rotation around the 'old' stance hip. The knee flexes to 15° to help cushion the shock and the ankle plantar flexes by 15° to allow ground contact. This LR is aptly named by the new nomenclature, and we can appreciate the damping of the vertical movement of the centre of gravity. Muscle activity in hip and knee extensors, also the ankle dorsiflexors, assists, and has been called 'eccentric contraction'. If the knee or ankle joint movement is faulty the patient vaults – a common fault while adjustment of new prostheses occurs (clearly due to excessive rise of the centre of gravity with the step). In *Figure 2.9(c)*, *mid-stance* (MST), 10–30% of the gait cycle, we see weight being fully accepted by the stationary foot and the body progresses over it. The hip and knee are in extension, the ankle is still in neutral with the foot in ground contact. At IC the knee joint was extended, it then flexed during LR and now again is at full extension (MST).

The centre of gravity has been raised to its fullest extent at this 'top-dead-centre' (*Figure 2.9(c)*) and the weight has also shifted towards this stance foot (*Figure 2.7*). Muscle activity is surprisingly little, showing a great concern to conserve muscle energy. Hip abductors are active on the stance side to prevent the swinging leg hemipelvis from dropping, thereby stopping swing-foot clearance. The ankle plantar flexors, particularly the gastro-soleus complex, are beginning to fire as and they are preparing for *terminal stance* (TST; *Figure 2.9(d)*), 30–50% of the cycle. This period is defined as starting when the body moves forward in relation to the support foot. The hip and knee remain extended, and the heel is rising as the gastro-soleus contracts strongly for a 'final push' (not the 'push-off' of the old nomenclature).

This is followed by *pre-swing* (PS; *Figure 2.9(e)*), 50–60% of the cycle. PS is a transitional phase where double support has occurred (assisting balance) and unloading of the limb occurs rapidly to allow this to become the new swing-leg. The hip is now extending, but the knee starts flexion, reaching 35°, and the ankle is fully plantar-flexed at 20°. The gastro-soleus is now silent, but ileopsoas is now contracting strongly, and the foot dorsiflexors contract to prepare for the swing phase.

The frequency of succession of left and right steps is cadence. One walking cycle (from left heel contact to next *left* foot fall) is the *stride* length; the step length is left foot contact to *right* foot contact at the *next* foot fall. The combination of cadence and stride length determines speed – we increase our speed by (usually) increasing our stride length.

Kinetics

The study of forces that produce or change motion is called kinetics. The initiating engine providing the mechanical energy is muscle activity, and although the muscles are active for minimal periods, we nevertheless are constantly using our muscles to control joint position. We provide our intrinsic stability by resisting gravity, which would tend to make us collapse like a bag of bones, simply by balancing one body segment upon another. Movement requires alteration of the state, and muscles control that change. Our objective is to stabilise our joints quickly in a new, stable position. Unfortunately the hip joint is too offset to allow the centre of mass to be easily placed above the hip. In *Figure 2.10* we see the moments acting about a hip. The forces are BW (body weight) and AM (abductor muscles). If BW is balanced by AM to hold the hip in one position, and if b = 2a, then AM = 2BW and the total load is 3BW. It can be reduced by shortening the moment arm 'b' — moving the trunk over the hip (which explains the osteopathic hip walk). If the patient is to put a stick in the opposite hand and push down on it, then again he can reduce the lever-arm 'b' by moving the opposite pelvis and body weight towards the centre of the hip joint. He can also reduce BW by dieting!

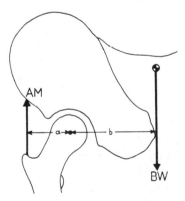

Figure 2.10. Compressive force on the hip joint. BW = body weight; AM = abductor muscles; ab = moment arms.

In the gait laboratory these forces can often be directly calculated, and tend to confirm our explanation of the gait events as described above. Future kinetic calculations on patients undergoing joint replacements or corrections of deformity may be helpful. Andriachi has shown an important predictive use of gait study in calculating the adducting moments at the knee in patients with medial-compartment osteoarthrosis. Apparently similar patients, according to age, size, severity of symptoms etc., were found to have high or low adducting moments at their knees. Both groups had a high tibial osteotomy as treatment; those in the high adducting-moment groups had a worse result than those with lower moments. Clearly it can be proposed that furthur examples of direct kinetic measurement will have effects upon patients and their care. Bio-mechanical considerations are always necessary in any treatment system, be it surgery, orthoses and physiotherapy, even concerning the use of drugs which have an effect on the neuromuscular or skeletal system.

Our concern is to understand and facilitate human walking, to discover the possible disabilities during a walk, and propose benefits from forms of treatment, by direct or indirect treatment. With the advent of simple energy-equivalent tests (e.g. the Physiological Cost Index (PCI), MacGregor 1981) we can now begin to audit our results. If the PCI can be shown to lessen with any treatment, then the patient must have gained, literally. A reduction implies a lessening of his energy expenditure, and our task is to achieve this if at all possible. Measurement of the PCI could become as routine as a haemoglobin estimation, although at present it can be performed only in a gait laboratory environment.

References

Chadwick, C. et al., (1985). JBJS(A), **67**, 1188–94.

Gracovektsky, S.A. and Lacano, S. (1986). Energy transfer in the spinal engine. *Journal of Biomedical Engineering*, **9**, 99–114.

Inman, V.J. (1981). *Human Walking*. Williams & Wilkins, Baltimore and London.

MacGregor, J. (1981). The evaluation of patient performance using long-term ambulatory monitoring technique in the domiciliary environment. *Physiotherapy*, **7**(2), 30–33.

3 Applied Gait Assessment

P.B. Butler

The biomechanics of gait have been examined in Chapter 2. We examine here ways in which the therapist may approach gait assessment and the techniques that are available. The process of gait assessment may be divided into three stages:

- The gait itself is examined and analysed.
- One or more theories are formulated to explain particular features of the patient's gait and a solution is proposed. This is probably the most important stage. Full consideration must be given to all the implications of the proposal, a point which will be considered in greater depth in a later example. The solution may include therapy, surgery or orthotic prescription.
- In the experimental stage the solution is put into practice and the gait reanalysed.

This process can be illustrated by a flow diagram, and ideally the analytical process will continue until a satisfactory end-point is reached (*Figure 3.1*). This may be achieved almost immediately by, for example, the provision of a walking aid, or may involve a much longer time-scale if extensive therapy is required.

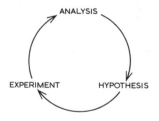

Figure 3.1. Flow diagram of gait assessment.

Components of gait assessment

There are four main areas involved in gait assessment:

- Kinematics: monitoring gait patterns.
- Kinetics: measurement of forces.
- Electromyography: monitoring muscle activity.
- Efficiency: monitoring performance, for example by speed and heart rate.

Preliminary assessment

Analysis of a patient's gait should first be put into its context. A careful history will reveal what the patient finds to be his major problems, the duration and degree of his signs and symptoms, particularly pain, and the effect of these on his lifestyle. All aspects of mobility thus become a part of gait assessment and will include rising from sitting, and climbing stairs. It is important to discover the patient's own solutions to his problems, as these can give valuable guidance about profitable areas of experimental solutions.

Example 1   A patient stated that she found walking easier when carrying her shopping bag in the right hand. Examination revealed weak right hip abductors and a positive Trendelenburg sign. Carrying a weight in the right hand reduced the moment at the hip joint without the compensatory body sway otherwise involved (*Figure 3.2*).

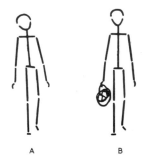

Figure 3.2. A. Mid-stance right leg: compensatory body sway used to reduce moment at the right hip joint. B. Mid-stance right leg: weight of shopping bag eliminates compensatory movement.

Following the functional history the patient is examined and the range of movement of the limbs and spine recorded, together with sensory status and proprioception, muscle power and tone, and degree and type of pain. It should be remembered that the range of movement during walking can often differ considerably from that found on examination of the patient.

Equally important is examination in standing. The posture may be observed together with the effect of the upright position on muscle tone or weakness. The patient is asked to stand first on one leg and then on the other, revealing problems of balance and control, or of isolated muscle weakness. A note is made of the walking aids used. Inspection of the shoes — the uppers, inside and soles — can give many useful clues about walking patterns.

Gait assessment continues using each of the four aspects as appropriate for each patient.

Kinematics

This is the study of *gait patterns* and *geometry* of walking. The key to this is observation, which is made easier and more successful by a visual recording of the gait. This recording serves two functions: first, it permits detailed analysis at the time of assessment and, second, it provides a permanent record for later comparison, perhaps at intervals of one year or more.

Visual recording

Video is a readily available means of visual recording which is relatively inexpensive. It permits immediate replay, so enabling the three stages of assessment to take place immediately. Thus the effect of an experimental solution, such as a walking stick or an orthosis, can quickly be analysed. The facility for slow motion replay allows analysis to be more detailed and accurate than visual observation alone. Video has the further advantage of being an electronic system, so enabling other electronically monitored physiological or physical data to be mixed directly for display on the video screen. An example of such data is the ground reaction force.

Many therapists, however, will not have access to visual recording equipment. They will need to develop expertise in gait analysis while the patient is walking at normal speed, and to do so quickly for patients who have a low exercise tolerance.

Written records

It is essential to note findings in gait analysis for future reference and this may be done in written form, by some diagrammatic means, or by a graphical notation such as Benesh Movement Notation (McGuinness-Scott, 1982).

Observations of the patient

Observation and analysis should be made in three planes — sagittal, coronal and horizontal (overhead) — although often it will be possible to use only the first two. The patient should be observed from the right and left lateral view, from the front and from behind and if possible from overhead. Close-ups can provide much specific information, and the therapist without visual recording facilities should be prepared to look closely at particular joints, walking alongside the patient if necessary.

Initial analysis

When commencing the analysis it is helpful first to make an overall judgement about the gait which can provide many clues.

Example 2   A 10-year-old girl presented with an uncertain, hesitant appearance when walking barefoot and a happy confidence when in shoes. She had idiopathic tightness of the tendo calcaneus and so was unable to put her heel to the ground when walking barefoot (*Figure 3.3(a)*). She thus had a small support area with consequent decrease in balance and confidence. The heel height of her shoes (which she had chosen herself) compensated exactly for the tightness of her tendo calcaneus, resulting in a steady confident walk with increased step length (*Figure 3.3(b)*).

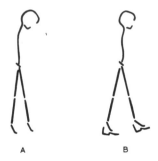

A   B

Figure 3.3. (a) Toe-stepping gait caused by idiopathic tightness of the tendo calcaneus. (b) Heel height of shoes compensates for tightness of tendo calcaneus.

Further analysis

There are three main aspects to be considered when analysing gait:

- The sequence in which events occur.
- The range of movement of the joints.

• Closely associated with these is the timing in which events occur.

Thus, in the lateral view the sequence of events which form one stride can be noted and the positions of the arms, head, trunk and legs observed. A simple example of disturbed sequence is the patient who has a toe strike before putting the foot flat, and then goes to toe-off. Inspection of range of motion during walking will reveal such abnormalities as a flexion deformity. A deformity in one joint almost always creates a compensatory movement in another joint in the same plane. For example, a fixed flexion deformity at the knee will result in flexion at the hip during walking to keep the body mass over the base of support (*Figure 3.4*). Similarly, a fixed flexion deformity at the hip will result in a flexed knee. This highlights an important aspect of gait assessment, namely that of isolating cause from effect, and correct interpretation will lead to successful recommendation.

Figure 3.4. Fixed flexion of knee with compensatory flexion of hip to keep the body mass over the base of support.

Example 3a A 12-year-old boy with spastic cerebral palsy was noted to walk on his toes with grossly hyperextended knees. Examination showed that he had bilateral tight tendo calcaneus, a normal range of knee flexion with slight hyperextension and adequate musculature. Gait analysis showed that his problems were twofold:

• A control problem imposed by his cerebral palsy giving imbalance between his dorsal and plantar flexors and causing him to have an equinus. The plantar flexors contracted, so limiting his range of movement.
• This limited ankle range gave a mechanical problem of joint movement pattern.

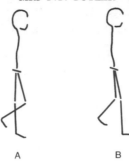

A   B

Figure 3.5. (a) Equinus resulting in abnormal moments and pushing knee into hyperextension. (b) Use of a correctly adjusted fixed ankle foot orthosis overcomes this problem and a more normal gait results with a reduction of knee stress.

The effect of the equinus was to produce abnormal moments which pushed the knee into hyperextension (*Figure 3.5(a)*). Stretching of the tight plantar flexors and use of a correctly-adjusted fixed ankle foot orthosis (Butler and Nene, 1991) resulted in a more normal gait with a reduction of knee stress (*Figure 3.5(b)*).

Example 3b A 7-year-old boy with muscular dystrophy presented with a similar problem at first view. He had a toe-stepping gait with minimal tightness of the tendo calcaneus, normal knee range but weak quadriceps muscles. However, this child's problems were very different from the preceding case, being:

- The limited range of movement at his ankle.
- Stabilisation of a multi-segmented structure (the leg) because of weak musculature.

Elongation of the tendo calcaneus had been considered, but the necessity of considering all the implications of a solution is shown very clearly here. This child was using a dynamic equinus to produce an extending moment to stabilise his knee during stance phase and so compensate for his quadriceps weakness. If this facility were removed by tendon elongation, it is very probable that he would not then have sufficient knee stability to walk at all (Khodadadeh *et al.*, 1986). This child required careful follow-up to ensure that he did not develop knee flexion deformity.

Example 4 An elderly man with an arthritic right knee and severely restricted flexion was noted to walk with circumduction of the right leg in swing phase and lateral tilting of the trunk to the left. He had elected to compensate in this way for his inability to clear the right foot from the ground by the normal knee flexion (*Figure 3.6(a)*). Another patient with a similar problem – an ankylosed right knee in a 35-year-old man following a road traffic accident – opted to use increased plantar flexion of the left ankle to clear the right leg (*Figure 3.6(b)*). The elderly man found that he was more stable using circumduction rather than by rising onto his toe, and with his slower gait the method he adopted was more energy efficient. The younger man preferred the appearance of rising onto his toe and accepted the slight increase in energy cost. Each patient will instinctively make use of the available options in his own preferred way.

Observation of the anterior and posterior views will reveal such problems as increased lateral trunk sway and deformities of the hip, knee and subtalar joint in the coronal plane. Width of base can be noted.

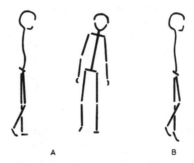

A   B

Figure 3.6. (a) A fixed flexion deformity at the right knee prevents normal swing-through. Circumduction and lateral tilt are used to compensate for loss of knee flexion and to clear the foot. (b) Fixed knee flexion in this patient is compensated by increased plantar flexion.

Example 5 A lady with long-standing rheumatoid arthritis complained of pain in the left knee on weight-bearing. Gait analysis showed an abnormal range of motion. There was laxity of the medial collateral ligament with joint instability giving a deforming moment about the knee at mid-stance (*Figure 3.7(a)*). Examination had shown this deformity to be fully correctable, and an orthotic solution was proposed. An orthosis applying three-point fixation held the knee in correct alignment, and pain was reduced on weight-bearing (*Figure 3.7(b)*).

The overhead view provides additional information about horizontal rotations to that obtained from the other views (*Figure 3.8(a)*).

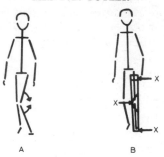

Figure 3.7. (a) Left mid-stance: instability of the knee gives a deforming moment about the knee. (b) Left mid-stance: an orthosis applying three-point fixation (xxx) holds the knee in the correct position.

Example 6 A child with cerebral palsy wore out his shoes in one month on the antero-medial aspect. Physical examination revealed limitation of rotation and fixed flexion deformity of the hips. Gait analysis in shoes showed:

- A control problem imposed by the cerebral palsy with muscle imbalance at the hips leading to muscle contractures.
- This resulted in an absence of extension and subsequent effect on step length.

Step length is a combination of forward motion of the swing-leg (hip flexion) and extension of the stance leg (hip extension). The fixed flexion deformity in this child meant that step length was greatly reduced. Swivelling on the forefoot (foot/ground interface)

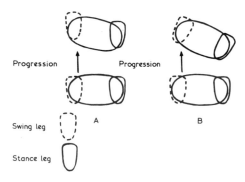

Figure 3.8. (a) Normal situation: pelvis viewed from above. (b) Step length is generated here by swivelling at the foot–ground interface. This compensates for absence of hip extension/rotation.

enabled the swing leg to be placed further ahead (*Figure 3.8(b)*). However, the penalty for this was wear of the shoes.

It is useful to take measurements of particular features of gait, such as abnormal joint angles. Step and stride length can be measured, providing valuable follow-up information.

A simple and convenient method of measuring step length is to stick paint-soaked felt pads to the patient's shoes. Two rectangles of orthopaedic felt approximately 1.5cm × 1cm are stripped of the surface felt until 2—3mm thick. This provides an absorbent surface for the paint. Washable water colour is used, a different colour for right and left shoes. The pads are stuck to the *front* edge of the heel (*Figure 3.9*) and not on the posterior edge, which may cause the patient to slip. The patient walks across a washable floor or length of paper. A distance of at least 6m (20ft) permits the patient to achieve a normal stride and to exclude the last few decelerating steps, the middle section being measured. The time taken for the events of one stride will supply further information on the nature of the patient's problems. It includes comparison of the duration of swing and stance phase on each leg. Thus, a patient with a painful hip may present with a pain-avoiding (antalgic) gait and have a shorter stance phase on the affected leg.

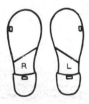

Figure 3.9. To show optimal position of paint-soaked pads for measuring step length. On heels *if heel strike obtained; on* lateral border *if no heel strike.*

Kinetics

This is measurement of the *forces* involved in walking. There are two types of force to be considered:

- The external forces such as the ground reaction force.
- The internal forces of the body, such as individual muscle forces which are, at present, largely unquantifiable during gait.

Ground reaction force

The ground reaction force can be measured, and force platforms (force plates) are used to monitor both the horizontal and vertical components. The patient walks over a force platform, set flush into a walkway, and the components of force, which are equal and opposite to that exerted by the patient, are registered. A vector of this ground reaction force can then be constructed (*Figure 3.10*; Stallard, 1987).

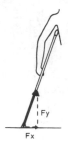

Figure 3.10. Ground reaction vector to a crutch. Fy = vertical component; Fx = horizontal component.

In example 5 (p. 45) the lady with an unstable rheumatoid knee will have a ground reaction vector, as in *Figure 3.11(b)* with a large valgus-deforming moment acting about the joint. The effect of the orthosis can also be seen (*Figure 3.11(c)*). This is an extreme example, but even subtle changes in force can result in the ground reaction vector passing to one side or the other of the joint centre, so changing the direction of the moment. Such changes may be apparent to the experienced eye without the use of force

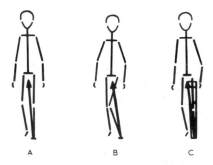

Figure 3.11. (a) Normal ground reaction vector mid-stance left leg (Note: Vector passes slightly medial to knee joint axis.) (b) Instability of the knee, left mid-stance: large deforming moment about the knee. (c) Orthosis controls knee instability and a normal vector results.

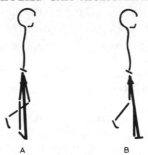

Figure 3.12. Boy with spastic cerebral palsy. (a) Vector passes in front of knee, producing a large knee-extending moment. (b) Correctly adjusted fixed ankle foot orthosis. Vector passes through knee joint.

monitoring, but there will be many occasions when the changes are detected only with this type of instrumentation, particularly for the beginner in such studies.

Reference back to the two cases involving hyperextended knees (examples 3a (p. 43) and 3b (p. 44) will show how important monitoring ground reaction force can be. In example 3a, the boy with spastic cerebral palsy, the vector was seen to pass well in front of the knee (*Figure 3.12(a)*) which produced a very large knee-extending moment, so causing abnormal stresses in the knee. However, despite apparently similar kinematics, example 3b, the boy with muscular dystrophy, had a vector which passed through the centre of the knee thus eliminating any moment (*Figure 3.13*). In his case, surgery would almost certainly have caused the vector to pass behind the knee joint centre, thus producing a knee-flexing moment which his weak quadriceps would have difficulty in opposing (Khodadadeh et al., 1986).

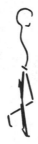

Figure 3.13. Boy with muscular dystrophy. Vector passes through knee joint centre. Surgery to elongate the tendo calcaneus could cause the vector to pass behind knee and muscles are not strong enough to counteract this.

The therapist should be aware of the forces involved in gait and their possible effects, although their measurement and interpretation are specialties.

Electromyography

This is a rapidly expanding field in which *muscle activity* is monitored during joint movement and walking. Again, it is a specialised area and requires instrumentation. It is possible to monitor the phasic activity of various muscles and to discover which muscles work in stance or swing phase and at which parts of the phase. This can then be related to the kinematic and kinetic data, which may help to determine whether it is, in fact, appropriate for a particular muscle group to be active when it would normally be quiescent. There may, for example, be a hip-flexing moment at a phase in the gait cycle when an extensor moment is more normal. Such a hip-flexing moment may need, therefore, to be balanced by hip extensor activity.

Example 7 Assessment of a young man with early muscular dystrophy showed that he had a typical myopathic posture, with fixed flexion deformities of 15° at the knees and 10° at the hips with weakness of his hip and knee extensors (*Figure 3.14(a)*). Because of the weakness of his extensors this patient needed to place the body mass of his head, trunk and arms through or behind his hip joints. He attempted to achieve this by extending his spine, although his flexion contractures made it more difficult. His ground reaction vector showed that, despite his extended spine, the origin of the vector was forward on his feet and the vector passed in front of his hip, thus producing a hip-flexing moment (*Figure 3.14(b)*). Electromyographic studies of his hip extensors and quadriceps confirmed that he did not quite succeed in placing his body mass behind the hip axis. He therefore needed and demonstrated considerable extensor muscle action during all phases of gait (*Figure 3.14(c)*). Follow-up of this patient included ensuring that his hip and knee flexion contractures did not increase, as this could prevent his walking.

Efficiency of gait

The efficient nature of walking, as demonstrated by energy cost, has been described. There are two main parameters of efficiency of gait, *speed* and *energy expenditure*. A further aspect which will

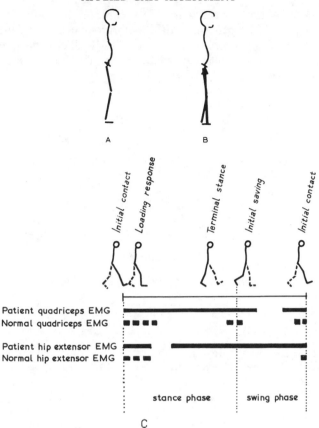

Figure 3.14. (a) Typical myopathic posture: extension of spine to place mass of head, trunk and arms near hip joints. (b) Vector passes in front of hips. (c) Electromyographic studies showed extensor muscle action in all phases of gait in this patient.

also be considered is endurance, based on measurements of both speed and heart rate.

Speed

Speed is easily calculated from the time taken to walk a measured distance, for example 6m (20ft). In a gait laboratory this measurement will be automated, but it can easily be accomplished in a ward or department by using a stop-watch. The patient is asked to walk at his normal speed. Results are more reliable if timings are taken after the second length is completed, so that familiarity with the test is ensured, although this may not be possible in patients with low exercise tolerance.

Example 8 A 12-year-old was assessed before and after calcaneal osteotomy with lengthening of the tendo calcaneus, with a 7-month interval between assessments. She walked five lengths of 20ft with a short rest between each length. The results showed an increase in speed of 46% (*Figure 3.15*).

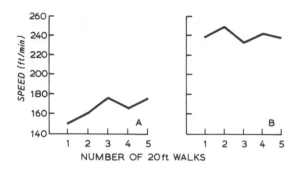

Figure 3.15. (a) Pre-operative speed over five walks. (b) Postoperative speed over five walks.

Heart rate

Heart rate has been shown to be a reliable parameter of energy expenditure (Astrand and Rhyming, 1954; Rowell *et al.*, 1964) and to increase linearly with work load at submaximal levels (Bengtsson, 1956; Bradfield *et al.*, 1971; Poulsen and Asmussen, 1962; Wahlund, 1948). It is preferable in a clinical context to the assessment of energy expenditure by oxygen uptake, which usually involves wearing a nose-clip and breathing through a mouthpiece with collection of expired air. Heart rate is not a quantitative method of energy cost and, indeed, at this time no reliable or reproducible measurement method exists. When combined with speed and cadence (number of steps per minute) it provides a useful baseline in gait assessment (Butler *et al.*, 1984a; Khan *et al.*, 1975; Stallard *et al.*, 1978).

Factors other than energy expenditure can affect heart rate, the most notable being emotional stress. It is recognised, however, that this diminishes markedly when work is undertaken (Astrand and Rhodahl, 1970). The effects of both emotional stress and other factors, such as ambient temperature, which affect heart rate, can also be diminished by careful control of the environment in which tests are performed.

Example 9 A paraplegic patient with a low lumbar lesion was prescribed a ParaWalker (*Figure 3.16*; Butler *et al.*, 1984b), as an interim learning device, after which it was considered that he

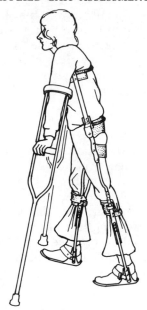

Figure 3.16. ParaWalker: this can provide effective low energy reciprocal, as opposed to swing-through, ambulation with crutches for patients with spinal cord lesions of L1 and above.

might be able to graduate to knee—ankle—foot orthoses (KAFOs or long-leg calipers) only. The change to KAFOs was monitored carefully over a series of weekly assessments, starting with an initial assessment in a ParaWalker. Heart rate was monitored by telemetry (*Figure 3.17(a)*). When the patient's performance had

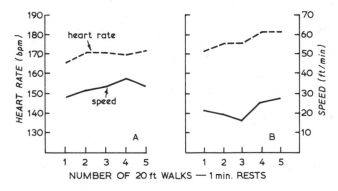

Figure 3.17 Monitoring heart rate. (a) Trial 1: ParaWalker and crutches. (b) Trial 2 (3 months later): Knee—ankle—foot orthoses (KAFOs) and crutches.

reached a plateau, assessment showed that ambulation was costing 10 beats per minute (b.p.m.) more than with a ParaWalker (*Figure 3.17(b)*). Inclusion of speeds in these two tests made a more complete measure of efficiency. It is clearly seen that he walked 20% slower in KAFOs. On this basis a decision was taken to return him to a ParaWalker.

Endurance
Monitoring speed and heart rate can provide useful information in the less heavily handicapped patient. If a patient with near normal exercise tolerance is requested to walk continuously, a more representative picture of his problem may emerge.

Example 10 Two comparative trials were made of a patient walking consecutive 80ft lengths until tired, one without orthoses and one after 5.5 months' practice with bilateral plastic below-knee fixed-ankle orthoses. The improvement in speed, heart rate and distance walked is shown in *Figure 3.18*.

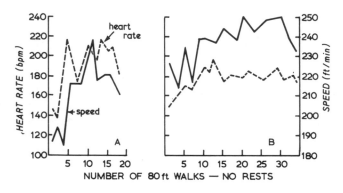

Figure 3.18. Monitoring endurance. (a) Trial 1: No orthoses. (b) Trial 2 (6 months later): Bilateral ankle–foot orthoses (AFOs). Endurance test showed improvement in speed, heart rate and total distance walked.

Conclusion

Many of the patients seen by a therapist will benefit from gait assessment. The more complex problems may need the help and advice of a gait laboratory, but in both these and the more straightforward cases much useful data can be obtained by following the preceding guidelines. It is necessary to approach gait assessment in an organised manner, and to retain the concept of analysis, formation of hypothesis and experiment. There is no substitute for thought, practice and experience, and what appears to be the solution with the first impression may well require further assessment and analysis.

References

Astrand, P.O. and Rhyming, I. (1954). A nomogram for calculation of aerobic capacity (physical fitness) from pulse rate during submaximal work. *Journal of Applied Physiology*, **7**, 218.

Astrand, P.O. and Rhodahl, K. (1970). *Textbook of Work Physiology*. McGraw Hill, New York.

Bengtsson, E. (1956). The working capacity in normal children evaluated by submaximal exercise on the bicycle ergometer and compared with adults. *Acta Medica Scandinavica*, **154**, 91–109.

Bradfield, R.B., Paulos, J. and Grossman, L. (1971). Energy expenditure and heart rate of obese high school girls. *American Journal of Clinical Nutrition*, **24**, 1482–1488.

Butler, P.B., Engelbrecht, M., Major, R.E., Tait, J.H., Stallard, J. and Patrick, J.H. (1984a). Physiological cost index of walking for normal children and its use as an indicator of physical handicap. *Developmental Medicine and Child Neurology*, **26**, 607–612.

Butler, P.B., Major, R.E. and Patrick, J.H. (1984b). The technique of reciprocal walking using the hip guidance orthosis (hgo) with crutches. *Prosthetics and Orthotics International*, **8**, 33–38.

Butler, P.B. and Nene, A.V. (1991). The biomechanics of ankle foot orthoses and their potential in the management of cerebral palsied children. *Physiotherapy*, **77**(2), 81–88.

Khan, A., Thomasson, H. and Rose, G.K. (1975). A method for assessing the physiological cost of doing work in handicapped children. *Developmental Medicine and Child Neurology*, **17**(6), Supplement 35, 159–160.

Khodadadeh, S., McClelland, M.R., Patrick, J.H., Edwards, R.H.T. and Evans, G.A. (1986). Knee moments in Duchenne Muscular Dystrophy. *The Lancet*, 6 Sept., 544–545.

McGuinness-Scott, J. (1982). *Benesh Movement Notation*. Chartered Society of Physiotherapy, London.

Poulsen, E. and Asmussen, A. (1962). Energy requirements of practical jobs from the pulse increase and ergometer test. *Ergonomics*, **5**, 33–36.

Rowell, L.B., Hayler, H.L. and Wang, Y. (1964). Limitations to prediction of maximal oxygen uptake. *Journal of Applied Physiology*, **19**, 919.

Stallard, J. (1987). Assessment of the mechanical function of orthoses by force vector visualisation. *Physiotherapy*, **73**(8), 398–402.

Stallard, J., Rose, G.K., Tait, J.H. and Davies, J.B. (1978). Assessment of orthoses by means of speed and heart rate. *Journal of Medical Engineering and Technology*, **2**(1), 22–24.

Wahlund, H. (1948). Determination of physical working capacity; physiological and clinical study with special reference to standardisation of cardio-pulmonary functional tests. *Acta Medica Scandinavica Supplement*, **215**(132), 1–78.

Bibliography

Carlsoo, S. (1972). *How Man Moves*, William Heinemann Limited, London.
Inman, V.T., Rawlston, J.H. and Todd, F. (1981). *Human Walking*, Williams and Wilkins, Baltimore.
Winter, D.A. (1987). *The Biomechanics and Motor Control of Human Gait*, University of Waterloo Press, Waterloo, Ontario.

4 Bone and Joint Pathology

A.J. Darby

Bone

Bone is a uniquely versatile tissue combining strength, elasticity and adaptability. Besides its ability to mould its structure to accommodate long-term stresses (*Figure 4.1*), it is continually remodelling and renewing itself by the cellular processes of osteoclastic resorption and osteoblastic formation. Manipulation of these opposing cellular processes enables the skeleton to grow throughout childhood and to repair itself following injury. Failure of the normal controlling mechanisms for resorption and formation leads to the commonest disease of bone — osteoporosis; this failure is also involved in congenital and neoplastic disorders. In addition, bone acts as a reservoir for calcium and other ions essential for the function of most other organs of the body.

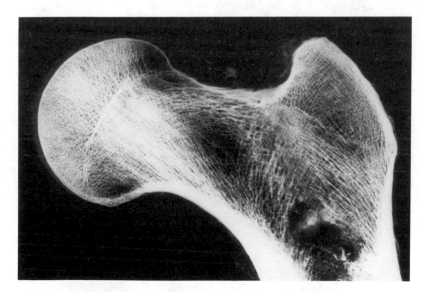

Figure 4.1. Radiograph of a slice through a femoral head showing the stress orientated trabecular pattern of the bone.

In spite of its strength, bone is subject to all the various pathological processes that affect other tissues of the body. The most important of these for our purposes are infection, so-called metabolic bone disorders and tumours.

Pyogenic infections

Infection of bone, osteomyelitis, may be caused either by blood-borne bacteria or by the direct bacterial contamination of bone during surgery (*Figure 4.2*) or following severe trauma. In children, acute osteomyelitis commonly occurs in the metaphyseal region, because this is the most vascular part of the growing bone. In adults, infection of the spine is not uncommon and is often associated with urinary tract infection which, in men, may follow

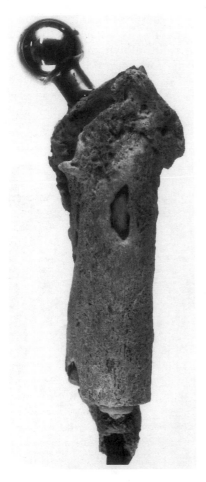

Figure 4.2. The upper end of the femur after chronic infection of a femoral prosthesis. The granular surface is due in part to the formation of an involucrum. The hole drained pus from a central abscess cavity to a discharging skin sinus.

prostatectomy. Patients who are receiving steroids or immuno-suppressive therapy are particularly prone to osteomyelitis. Joint replacement surgery also leads to infection in a small percentage of cases.

Bacterial proliferation starts in the bone marrow of the medullary cavity. The ensuing inflammatory reaction together with the production of bacterial toxins causes death of both soft tissues and bone. Pain and pyrexia are early features of the disease, but the other signs of inflammation — swelling and redness — develop later, if at all, depending on the site of the lesion and the virulence of the organism.

Diagnosis of osteomyelitis may often be made confidently by a combination of clinical and radiological signs, but biopsy is essential to confirm the diagnosis. In a readily accessible site this may be by curretage to remove all the affected tissue. In areas such as the vertebral column, needle biopsy under X-ray control is quicker and easier. Antibiotic treatment can be started immediately after the biopsy and altered if necessary, following sensitivity tests on the bacteria isolated in the laboratory.

In the absence of prompt antibiotic treatment, chronic osteo-myelitis develops with the formation of an abscess cavity. Pus may track along the marrow cavity, but in children the growth plate usually acts as a barrier preventing spread into the epiphysis and the joint cavity. Pus may also travel through the vascular channels of the cortex to the periosteal surface. Here it lifts up the periosteum and stimulates it to form a shell of new bone called the *involucrum*. Later the periosteum itself is breached and a sinus may develop, communicating between the medullary cavity of the bone and the skin surface and causing a persistent purulent discharge. The defect in the bone at this point is called a *cloaca*.

Areas of necrotic bone are recognised as such by the body and attempts are made to remedy the situation. Osteoclasts are attracted from the neighbouring viable bone and begin to resorb the dead bone. As this process of resorption continues, the dead bone becomes completely separated from the living bone and is then known as a *sequestrum*. With continuing osteoclastic activity, the sequestrum itself is often divided into smaller fragments which may be extruded through the sinuses to the skin surface.

At any stage of the disease the patient is at risk of dying from septicaemia. Established chronic osteomyelitis can be very resistant to treatment and two important, potentially fatal, complications can occur. One is the development of secondary amyloidosis with involvement of many organs, particularly the kidneys, leading to chronic renal failure. The other is the appearance of squamous carcinoma of the chronically irritated skin around the edge of a sinus. Fortunately both these complications are rare.

Tuberculous osteomyelitis

With the advent of antituberculous drugs and BCG vaccination, tuberculosis is now fortunately rare, although the spread of AIDS may well cause it to assume greater prominence in the future. Tuberculosis can affect any part of the skeleton, but nearly half the cases involve the spine, where the condition is known as Pott's disease. In developing countries and among immigrants children are commonly affected, but in Britain it is usually a disease of adults.

Infection most commonly starts in the vertebral body near the disc. Progression is slower than in pyogenic infection and, because the necrotic bone can be resorbed almost as fast as it is produced, only small sequestra are formed. Spread of the infection beneath the periosteum often leads to paravertebral abscess formation, which can be seen radiologically, and to involvement of adjacent vertebrae. Angular kyphosis is caused by bone destruction and collapse of the anterior portion of one or more vertebral bodies.

Other infections

Syphilis, both congenital and acquired, may affect the skeleton. There is irregular new bone formation, often periosteal, and patchy destruction and replacement of bone by fibrous granulation tissue.

In sheep farming areas, hydatid disease of bone is still seen occasionally. Immunocompromised patients are subject to a variety of otherwise rare fungal infections.

Metabolic bone disease

There are four commonly recognised metabolic diseases of bone: osteomalacia, osteoporosis, hyperparathyroidism and Paget's disease.

Osteomalacia

Osteomalacia, known as rickets in children, results from a lack of the active metabolite of vitamin D, 1,25-hydroxycholecalciferol (1,25 $(OH)_2D$), which is necessary for bone to mineralise properly as well as enhancing calcium absorption from the gut. The two sources of vitamin D are in the diet and in the skin by the action of ultraviolet light from the sun. 1,25 $(OH)_2D$ is formed by further metabolism in the liver and kidney. Its presence is necessary for calcification of the growth plate in children, without which longitudinal growth of bones cannot occur, and bone also fails to mineralise completely. In children, who are making bone rapidly, this can lead to bending and deformity of the bones. In adults the poorly calcified bone is weak and multiple microfractures cause pain.

Diagnosis is usually possible by examination of serum bio-chemistry, and treatment is by oral vitamin D.

Osteoporosis

Osteoporosis is a reduction in the density of the bone and the amount of both cancellous and cortical bone may be decreased. It may be either localised or generalised. The most common cause of localised osteoporosis is immobility, following a fracture, for example, or adjacent to an inflamed joint.

Generalised osteoporosis is the commonest of all bone diseases. It is caused by an imbalance between the normal processes of bone resorption and formation. All adults lose bone slowly with age but this loss is accelerated in women after the menopause because of the decrease and eventual cessation of oestrogen production by the ovaries. This decrease in bone density is accompanied by a decline in bone strength and leads in a high proportion of women to fractures.

Vertebral collapse fractures account for most of the loss of height seen in elderly women. Anterior collapse of the thoracic vertebrae causes kyphosis, the so-called 'dowager's hump'. More important is fracture of the neck of the femur. The stress of surgery and sometimes prolonged immobility is a major cause of morbidity in the elderly and many patients die within a year of fracture.

In men, osteoporosis tends to occur at a more advanced age, probably due to a more gradual decline in levels of male sex hormones. In younger people, steroid therapy is an important cause of osteoporosis but the mechanism for this is poorly under-stood. Thyrotoxicosis is another hormonally mediated cause of osteoporosis.

Treatment of osteoporosis is as yet controversial and largely unsatisfactory, but most postmenopausal osteoporosis could probably by prevented by hormone replacement therapy.

Hyperparathyroidism

Parathyroid hormone (PTH) helps maintain the level of serum calcium in two ways. It increases the amount of osteoclastic relative to osteoblastic activity in bone, thus releasing some of the skeleton's calcium stores into the blood. Less directly it increases calcium absorption from the gut by facilitating renal production of 1,25 $(OH)_2D$. Excess production of PTH is usually caused by a benign tumour, adenoma, of one of the four para-thyroid glands, so-called primary hyperparathyroidism. Less commonly, secondary hyperparathyroidism results from an attempt by all four glands to counteract calcium depletion due to chronic renal failure.

In both cases the effect on the skeleton is to increase the amount of skeletal remodelling. Although regional variations occur, there is an overall tendency towards osteoporosis. Thanks to earlier diagnosis and treatment, severe hyperparathyroidism is now rare, but in earlier days it was an important cause of renal stones due to prolonged hypercalcaemia. Treatment is directed to the cause of the disease, either surgery to the parathyroid glands or medical treatment for hypercalcaemia and/or renal disease.

Paget's disease

Although usually included with the metabolic bone disorders, unlike the others Paget's disease is not a generalised disorder and there is increasing evidence that it may be of viral aetiology. Its incidence varies widely throughout the world. Almost unknown in Asiatic countries, it affects about 10% of the elderly population in Britain. Fortunately, in most people it is asymptomatic and is diagnosed as a chance finding on X-ray.

The pelvis and lumbar vertebrae are most commonly involved. Usually only a part of one bone is affected and the abnormal area gradually increases in extent over the years. In severe cases there may be gross deformity and involvement of many bones.

The disorder starts as an area of intense but unco-ordinated bone remodelling. Giant osteoclasts are found on microscopic examination of bone and the lesion is predominantly lytic on X-ray. As the disease progresses, what was originally lytic becomes filled in with an excess of irregularly laid-down woven bone, which appears sclerotic on X-ray, and new areas of lysis develop (*Figure 4.3*). The disorganised remodelling of bone often leads

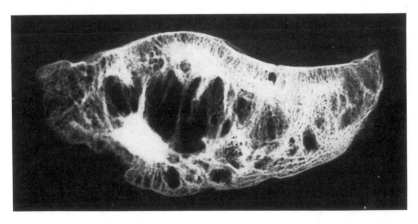

Figure 4.3. Radiograph of a slice of a patella affected by Paget's disease. The trabecular pattern is disorganised with irregular thickening and areas of sclerosis and lysis of bone.

to expansion and deformity. The normal demarcation between cortical and cancellous bone is lost and, because much of the new bone formed is weak woven bone, bowing and fracture of long bones may occur. Even without fracture the affected area may be the source of persistent pain. The most serious, but fortunately rare, complication is the development of a sarcoma in the pagetic bone (*Figure 4.4*). Such tumours are usually highly malignant and survival is seldom longer than a year.

Treatment is directed at stopping the abnormal osteoclastic activity. If this can be achieved, the rest of the remodelling

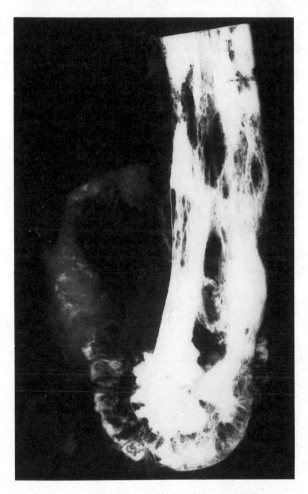

Figure 4.4. Radiograph of a slice of the lower femur. The whole of the specimen is involved by Paget's disease. At the distal end a sarcoma has developed and has grown through the cortex into the soft tissues.

abnormality is usually aborted and the disease progression may be halted or even partially reversed. Drugs used include the hormone calcitonin and the group of agents known as bisphonates.

Tumours of bone

By far the commonest form of tumour involving bone is metastatic carcinoma. This often involves multiple sites, and radio-isotope scanning is the most efficient method of detecting bone metastases. The most common primary sites for tumours metastatic to bone are breast, lung, thyroid, kidney and prostate.

Primary tumours of bone may be either benign or malignant and are classified according to their presumed cell of origin (*Table 4.1*). However, in some cases this may be uncertain and any classification will reflect areas of ignorance and controversy. *Table 4.1* is by no means complete, but includes most of the important categories of bone tumour.

Table 4.1. Classification of primary bone tumours.

Cell type	Benign	Malignant
Osteoblastic	Osteoid osteoma	Osteosarcoma
	Benign osteoblastoma	
Cartilaginous	Osteochondroma (exostosis)	Chondrosarcoma
	Enchondroma	
	Chondroblastoma	
Fibrous	Fibrous cortical defect	Malignant fibrous histiocytoma
	Non-ossifying fibroma	Fibrosarcoma
Unknown	Giant cell tumour	Ewing's sarcoma
		Adamantinoma
Marrow	Plasmacytoma	Multiple myeloma
	Eosinophilic granuloma	Lymphoma
Vascular	Haemangioma	Haemangioendothelioma
		Angiosarcoma
Notochordal		Chordoma

Most benign tumours tend to affect children and young adults. Malignant tumours, by contrast, arise in middle-aged and elderly patients with the exception of Ewing's sarcoma, which is commonest in childhood, and osteosarcoma, which affects teenagers and young adults. Space allows only a brief description of selected tumours.

Osteoblastic tumours

Osteoid osteoma produces a rounded mass of poorly formed osteoid trabeculae which never exceeds 2cm in diameter (*Figure 4.5*). It is often associated with persistent nagging pain. The surrounding

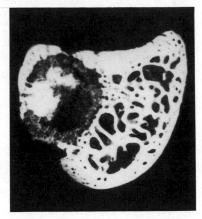

Figure 4.5. Radiograph of a slice of rib containing an osteoid osteoma. The tumour occupies the left half of the specimen.

bone reacts by sclerosis which may obscure the lesion on plain X-ray, but it shows as an intense hot spot on isotope scanning.

Benign osteoblastoma is similar in histology to the osteoid osteoma but is larger and lacks a sclerotic reaction. It occurs most frequently in the vertebral column and complete removal may be difficult. Although benign, tumour recurrence following inadequate surgery may cause serious local problems.

Osteosarcoma is the most important of the bone-forming tumours. It arises in the metaphyseal region of long bones, particularly the distal femur and proximal tibia. Although a tumour of osteoblasts, the amount of mineralised bone produced is variable and radiographs show a mixed pattern of lysis and sclerosis. Tumour growth is rapid and aggressive and early invasion through the cortex produces a soft tissue mass. Even when impalpable on clinical examination, this soft tissue extension is usually visible on the radiographs and is well seen on a CAT scan.

Although osteosarcoma may present at any age, it is predominantly a tumour of teenagers and young adults. Most such tumours arise spontaneously, but in older persons osteosarcoma may arise following radiotherapy to the affected site or as a complication of Paget's disease of bone (*Figure 4.4*). The long-term prognosis is not good, but five-year survival has improved with a combination of aggressive chemotherapy and either amputation or prosthetic replacement of the affected bone.

Cartilaginous tumours

Osteochondromas, or *exostoses*, as they are often known, may be single or multiple. Multiple osteochondromas are inherited as a Mendelian dominant condition. The tumour is essentially a defect of bone development and consists of a bony lump with a cap of cartilage. The lump protrudes from the bone surface and continues to grow until skeletal maturity, at which point the cartilage cap becomes completely ossified and only the bony mass remains. Surgery is necessary for cosmetic reasons or for symptoms caused by local pressure effects. Because of a small risk of malignant change, excision is also recommended if an exostosis recommences growth or becomes painful in adult life.

Enchondromas, by contrast, are composed entirely of cartilage. They are most frequent in the small bones of the hands and feet (*Figure 4.6*). They may also be single or multiple but, unlike multiple exostoses, multiple enchondromas are not inherited. The condition of multiple enchondromas, or enchondromatosis, is also known as Ollier's disease or, when combined with soft tissue haemangiomas, as Maffucci's syndrome.

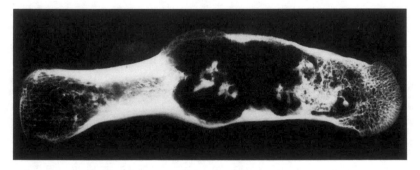

Figure 4.6. Radiograph of a slice of metacarpal containing a cartilaginous tumour. The tumour is expanding the bone and contains areas of calcification.

Malignant transformation of an enchondroma into a chondrosarcoma happens more frequently than does similar change in an exostosis, but is still rare. Not surprisingly, malignant change is commoner in patients with Ollier's disease because of the increased number of tumours at risk, but it is still unusual. However, in Maffucci's syndrome malignant disease occurs in about half of patients, either as chondrosarcomatous change in a chondroma or as tumours arising in other organs.

Chondrosarcomas may arise in any part of the skeleton and at any age but are most frequent in the middle-aged and elderly. They usually arise *de novo* but, as indicated above, may be secondary to pre-existing lesions. Radiologically they appear as expanding osteolytic lesions with areas of calcification. They are usually slowly growing tumours and metastasis occurs late if at all. Because of this a cure is possible if a correct diagnosis is made at first presentation and the tumour is excised completely. Otherwise, recurrences may be difficult to remove in their entirety and death may result from local invasion or late metastasis.

Fibrous tumours

Fibrous cortical defect is very common as an incidental X-ray finding in children and resolves spontaneously. *Non-ossifying fibroma* is a very similar but larger lesion that fails to resolve and continues growing. It may be the cause of pathological fracture. Cure is effected by simple curettage and, if necessary, bone grafting.

Malignant fibrous histiocytoma is a recently described tumour occurring most often in the elderly. It is composed of a mixture of cells with fibroblastic and histiocytic (macrophagic) characteristics. It is usually of high grade malignancy and metastasizes early. Some tumours respond to chemotherapy. *Fibrosarcoma* is a closely related tumour, but lacks a histiocytic element. Many tumours are comparatively low grade and the prognosis is correspondingly better.

Tumours of unknown origin

Giant cell tumour contains numerous multinucleated giant cells, osteoclasts (it is also known as *osteoclastoma*). However, the predominant cell type in this tumour is a mononuclear cell of uncertain origin. It never occurs in a bone that is still growing and it always involves the epiphyseal region of the bone (*Figure 4.7*). Like osteosarcoma, it is common in the distal femur and proximal tibia. Unlike osteosarcoma, it is benign. It is almost always cured by complete excision and metastases are extremely rare and may themselves often be cured by surgery alone.

Ewing's sarcoma is also of unknown cell origin. It is commonest in children but can occur in adults. It used to be rapidly fatal, with widespread metastases, but some improvement in survival has been achieved by modern chemotherapy.

Marrow tumours

Eosinophilic granuloma is derived from cells related to the macrophage family. It is usually a solitary tumour presenting in childhood. Many cases undergo spontaneous resolution and provided there is no risk of pathological fracture it may be treated conservatively. Otherwise simple curettage or low-dose radiotherapy may suffice. Unfortunately, some patients have a progressive form of the disease with involvement of multiple bones and these may require chemotherapy. When this occurs with pulmonary and pituitary involvement it is known as *Hand—Schüller—Christian*

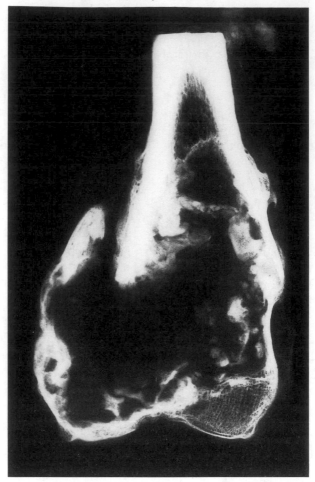

Figure 4.7. Radiograph of a slice through a giant cell tumour of the distal femur. The tumour has destroyed much of the epiphyseal region of the bone and the expanded cortex has fractured.

disease. A rare, widely disseminated form of the disease in infancy (*Letterer–Siwe disease*) is usually rapidly fatal.

Multiple myeloma is the commonest malignant tumour of bone. The neoplastic proliferation of the plasma cells is seen on X-ray as numerous lytic lesions throughout the skeleton. In the skull it produces the characteristic 'pepper-pot' appearance. All the malignant cells secrete the same abnormal immunoglobulin molecule which is seen as a monoclonal band on serum electrophoresis. Complications include the development of systemic amyloidosis and renal failure. The malignant cells crowd out the normal antibody-producing cells of the marrow and death due to infection is common.

Joints

Diseases of joints may be conveniently classified as degenerative, inflammatory, infective and metabolic.

Osteoarthritis

Osteoarthritis or degenerative arthritis is the commonest joint disease. Most cases are of unknown aetiology but some are secondary to other disorders of the joint or neighbouring bone. It is common in weight-bearing joints and may in some instances be started by simple 'wear and tear'.

The first changes seen are degeneration and fissuring of the articular cartilage. This progresses to loss of cartilage and exposure of the subchondral bone. This is recognised by diminution of joint space on the X-ray. The altered stresses on the bone caused by this loss of cartilage lead to disturbance of the normal bone remodelling activity. The exposed bone becomes sclerotic. Localised areas of fibrous replacement of bone are seen as 'cysts' on X-ray. Elsewhere, usually at the joint margin, excess production of bone forms osteophytes and the whole contour of the bone end is distorted (*Figure 4.8*).

Rheumatoid arthritis

Unlike osteoarthritis, where the disease process appears to be initiated in the articular cartilage, rheumatoid arthritis starts as an inflammation of the synovial membrane. In the early stages this causes thickening of the synovium which, together with a fluid exudate into the joint cavity, appears as painful swelling of the joints on clinical examination and an increase of the joint space on X-ray. Later, inflammatory granulation tissue destroys the bone at the joint margin (marginal erosions on X-ray). This tissue then grows over the joint surface, where it is known as *pannus*, and destroys the articular cartilage. If untreated, fibrous union or ankylosis of the joint may follow. It is the combination of bony and cartilaginous destruction together with fibrosis that leads to the deformities seen in advanced rheumatoid arthritis.

Infective arthritis

Acute infective arthritis is a rare complication of infection elsewhere in the body. Unless diagnosis and treatment are rapid, it may progress within a few days to extensive destruction of

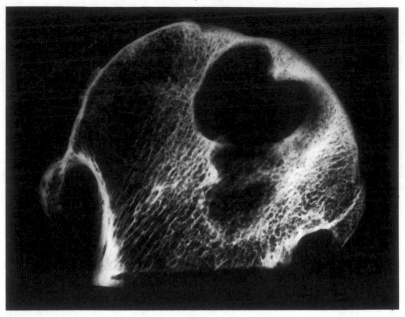

Figure 4.8. A slice through an osteoarthritic femoral head. The weight-bearing region is sclerotic; cyst formation is well developed and there are small marginal osteophytes.

the articular cartilage and subchondral bone. This is followed inevitably by the development of secondary osteoarthritis.

Chronic infective arthritis may result from infection by organisms of low virulence following joint replacement, or be tuberculous in origin.

Metabolic arthritis

The principal metabolic cause of joint disease is *gout*. Gout is a disorder of purine metabolism and most patients have a raised serum urate level. Periodically precipitation of urate crystals in synovial fluid causes an acute inflammatory reaction with swelling and severe pain. The diagnosis can be confirmed by identification of urate crystals in the joint fluid by microscopical examination using polarised light.

Bibliography

Ball, J. (1986). Aetiology and pathology of osteoarthrosis. In *Copeman's Textbook of the Rheumatic Diseases*, ed. J.T. Scott. Churchill Livingstone, pp. 821–845.

Bullough, P.G. and Vigorita, V.J. (1984). *Atlas of Orthopaedic Pathology*. Gower Medical Publishing.

Cormack, D.H. (1987). Ch 12, Bone; Ch 13, Joints. In *Ham's Histology*, J.B. Lippincott Co, pp. 273–323, 324–338.

Dahlin, D.C. and Unni, K.K. (1986). *Bone Tumors*. 4th edition, C.C. Thomas.

Gardner, D.L. (1986). In *Copeman's Textbook of the Rheumatic Diseases*, ed. J.T. Scott. Churchill Livingstone, pp. 821–845.

Revell, P.A. (1986). *Pathology of Bone*. Springer-Verlag.

5 Childhood Disorders of the Hip and Inequality of Leg Length

G.A. Evans and V. Draycott

Congenital dislocation of the hip

Epidemiology

Congenital dislocation of the hip occurs more frequently in females than males with a ratio of 3:1 at neonatal diagnosis. The reported incidence at birth is between three and five cases per thousand live births. The left hip is affected more frequently than the right, and it is bilateral in 20% of cases (*Figure 5.1*). Familial and environmental factors predispose to this condition. It is probable

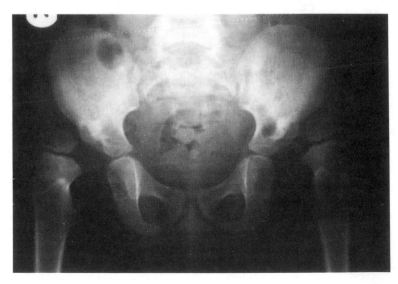

Figure 5.1. Bilateral dislocation of the hips in a 3-year-old child. It is associated with acetabular dysplasia and a straight femoral neck-shaft angle due to excessive anteversion.

that the most important familial factor is excessive generalised joint laxity, and if one parent has suffered from congenital dislocation the risk of presentation in a child is 12% (sons 6%, and daughters 17%) (Wynne-Davies, 1973). Antenatal environmental factors associated with an increased incidence of a dislocation are first-born child, breech presentation, and lack of amniotic fluid.

It is possible that intra-uterine compression, foetal position, or a combination of the two, results in a dislocation in those babies with a genetic predisposition. The joint laxity may be further increased in the perinatal period by maternal hormones responsible for relaxing the ligaments of the birth canal crossing the placenta and affecting the baby. In the post-natal period it is known that the majority of unstable hips undergo spontaneous resolution (Barlow, 1962). On the other hand if the hips are maintained in an unfavourable extended and adducted position spontaneous resolution does not occur, with the result that the incidence of dislocation appears much higher in societies in which it is customary to 'swaddle' infants.

Pathology
Neonatal hip instability varies in severity and has three different presentations:

- *Dislocation* — the femoral head is completely displaced from the acetabulum.
- *Dislocatable* — the femoral head is in the acetabulum but, with a provocative manoeuvre of backward pressure on the adducted thigh, it can be displaced from the acetabulum. Once the leg is released the femoral head usually reduces spontaneously.
- *Subluxation* — the femoral head has partial loss of articular contact but is not completely out of the acetabulum.

The shape of the femoral head and acetabulum is normal in the neonatal period, but persistence of the instability results in secondary anatomic abnormality. The acetabular labrum and capsule become deformed, and may be inverted between the head and acetabulum (limbus). When a dislocation has been present for a prolonged period, the inferior capsule and psoas tendon develop contractures, which prevent relocation of the femoral head. The femoral head begins to lose its spherical shape and the anteversion of the femoral neck tends to increase, rather than decrease as in the normally located joint. The acetabulum becomes shallow through lack of growth of its lateral and anterior margins (*Figure 5.1*). These features are progressive with the persistence of the dislocation. It is therefore important to diagnose and treat the condition at birth in order to prevent the development of the soft tissue and bony changes described, and to reduce the magnitude and morbidity of the treatment. Rarely, the dislocation may be present *in utero* and is usually associated with other joint problems such as arthrogryposis. In these circumstances the secondary changes will be present at birth.

Clinical presentation

All new-born children should be examined to try to identify dislocation or abnormal laxity of the hip. Frank dislocation is associated with shortening of the leg, a high-riding prominent trochanter, a relative emptiness of the femoral triangle, and telescoping on proximal pressure. The head can be felt to relocate on performing Ortolani's manoeuvre, which involves abducting and raising the flexed thigh forwards gently. Occasionally, on performing this manoeuvre the sensation of a click can be elicited from the joint. In the absence of displacement of the femoral head this is of no serious significance. With such neonatal screening, Barlow (1962) claimed that he was able to diagnose all cases in the new-born period and eradicate the late presentation of hip dislocation. However, in most centres world-wide, we have not been able to reproduce this success, and a minority of cases continue to present later in life. Apart from failure to recognise a neonatal dislocation, a further possible explanation is that the occasional neonatal subluxation, which is difficult to detect clinically, may result in progressive acetabular dysplasia and displacement of the femoral head (Kepley and Weiner, 1981). Examination of a new-born hip with ultrasound will possibly reduce the incidence of late presentation.

In the older child, the classical clinical signs of dislocation include limited abduction, a high greater trochanter, and relative femoral shortening. The dislocation is no longer reducible by the Ortolani manoeuvre. After the age of walking, there is a noticeable limp with a positive Trendelenburg test. Bilateral cases present with a symmetrical waddling gait, which may not be recognised as being abnormal until the child has grown out of the toddler age.

Treatment

The objective of treatment is to reduce the femoral head into the acetabulum without producing damage to it or its blood supply by forceful manoeuvres. The specific treatment depends on the age of the child at diagnosis. It is advantageous to start treatment in the neonatal period, before the onset of secondary soft tissue and bony changes. For this reason all children are screened for congenital dislocation as part of the neonatal examination, and at the developmental screening usually undertaken by the community physician at approximately 6 weeks and 6 months of age.

When the diagnosis is made in the *newborn*, the principle of treatment is to retain the hip in flexion and abduction, so that the femoral head is reduced in the acetabulum. The initial capsular laxity regresses, and after approximately 3 months' treatment the joint is stable, requires no further treatment, and the prognosis for a normal joint is excellent. Treatment usually starts once the diagnosis has been made, although in some centres it is deferred for 2−3 weeks because, as mentioned above, a large number resolve spontaneously and only the minority of hips with residual instability are then treated. There are many different devices available to maintain the flexed and abducted posture of the hips, and these include the Craig nappy splint, the Von Rosen splint, and the Pavlik harness. The former two splints tend to hold the hips in one position, whereas the Pavlik harness allows motion, but within a constrained range (*Figure 5.2*).

When treatment is started later, *up to 6 months of age*, the Pavlik harness achieves reduction in the majority of cases. When the harness is first applied the hip is still dislocated, but the active movement and kicking of the child within the constraints of

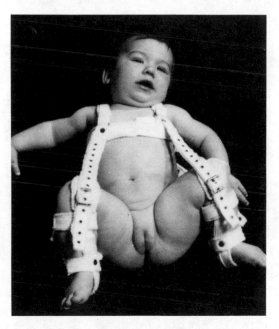

Figure 5.2. Pavlik harness applied.

the harness achieve a spontaneous reduction. The complications of this treatment in terms of damage of the femoral head are negligible. When successful, the reduction is achieved within 3 weeks, but the harness is usually retained for up to a further 6 months, depending on the appearance of the bony growth and remodelling on radiographic examination. The treatment described so far can be undertaken as an outpatient.

If diagnosed after *6 months of age*, or if any of the above-mentioned treatment has failed to achieve reduction, the child requires in-patient treatment. At this stage there is relative shortening of the soft tissues adjacent to the hip joint. Skin traction is therefore an important preliminary treatment to manipulative or operative reduction. This prevents excessive pressure on the head and damage to it following reduction. There are several different techniques of applying traction to the legs, some of which attempt to obtain reduction during the period of traction. Other forms, such as overhead divarication traction for 2 weeks (*Figure 5.3*) are used primarily to stretch the soft tissues, followed by a gentle manipulative reduction under general anaesthesia. This is called a 'closed reduction'. An arthrogram of the hip joint may be performed at the same time to demonstrate absence of soft tissue interposition between the femoral head and acetabulum. In a small child the majority of the femoral head and acetabulum are

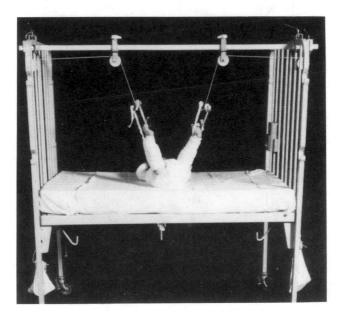

Figure 5.3. Gallows traction.

made of cartilage and do not show on a plain radiograph. If a closed reduction cannot be achieved (*Figure 5.1*) an operation is necessary to remove the obstructive factors and this is called an 'open reduction'. The most common obstructive factors are persistent contracture of the inferior capsule, a tight psoas tendon, and an inverted limbus. Once the reduction has been achieved, by either manipulation or operation, it is maintained by application of a plaster of Paris spica. The regime thereafter depends on the individual preference of the treating surgeon. In general terms, hip abduction is maintained by either a plaster cast or a splint until there is evidence of satisfactory bony remodelling of the joint on the radiograph. Plaster casts are changed at intervals depending on the rate of growth of the child, with short periods of physiotherapy at the time of admission for plaster change. Stiffness is more likely to be a problem after open rather than closed reduction.

Additional operative procedures may be required in an older child, when there is less potential for bony remodelling following reduction of a dislocation. It may be elected to correct either the excessive femoral anteversion, or the dysplasia of the acetabulum in order to improve the stability of the reduction while the leg is in the weight-bearing functional position. This reduces the need for prolonged splintage in abduction and flexion. The anteversion is corrected by derotation osteotomy of the proximal femur (*Figures 5.4(a)* and *5.4(b)*), and the acetabular dysplasia by a pelvic osteotomy, described by Salter, which tilts the acetabulum downwards, forwards, and laterally (*Figures 5.5(a)* and *5.5(b)*) (Salter, 1961). Following such surgery, the child is immobilised in a plaster spica for 6 weeks until the osteotomy has united, and then requires physiotherapy to assist progressive mobilisation. In the very occasional case presenting *after 3 years* of age, both the femoral and acetabular dysplasia may require surgical correction. The whole correction can be performed at one operation but there is an increased risk of postoperative joint stiffness.

Very occasionally a child may present for the first time during *adolescence* with a limp or discomfort in the hip due to subluxation and acetabular dysplasia (*Figure 5.6*). If the subluxation is irreducible, as is frequently the case at this age, the position is accepted and the cover of the femoral head improved with a pelvic osteotomy. At this age a Chiari osteotomy is appropriate, dividing the ilium immediately above the level of the head and displacing the lower fragment with the head medially under the cover of the upper fragment. The superior joint capsule remains between the articular surface of the femoral head and the exposed bone of the osteotomy surface (Chiari, 1974). Unlike the Salter osteotomy performed at a younger age, this does not place normal

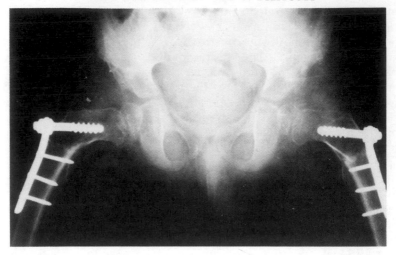

Figure 5.4(a). Open reduction and femoral derotation osteotomy to correct the anteversion (same patient as (Figure 5.1)).

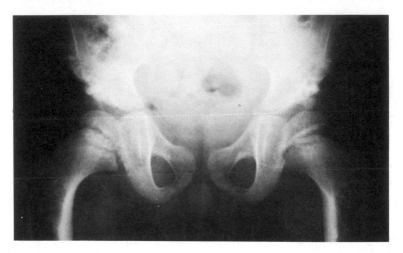

Figure 5.4(b). The surgical plate and screws have been removed, and the acetabulae are slowly remodelling as the child grows (Figures 5.1 and 5.4(a)).

articular cartilage over the head, and is therefore regarded as a salvage rather than a reconstructive operation. Sometimes a bony shell (Staheli, 1981) is constructed over the femoral head rather than performing the Chiari osteotomy. Following a period of immobilisation in plaster to allow the osteotomy to unite, the

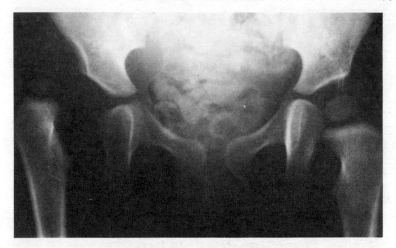

Figure 5.5(a). Unilateral dislocation in a 22-month-old-child.

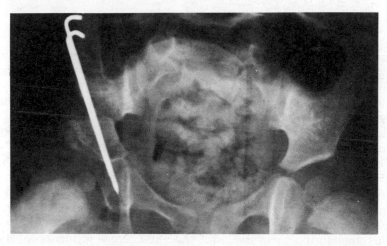

Figure 5.5(b). Following combined open reduction and a Salter pelvic osteotomy which turns the acetabulum over the reduced head (Figure 5.5(a)).

patient requires physiotherapy to mobilise the joint and to strengthen the abductor and extensor muscles.

Physiotherapy

Physiotherapy has only a small part to play in the early stages of the treatment, dealing mainly with the application of the various splints mentioned previously. As with all treatments, careful assessment should be made, looking for clinical signs

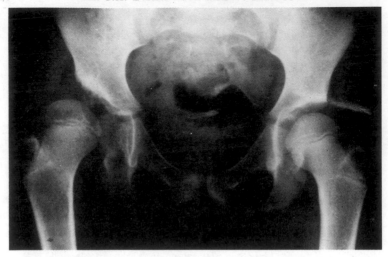

Figure 5.6. Adolescent child with subluxation of the femoral head and acetabular dysplasia.

such as limited range of abduction, apparent limb-length inequality and, in the child who has already begun to walk, looking for 'dipping' or toe-walking.

Should splintage not achieve its objective, hospital admission will be necessary, involving 2 weeks on traction. The purpose of the traction is to stretch the soft tissues around the hip joint prior to reduction, which may be either open or closed (*Figure 5.7*). During this time, if it is possible to get co-operation from the child, the physiotherapist should encourage active movements of the feet and isometric contractions of the quadriceps and gluteal muscles. It may mean that treatment takes the form of play, and parents and nurses should be encouraged to attempt to achieve this aim during their stay with the child. Once reduction of the hip has been achieved the child is immobilised in a plaster of Paris double hip spica for a minimum period of 6 weeks, which may extend to 10 weeks, depending upon the method of reduction used by the surgeon.

Once the plaster is bivalved then physiotherapy is of value. Exercises to regain mobility of the hips and knees, combined with strengthening of the muscles, especially the gluteals, are of vital importance. Wherever possible, mobilisation should include hydrotherapy. A gradual 'weaning' out of the plaster halves will take approximately 10 days, dependent upon each child's ability. Weight-bearing is commenced once the hips and knees are mobile and strong enough to allow a reciprocal gait, that is, at least 90° of

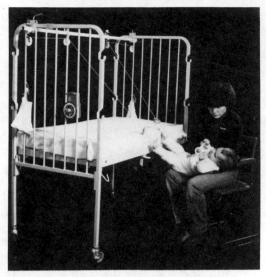

Figure 5.7. Baby on gallows traction allowing bonding with its mother.

hip and knee flexion, and the gluteal muscles are strong enough to prevent 'waddling'. Once walking has begun, it is important to discourage any asymmetry of gait which, if left uncorrected, may become habitual and lead to further acquired deformities.

Perthes' disease

Epidemiology

Perthes' disease is a transient ischaemic necrosis of the capital femoral epiphysis which occurs in children between the ages of 2 and 12 years, but mainly between 4 and 8. Boys are affected four times more frequently than girls and the condition is bilateral in approximately 12% of affected children. It was described almost simultaneously at the beginning of the twentieth century by Legg from the United States, Calvé from France and Perthes from Germany. There is no obvious pattern of inheritance. Many children appear to be undersized and skeletally immature at the time of developing Perthes' disease. There is also a slightly higher incidence of minor congenital anomalies in these children compared to a control population. It is speculated that there may be a congenital abnormality affecting skeletal development which in some ways makes the hip susceptible to Perthes' disease. However, the precise aetiology is unknown.

Pathology

The pathological process involves the death of part or the whole of the capital femoral epiphysis followed by gradual revascularisation of the area. The articular cartilage is normal or, at most, shows faint signs of degeneration in its basilar layers. At an early stage a radiograph will show flattening and increased density of the femoral head (*Figure 5.8(a)*). On microscopic examination there is pronounced necrosis of the bone with grossly distorted marrow trabeculae, and the bone fragments are of a soft consistency. Later the radiograph appears to show the femoral head broken up into areas that are relatively dense interspersed with areas of radiolucency. This represents the resorption of the dead bone with added areas of osteoid and new bone. The femoral head may become distorted, flattened, and extruded laterally from its normal location under the acetabulum. There is a gradual increase in the amount of living bone, and on the radiograph the femoral head usually regains its homogenous density over 2—4 years. In the meantime it may lose its normal spherical shape and become flattened superiorly. This is important as the final shape of the head influences the long-term prognosis of the joint. If the head remains spherical, even if it is slightly larger, the prognosis is good. Increasing loss of sphericity and congruity predisposes to a proportionate increase in the severity of secondary osteoarthritis during adult life.

Clinical presentation

The most frequently observed symptom is a limp, which may or may not be associated with pain in the groin and inner thigh. Occasionally, the pain may be referred to the distal thigh and knee. Muscle spasm is usually present and limits abduction and internal rotation of the hip. The absence of pyrexia, with normal haematological investigations, excludes the differential diagnosis of pyogenic arthritis or osteomyelitis of the femoral neck.

Treatment

Perthes' is a self-limiting condition and all affected femoral heads heal. The objective of treatment is therefore to try to minimise the deformity during the active stages of the disease in order to reduce the incidence of osteoarthritis during adult life. The age of onset of the condition and the amount of femoral head involved appear to be the two major prognostic factors. Children under 5 years usually do very well, especially if the femoral head is only partly necrotic. However, onset after 6 years of age, has a less favourable prognosis. When the child first presents, it is generally agreed that the appropriate treatment consists of bed rest and skin traction in order to relieve the muscle spasm and regain the

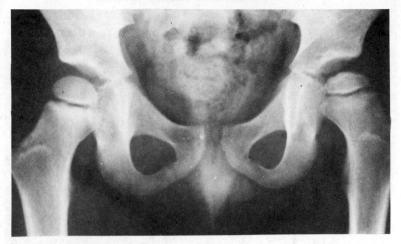

Figure 5.8(a). Early flattening and lateral displacement of the femoral head (right) due to Perthes' disease.

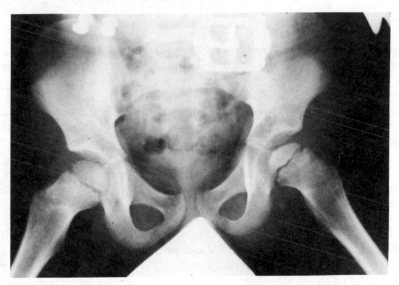

Figure 5.8(b). Femoral head 'contained' in the acetabulum by application of an abduction brace.

range of hip motion. An alternative to skin traction is resting the legs on slings and springs (Figure 5.9). The majority of children will have regained full abduction and internal rotation after 2–3 weeks' treatment. The management thereafter varies widely

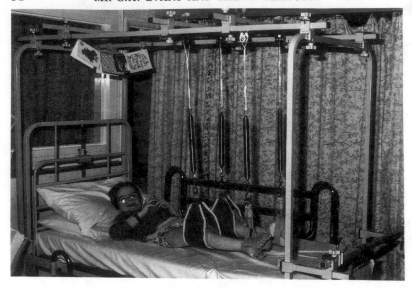

Figure 5.9. A child resting with his legs on slings and suspended by springs.

within Great Britain, and throughout the world. There has been a general trend to try to select the appropriate cases which would benefit from further treatment. For example, the prognosis for presentation under four years of age with partial head involvement, and without lateral displacement of the head, is excellent and does not justify the imposition of restricted activities or surgical intervention.

Although there are many different specific methods of managing Perthes' disease, there are two basic treatment principles, which may be applied individually or in combination. The first principle is *weight relief* and the second is *containment*. The latter principle refers to the fact that if the femoral head can be maintained deeply within the acetabulum during the soft vulnerable phase of the disease process, the acetabulum will function rather like a mould, and a more normal femoral head will result. Since it is the lateral and anterior portions of the capital epiphysis which become uncovered, the containment can be achieved by abduction and internal rotation of the hip. (*Figures 5.8(a)* and *5.8(b)*).

Non-weight-bearing treatment includes bed rest with or without traction, and was traditionally applied on a Robert Jones frame. Bed rest for longer than is necessary to regain motion in the hips is now no longer considered practical. Weight relief is also achieved with a Snyder sling. Ischial weight-bearing braces are not truly weight-relieving and on occasions may increase the pressure across the joint. The hip usually remains adducted with this brace and the results of treatment are inferior to those of containment methods. There are several methods of the treatment that rely on containment of the femoral head but allow weight-bearing. These include plaster casts to maintain the abduction, so-called broomstick or Petrie plasters (*Figure 5.10*); abduction splints and surgical intervention. There is probably little difference in the results of these containment methods and the choice will depend on the availability of an orthotist to undertake prompt delivery and repairs of a splint, and on the geographic and social factors which influence the indications for operative treatment. One type of abduction splint was developed at the Scottish-Rite hospital in Atlanta, USA, and allows the child to walk in abduction with minimal other restriction, to attend school and sit at his normal desk, and to play out of doors (*Figures 5.11(a)* and *5.11(b)*). This particular splint does not maintain internal rotation of the hip, but on weight-bearing there is usually a minimum of 20° flexion of the hip which achieves a similar cover of the anterior portion of the femoral head.

Surgical containment of the femoral head can be produced by either a proximal femoral varus derotation osteotomy (*Figure 5.12*) or by altering the acetabulum to provide further coverage with a Salter pelvic osteotomy. Surgery is more often indicated when the prognosis indicates that the healing phase may be prolonged, as in older children. It can also be used for

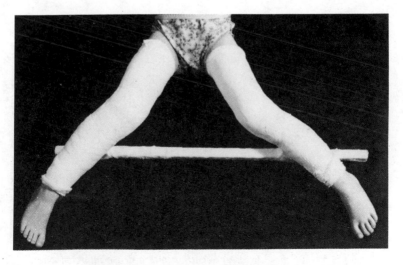

Figure 5.10. Petrie or broomstick plasters.

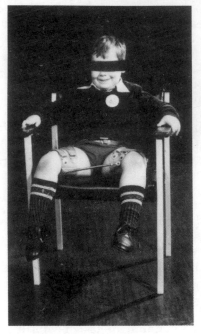

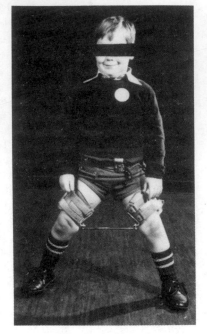

Figure 5.11(a). The Scottish-Rite brace (sitting).

Figure 5.11(b). The Scottish-Rite brace (standing).

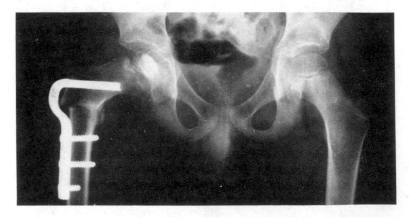

Figure 5.12. Perthes' disease presenting with a dense infarcted capital epiphysis which has been treated by femoral osteotomy.

ɔatients who will not tolerate a bracing programme. The range of movement must be almost normal prior to surgical treatment.

Physiotherapy

Providing the decision is made to institute active treatment, this may again be in the form of conservative or operative intervention. In both cases *containment* of the hip is the ultimate aim. Conservative measures may include both weight-bearing and non-weight-bearing means. If prolonged bed rest is advised as a method of non-weight-bearing the child must be taught all static exercises, particularly quadriceps and gluteals, together with resisted exercises to avoid muscle wasting. The Snyder sling may also be used; this allows the child to be mobile on axillary crutches and still remain non-weight-bearing on the affected side.

One method of weight-bearing with containment is the application of Petrie plasters (*Figure 5.10*). These are long leg plaster-of-Paris cylinders, with the knees flexed at approximately 15°. By attaching a broomstick at the lower end of the plaster cylinders, with the hips abducted 30° and internally rotated 20°, containment is achieved. This method does not allow reciprocal hip flexion and the child has to be taught to stand in the plasters, eventually becoming totally independent. Such children are readmitted to hospital at 3-monthly intervals, when the plaster is removed and a period of hip and knee mobilising begun, strictly non-weight-bearing. Hydrotherapy, once again, has proved invaluable at this time. Once a full range of movement has been regained, particularly in the knees, the plasters are reapplied and the child discharged. This procedure is repeated until, based on radiological findings, healing is complete.

Another method of weight-bearing treatment may be achieved by the wearing of the Scottish-Rite brace (*Figures 5.11(a)* and *5.11(b)*). The brace is custom-made by the orthotist and the child should be taught to be completely independent within the splint, leading as near normal a life as possible – some boys have been known to cycle while wearing the brace. Once the brace is fitted, the child has to be taught to balance in the abducted position, and from then on to progress to a reciprocal gait, making use of the universal joints on the abduction bar of the splint. In order to maintain an upright posture the child stands with flexed hips and knees, thus self-inducing containment of the femoral head. As long as the child is wearing the brace, the parents should be taught how to look after it, and be shown the exercises to be done with the child, daily, to maintain hip range and muscle power, particularly hip extensors.

Should surgical intervention be undertaken in the form of a femoral osteotomy (*Figure 5.12*) with plate fixation, the immediate

6 weeks' postoperative period is spent in a double hip spica, during which the child can be discharged home. On readmission, the plaster is bivalved and the child 'weaned' out of it over the first few days until full hip and knee joint range and power are regained. Weight-bearing is started once the child is able to control his leg.

Slipped upper femoral epiphysis

The term 'slipped capital femoral epiphysis' refers to a displacement of the femoral neck in relationship to the head, usually during adolescence. The femoral neck rotates externally and slides upward causing the radiological appearance of a femoral head which is displaced posteriorly and inferiorly (*Figure 5.13(a)*).

Epidemiology

Boys are more frequently affected than girls and, because of the delayed growth spurt in boys, the condition occurs on average about 2 years later than in girls. The age range for boys is 10–17 years, with an average of 11–12 years. The black population is apparently more frequently affected than the white population. The skeletal age is usually below chronological age, and approximately half the patients have body weight at or above the 95th percentile. The condition occurs bilaterally in approximately one-fifth of cases. There is occasionally a positive family history of the condition.

Aetiology

The precise aetiology is still unknown. The plane of separation is at the bone–cartilage junction of the growth plate and it is thought that there may be increased structural weakness at this site during the adolescent growth spurt. There are some interesting mechanical factors which have been observed. The growth plate normally changes from a horizontal to an oblique position during the early adolescent period and the periosteum of the femoral neck, which is the main stabiliser of the epiphysis, atrophies at the same time. In addition, there may be hormonal factors which relate to the balance of pituitary growth hormone and sex hormones. The sex hormones induce growth–plate closure at skeletal maturity, and growth hormone stimulates the proliferation of the cells of the growth plate. A frequent condition associated with slipped epiphysis is the adiposo-genital syndrome, a condition characterised by obesity and deficient gonadal development, which suggests that it may be due to excessive loading of the relatively weak growth plate. Less frequently, the condition occurs

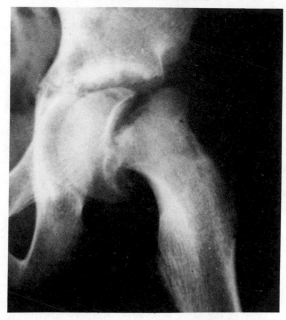

Figure 5.13(a). Displacement of the capital femoral epiphysis which occurred suddenly after a preceding history of an ache and occasional limp.

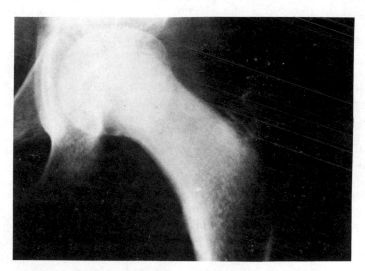

Figure 5.13(b). Improved position of the epiphysis as the result of skin traction applied with progressive abduction and internal rotation of the hip.

in very tall, thin boys, which may indicate a relative excess o: growth hormone and weakness of the rapidly proliferating growth plate. When the slip is bilateral and symmetrical, other conditions such as hypothyroidism should be excluded.

Clinical presentations
There are three classical presentations:

- The *acute* slip is the result of significant injury with no previous history of pain. It is usually severe enough to prevent weight-bearing.
- The *acute on chronic* slip presents with some aching in the hip or distal thigh for weeks or even months prior to an acute episode, as described above (*Figure 5.13(a)*).
- The *chronic* slip is the commonest presentation, the child complaining of a limp, pain, and loss of motion which may have been present for several weeks (*Figure 5.14(a)*). Occasionally, the only symptom is pain referred to the knee.

Examination reveals restriction of internal rotation and abduction, and as the thigh is flexed it tends to roll into external rotation and abduction. There is frequent shortening of the leg, which tends to lie in external rotation. Radiographic examination will confirm the diagnosis and indicate the severity of the displacement. In chronic cases there is remodelling of the inferior and posterior aspects of the femoral neck adjacent to the growth plate, which begins to develop a slight hook. The opposite hip should be examined carefully for early involvement, which may simply be a widening of the epiphyseal line.

Treatment
Once the diagnosis has been made, the child should not be allowed to weight-bear and arrangements should be made to admit the child directly to hospital for treatment. This is in order to prevent any further displacement. The child is placed in bed with skin traction on both legs in order to reduce spasm and relieve discomfort.

If the slip is acute the displacement can be corrected with skin traction, by slowly and progressively abducting and internally rotating the leg (*Figure 5.13(b)*). Alternatively, the reduction can be achieved by gentle manipulation under general anaesthesia. If the acute slip has been present for more than 2 weeks, there is considerable risk of avascular necrosis from manipulation, and because of this problem there is divided opinion as to whether manipulative treatment should be used at all. If an acute slip has occurred on a pre-existing chronic slip, it is important that the

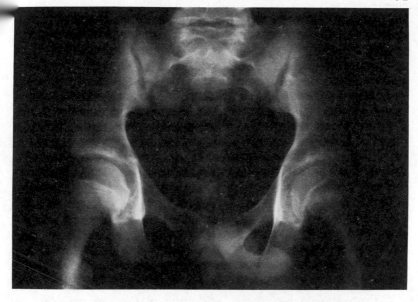

Figure 5.14(a). A chronic slip of the capital epiphysis (right). There is slight widening of the growth plate, and early upward displacement of the metaphysis.

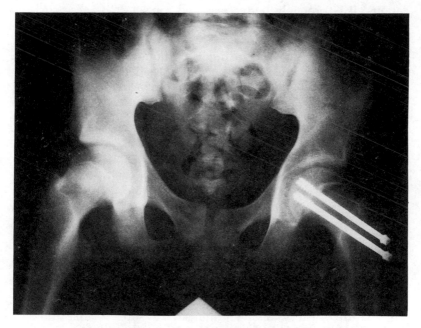

Figure 5.14(b). Surgical fixation of the epiphysis by insertion of screws which pass along the femoral neck and across the growth plate.

repositioning only reduces the acute aspect of the slip. The greater threat to the hip is avascular necrosis, and not incomplete reduction. Further displacement is prevented by surgical insertion of pins along the femoral neck into the epiphysis.

The objective of treatment in the child with a chronic slip is to stabilise the femoral head *in situ* and maintain the range of motion. This is usually preceded by a period of bed rest and traction, which relieves muscle spasm and synovitis, and apparently reduces the risk of the complication of chondrolysis. Further displacement is then prevented by operative insertion of pins or screws along the femoral neck into the epiphysis (*Figure 5.14(b)*). In cases with severe displacement this may be technically very difficult. Operations have been devised either to correct the displacement at the level of the open growth plate (Dunn's osteotomy) (Dunn and Angel, 1978), or to compensate for the deformity with a subtrochanteric osteotomy (Southwick, 1967) or intertrochanteric osteotomy (Griffith, 1976). There appears to be an increased risk of avascular necrosis with the former procedure, and of chondrolysis with the latter procedure.

If the opposite hip shows widening of the growth plate, or early slip, it should also be pinned. There is debate as to whether prophylactic pinning of the contralateral hip should be undertaken routinely. As pinning of the hip can be associated with complications, it is probably better reserved for selected cases such as those with predisposing hormonal abnormalities, for example the adiposo-genital syndrome.

The main complications of this condition and its treatment are avascular necrosis and chondrolysis. Avascular necrosis occurs as a result of tension and occlusion of the retinacular vessels passing along the femoral neck to the capital epiphysis. This causes necrosis and collapse of the femoral head with loss of sphericity. The potential for retaining a spherical head is very much poorer at this age than in young children with Perthes' disease, and usually results in secondary osteoarthritis during early adult life. Chondrolysis presents with acute pain and restricted motion of the hip joint. The precise cause is not known. There is a loss of articular cartilage, which is later replaced by fibrocartilage, which does not have the same properties of wear, and predisposes to secondary osteoarthritis. The initial treatment is to try to reduce the joint reaction with traction and salicylates, and to retain a range of motion with physiotherapy. This is followed by a prolonged period of non-weight-bearing and motion exercises. Despite this treatment the range of motion may be very limited. The natural history of even the severe slips is that they do well into middle life before the development of osteoarthritis, if there has been no avascular necrosis or chondrolysis. This therefore suggests that simple methods of treatment that decrease or eliminate the risk of avascular necrosis or chondrolysis should be most commonly used.

Following pin fixation of the femoral epiphysis the patient is encouraged to regain active control of the hip and, in particular, the ranges of abduction and internal rotation. When this has been achieved the child is allowed to weight-bear partially with the aid of crutches, and the decision to allow full weight-bearing will vary according to the degree of displacement and security of fixation. The growth plate usually fuses prematurely, which prevents any further possibility of displacement, and it is usual to remove the pins at this stage.

Physiotherapy

Following surgery, it is important that early assisted movements are given to the hip. Progressive exercises are given over the initial 10-day postoperative period, bearing in mind the need to maintain and, if possible, increase the muscle power of the unaffected leg, as the child, will have to be non-weight-bearing initially.

During the non-weight-bearing period it is important that the child continues with exercises to the affected hip. Isometric exercises for the gluteal and quadriceps muscles should be taught, together with maximum movement in all ranges at the hip joint. During treatment it is important to examine the sound hip at regular intervals as, occasionally, the contralateral epiphysis may slip; even during the postoperative period of bed rest. As the result of handling the patient on several occasions each day, it is often the physiotherapist who first detects this.

Coxa vara

Coxa vara is an abnormality of the proximal end of the femur which is characterised by a decrease in the neck shaft angle. This angle measures approximately 150° at 1 year and gradually decreases to 120° in the adult. A neck shaft angle of less than 120° in a child is arbitrarily labelled as coxa vara.

Aetiology

There are many different causes of coxa vara. *Infantile* coxa vara is regarded as a distinct entity and is characterised by having a triangular bone defect in the inferior part of the metaphysis of the femoral neck (*Figure 5.15*). It is sometimes bilateral but is not associated with any other developmental defect. Several reports

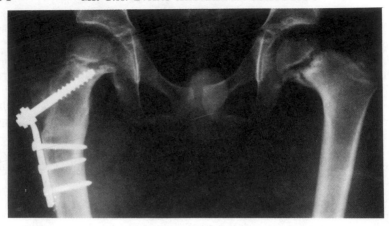

Figure 5.15. Bilateral coxa vara which has been corrected on one side by a valgus osteotomy. On the other side the triangular bone defect persists at the inferior margin of the metaphysis.

of a family history suggest that the condition has a genetic transmission.

Other focal forms of coxa vara include children with a congenital short femur, which may sometimes be associated with lateral bowing of the proximal femoral shaft and sclerosis on the concave side (Figure 5.16). In the more severe forms, a pseudoarthrosis may be present between the femoral neck and shaft, and this represents the minor end of the spectrum of congenital anomalies known as proximal focal femoral deficiency. Other causes of coxa vara include any skeletal disorder or dysplasia which results in softening or weakening of the bones. Examples include osteogenesis imperfecta, Morquio's disease, achondroplasia, and metaphyseal chondrodysplasia.

Clinical presentation
In infantile coxa vara the deformity is diagnosed when the child first walks, usually with a painless limp or waddling gait. Trendelenburg's sign is positive and hip abduction limited. The greater trochanter is elevated sometimes so that the tip of the trochanter impinges upon the ilium, resulting in marked gluteal deficiency. In unilateral cases there is usually a leg-length discrepancy.

Treatment
Treatment depends on the degree of deformity, the functional impairment, and the evidence as to whether the deformity is

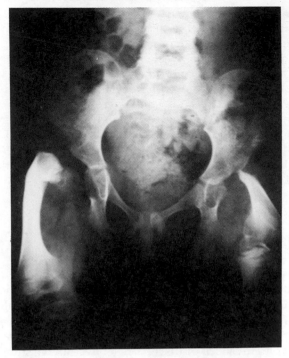

Figure 5.16. Congenital shortening of the femur with coxa vara. On the opposite side there is congenital absence of the femoral head and proximal shaft.

progressive. Conservative treatment may be employed in mild cases where the varus deformity is not progressing and the neck shaft angle approaches normal. However, in the majority of children with the infantile variety of coxa vara, early surgery provides the best opportunity to achieve a painless and fully mobile hip without further shortening of the limb. The indications for surgery are the presence of a vertical defect in the femoral neck, a neck shaft angle of less than 100°, and progression of the coxa vara, which may or may not be associated with discomfort. An intertrochanteric or subtrochanteric valgus osteotomy accompanied by internal fixation is the preferred form of treatment (*Figure 5.15*). The operative goal is to place the proximal femoral growth plate in a normal alignment, perpendicular to the resultant weight-bearing force acting across the hip joint. This in turn improves the hip abductor function, and reduces the leg length discrepancy. Postoperatively a plaster spica is applied for approximately 6 weeks until the osteotomy has united, and then mobilising and strengthening exercises are prescribed.

Physiotherapy

Treatment is based on the aim to preserve hip joint function. Following surgery the patient is usually immobilised in a plaster-of-Paris hip spica for 6 weeks. After this time the plaster is bivalved and gentle active assisted exercises are given to the hip and knee joints. Often the posterior half of the plaster is retained as a night splint until the child is able to control active leg movements adequately. Progressive non-weight bearing exercises are given, combined with hydrotherapy, until a full range of movement is achieved. Weight-bearing is started as soon as union of the osteotomy is confirmed radiologically and the patient is able to control the limb fully.

Inequality of leg length

Aetiology

The problem of leg-length discrepancy is common, despite the fact that the aetiological factors have changed considerably during the past 25 years. Prior to the advent of poliomyelitis vaccine, shortening due to the muscle paralysis of polio was the most common. Other causes of discrepancy have now assumed greater importance, and may result in either shortening or lengthening of a limb. A short leg may be caused by a congenital abnormality (*Figures 5.17(a)* and *5.17(b)*), infection of bone and joint, and fractures of the long bones, especially those which result in damage and tethering of the growth plate. Neurological conditions, such as spinal dysraphism and spastic hemiparesis, may also sometimes cause significant shortening. Overgrowth of the limb may be associated with a haemangioma or arteriovenous malformation, neurofibromatosis, and fibrous dysplasia. Rarely, significant overgrowth may occur due to stimulation of bone growth following fracture of the femur or tibia, or the stimulus of osteotomy and subsequent plate removal.

Clinical presentation

The child may present with a limp, and other symptoms or signs which relate to the aetiology of the discrepancy. The inequality of leg length does not cause pain. When standing with both feet flat on the floor there is a pelvic obliquity and compensatory scoliosis, which the child tolerates without symptoms (*Figure 5.17(a)*). Alternatively, the child can stand with a level pelvis either by flexing the knee on the longer leg or by weight-bearing on the forefoot of the shorter leg. If the condition is not associated with weakness or derangement of the joints, the gait may appear

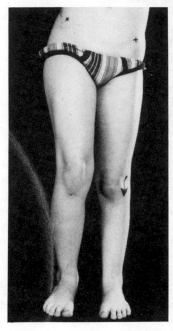
(a)

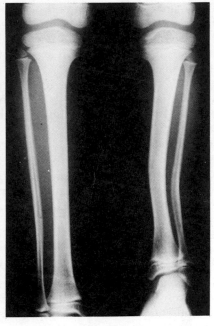
(b)

Figure 5.17(a). Inequality of leg length. The child stands with pelvic obliquity and compensatory scoliosis.

Figure 5.17(b). Radiograph showing the short and slightly bowed tibia and fibula.

remarkably normal. The child frequently vaults on the forefoot of the short leg in order to compensate for the discrepancy.

Treatment

The most significant factor in deciding the appropriate management is the degree of discrepancy. Differences of less than 2cm are usually accepted by the patient and can be treated by non-surgical methods, such as a shoe-raise. At the other end of the scale, any projected inequality exceeding 20cm is usually in excess of the amount that any combination of operations can be effectively or predictably employed to equalise. The only exception is when surgical conversion (amputation or disarticulation) and application of a prosthesis are employed. For the most part, therefore, only discrepancies between 2 and 20cm warrant serious consideration for surgical equalisation. These are not rigid figures and they represent only practical guidelines, which may be modified by the many other factors involved in the aetiology of the discrepancy. It is assumed for the purpose of the following discussion that the problem is a true discrepancy of length, rather than an apparent shortening or lengthening of the limb produced by a fixed adduction or abduction contracture, respectively, at the hip.

In addition to the severity of the discrepancy, other factors which influence the nature and timing of treatment include the skeletal age, anticipated adult height, and sex. The progression of discrepancy can be measured accurately by taking serial radiographs known as grid films or scanograms. These also allow assessment of the relative discrepancy within the femur and tibia. Serial radiographs of the hand will allow an assessment of bone age and development, which may precede or lag behind chronological age by up to 2 years. Serial measurement of height on a percentile chart will allow prediction of the anticipated adult height. These measurements are important to help decide the most appropriate treatment, and to monitor the effect if started prior to skeletal maturity.

Surgical equalisation of limb length can be achieved either by shortening the long side, lengthening the short side, or utilising a combination of shortening and lengthening.

A limb can be shortened in one of three ways:

- The growth plate of the distal femur, or proximal tibia and fibula, can be arrested prematurely by epiphyseodesis (Phemister, 1933).
- The same centres can be arrested temporarily or permanently by epiphyseal stapling (Blount, 1958).
- The femur or tibia (or both) can be shortened by resection of bone.

Epiphyseodesis is performed on the longer leg at an appropriate time prior to skeletal maturity and, if successful, the short limb continues to grow and will exactly correct the discrepancy by the completion of growth. It is critical to time the operation correctly and this depends on the information gained from serial pre-operative grid films and bone-age assessment. Epiphyseodesis is usually reserved for discrepancies not exceeding 5cm. It is a relatively simple operation, without significant complications, and the rate of acceptable correction is high. Stapling of the epiphysis has a similar effect and convalescence is more rapid. Theoretically, the principal advantage that this operation offers over epiphyseodesis is that the operation can be reversed by removal of the staples if overcorrection is occurring. However, practical experience has shown that the response of the growth plate to staple removal is not predictable and the reliability of this procedure is not really proven. The operation is also technically demanding and if the staples are not inserted in precisely the correct site there is a risk of producing asymmetrical growth arrest and deformity. Unlike the former two procedures, bone-shortening operations can be used during or after completion of growth. Up to 6cm of subtrochanteric bone can be resected from the femur without permanent weakening of the thigh or hip, and even more bone can be resected at a midshaft shortening. Shortening below the knee requires resection of a portion of tibia and fibula. These operations are usually associated with internal fixation of the bone fragments.

Correction of inequality can also be achieved by lengthening of bone. The method which has remained most consistently acceptable is osteotomy followed by gradual distraction. The technical steps include an osteotomy, application of a mechanical distraction device, and gradual distraction of 1mm per day (*Figure 5.18*). Electromyographic study of the lengthened muscles indicates that a 10% lengthening of the bone's initial length is a safe limit, with 15% being the absolute maximum. Slow lengthening protects the soft tissues, in particular the peripheral nerves, and during distraction daily clinical assessment should

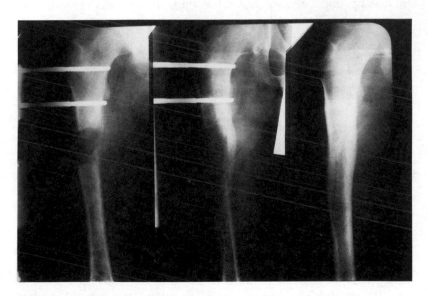

Figure 5.18. Three stages in the lengthening of a femur. Initially, the fixator is distracted, drawing out bone between the osteotomy surfaces. Once the desired length is achieved the fixator is locked and later dynamised to allow progressive strengthening of the new bone. Finally, the fixator is removed.

be performed to exclude early or minor neuropraxia. If present, further distraction is temporarily discontinued until nerve function has recovered, and then further gradual lengthening is usually possible until the desired lengthening is achieved. Clinical guidelines which are helpful in governing the rate of distraction are the degree of pain, the development of sensory or motor neurologic deficit, alterations in local circulation, and any significant elevation of the diastolic blood pressure. The lengthening operations are more extensive surgical interventions, and are accompanied with greater morbidity, than the shortening operations. Lengthening is therefore reserved for patients who either have a short stature and would be unsuitable for shortening, or have a discrepancy which cannot reasonably be corrected by shortening procedures alone. The soft tissue constraints and potential complications are greater for congenital shortening than for acquired shortening due to a fracture or for the symmetrical dwarfing of a skeletal dysplasia, such as achondroplasia.

The techniques of lengthening continue to develop and several different external fixators are available. In principle, the shaft of a bone is divided carefully to minimise damage to its blood supply and periosteum, and distraction of the external fixator is delayed for 2 weeks. Healing callus starts to form and then fills the increasing gap between the bone ends during distraction. This technique has been called callotasis (De Bastiani et al., 1987). The patient continues to weight-bear. When using the orthofix external fixator, which is a monolateral device with screws passing into the bone (Figure 5.18), once the desired length is achieved it is locked for 1 month. Following this period it is unlocked to allow loading of the bone along its axis (dynamisation), until it has gained sufficient strength to allow safe removal of the fixator. A circumferential external fixator attached to thin pins which transfix the whole limb is more versatile in the complex cases which also require correction of deformity (Ilizarov, 1990). Both types of fixator can usually be removed in the out-patient clinic, and it is prudent initially to protect the lengthened femur by partial weight-bearing or the lengthened tibia by weight-bearing in a plaster gaiter.

Lengthening may also be performed by distraction across a growth plate, but the continued function of the growth plate at the completion of treatment is not predictable. This technique, called chondrodiatesis, is used less frequently than callotasis and usually for children within a year of skeletal maturity (Aldegheri et al., 1989).

There is one situation where the *cause* of discrepancy may be remedied. Following a fracture across the germinal layer of the growth plate a bony tether sometimes forms between the

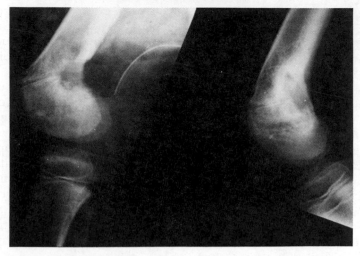

Figure 5.19. (left) Postoperative appearance following resection of a bony tether; (right) the appearance nine months later showing continued growth of the femur and realignment of the growth plate to a more normal transverse position.

epiphysis and metaphysis. This retards growth, and if the tether is not central it causes angular deformity. An operation may be performed to resect the bony bridge or tether and this was first described by Langenskiold (1981). The surgical defect created is then filled with inert material, such as a fat plug or bone cement, in order to prevent the bone from growing into the defect and retethering the growth plate (*Figure 5.19*).

Minor angular deformities will correct spontaneously with further growth (*Figure 5.19*) and the operation may be of benefit for tethers which affect up to 40% of the growth plate. Following this procedure the leg is initially protected in a plaster, and subsequently physiotherapy is required to mobilise and strengthen the limb. A brace is sometimes applied to protect the leg until the weakened area of bone has remodelled.

Physiotherapy

Leg shortening

- Following epiphyseodesis, the child is immobilised in a removable knee-extension splint. This allows the physiotherapist to begin active knee flexion on the second postoperative day, together with static quadriceps exercises. The splint is worn at all times other than during physiotherapy sessions. On approximately the sixth day, when 90° of flexion should have been achieved, a plaster-of-Paris cylinder is applied for a further three weeks, and the patient discharged. On admission the plaster is removed and knee mobilisation recommenced. Initially, the knee is often very stiff and a great deal of encouragement is needed. It can help to involve the child in the treatment by charting the joint range daily – the child being responsible for filling in the chart. Hydrotherapy should be used whenever possible. Full weight-bearing without the plaster is commenced once the quadriceps are strong enough to control the knee, and the joint range is at least 90°.

It is important to point out to the child and the parents that at the end of the 4 weeks the limb length will be exactly the same as pre-operatively and a shoe raise – if worn previously – will still be necessary. This often leads to disappointment, but when the explanation is such, namely the attempt to compensate by reducing the growth on the sound side as the short limb catches up both patient and parents will accept the need for the shoe raise, reducing in size as growth becomes complete.

• Leg shortening can also be achieved by simple resection of the bone – either femoral or tibial, on the longer side, with internal fixation. Immediately postoperatively, a system of slings and springs is applied to both legs with the intention of relieving any muscle spasm and encouraging free movements. These are used for approximately 5 days and then discarded during the day as more intensive physiotherapy is given, including beginning non-weight-bearing on axillary crutches. The slings and springs may be worn for a further week at night until the child is confident in controlling the limb.

Leg lengthening   This is carried out by means of a distraction device. Close observation of the limb is of vital importance post-operatively, and the physiotherapist should be aware of the complications, such as interference with blood and nerve supply to the limb. During the period of active lengthening, intensive physiotherapy is necessary to stretch the soft tissues around the site and maintain the length of the surrounding muscles, parallel with the bone length. In *lengthening of the femur*, it is vital to maintain full extension of the knee to avoid postero-lateral subluxation of the tibia as the hamstrings become tighter relative to the increasing length of the underlying femur. Tensor fascia lata may also prove extremely difficult to stretch in parallel, thus producing a 'valgus knee'. A full-length plaster-of-Paris night splint should be worn throughout the treatment to help to maintain knee extension. Intensive exercises are also given to maintain a range of movement at the knee joint. In *lengthening the tibia*, the posterior tibial group of muscles must be stretched frequently to prevent a secondary equinus deformity of the foot. With the 'Callotasis' technique of lengthening, the patient is encouraged to weight-bear with the aid of crutches.

References

Aldegheri, R., Trivella, G. and Lavini, F. (1989). Epiphyseal distraction: chondrodiatasis. *Clinical Orthopaedics and Related Research*, **241**, 117–127.

Barlow, T.G. (1962). Early diagnosis and treatment of congenital dislocation of the hip. *Journal of Bone and Joint Surgery*, **44B**, 292–301.

Blount, W.P. (1958). Unequal leg length in children. *Surgical Clinics of North America*, **38**, 1107–1123.

Chiari, K. (1974). Medial displacement osteotomy of the pelvis. *Clinical Orthopaedics and Related Research*, **98**, 55–71.

De Bastiani, G., Aldegheri, R., Renzi-Brivio, L. and Trivella, G. (1987). Limb lengthening by callus distraction (callotasis). *Journal of Pediatric Orthopedics*, **7**, 129–134.

Dunn, D.M. and Angel, J.C. (1978). Replacement of the femoral head by open operation in severe adolescent slipping of the upper femoral epiphysis. *Journal of Bone and Joint Surgery*, **60B**, 394–403.

Griffith, M.J. (1976). Slipping of the capital femoral epiphysis. *Annals of the Royal College of Surgeons England*, **58**, 34–42.

Ilizarov, G.A. (1990). Clinical application of the tension-stress effect of limb lengthening. *Clinical Orthopaedics and Related Research*, **250**, 8–26.

Kepley, R.F. and Weiner, D.S. (1981). Treatment of congenital dysplasia–subluxation of the hip in children under one year of age. *Journal of Pediatric Orthopaedics*, **1**, 413–418.

Langenskiold, A. (1981). Surgical treatment of partial closure of the growth plate. *Journal of Pediatric Orthopaedics*, **1**, 3–11.

Phemister, D.B. (1933). Operative arrestment of longitudinal growth of bones in the treatment of deformities. *Journal of Bone and Joint Surgery*, **15**, 1–15.

Salter, R.B. (1961). Innominate osteotomy in the treatment of congenital dislocation and subluxation of the hip. *Journal of Bone and Joint Surgery*, **43B**, 518–539.

Southwick, W.O. (1967). Osteotomy through the lesser trochanter for slipped capital femoral epiphysis. *Journal of Bone and Joint Surgery*, **49A**, 807–835.

Staheli, L.T. (1981). Slotted acetabular augmentation. *Journal of Pediatric Orthopaedics*, **1**, 321–327.

Wynne-Davies, R. (1973). *Heritable Disorders in Orthopaedic Practice*. Blackwell Scientific Publications Limited, Oxford.

Bibliography

Bennet, G.C. (ed.) (1987). *Pediatric Hip Disorders.* Blackwell Scientific Publications, Oxford.

Evans, G.A. (1985). *Current Operative Surgery: Orthopaedics and Trauma,* Ed. S.P.F. Hughes. Baillière Tindall, London.

Lovell, W.W. and Winter, R.B. (1990). *Pediatric Orthopedics,* Ed. R.T. Morrissy J.B. Lippincott Co, Philadelphia.

6 Examination and Assessment of the Spine and Peripheral Joints

K. Major

Introduction

Examination may be divided into two parts, subjective and objective.

Subjective
This is a detailed question and answer session tailored to elicit as much relevant information as possible about the patient's problem(s) and medical history. This then can be used as a framework to plan the objective part of the examination.

Objective
A series of tests designed to elicit measurable indicators, its aim being to reproduce a relevant sign of an appropriate structure in relation to the patient's symptoms, in either peripheral or spinal problems. The objective may be expanded or contracted as the patient's tolerance will allow.

The following sections have been arranged so that the subjective written below is common to all joint examination. A spinal objective examination is then taken as a whole and features specific to each area are discussed. Assessments for each peripheral area are written separately.

Subjective examination

Social history
After the necessary introductions, it is useful to establish a brief social history, including age, occupation and any hobbies or regular activities. The therapist then needs to know whether or not the patient is currently at work, or able to participate in a chosen sport or pastime. This gives some indication of the severity

of the patient's present condition, and an idea of future physical requirements. Also, where necessary, look into home conditions and the support available from relatives.

Present problem (body chart)

It is useful to establish the patient's presenting problem. The exact area involved, and the *patient's* description of symptoms, including frequency, depth and intensity, are all-important factors which are recorded on a body chart. Other features to be noted are any associated symptoms, such as altered (e.g. pins and needles) or reduced sensation. Remember to ask about the presence of symptoms in other parts of the body so that unaffected areas can be recorded ($\sqrt{}$).

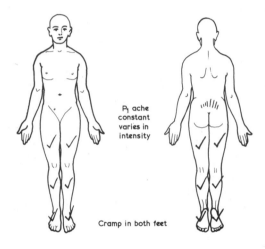

P₁ ache
constant
varies in
intensity

Cramp in both feet

Figure 6.1. Area P₁ ache constant varies in intensity.

The use of a body chart allows a visual appreciation of the patient as a whole, and the information above will give the therapist a brief impression of the patient's view of his complaint.

Symptom behaviour

The behaviour of the symptoms must then be interpreted, which is most easily done by taking two lines of questioning.

Aggravating/easing factors   The aim of questioning is to establish the complexity of forces required to bring on the symptoms – whether or not their severity curtails activity, and how the patient goes about reducing the symptoms (for example, whether a specific position or movement is necessary). It is important to note the time taken to provoke the symptoms in relation to the time taken to ease them. The therapist can then assess the irritability of the condition.

A brief appraisal of an average 24 hours   It is useful to begin at night, and ask if there is any change in the patient's sleep pattern, which gives an indication of the severity of the problem. If sleep is disturbed, this highlights possible positioning problems for which advice will be needed. On waking in the morning, does the patient have any symptoms, or do these start on getting out of bed? How does this compare with the night before? Does the patient suffer any stiffness, and if so how long does it last?

How do the symptoms vary through the day? They may improve with gentle activity, or worsen as the day goes by, or they may be present only with certain activity and then resolve quite quickly. How do the symptoms in the evening compare to those experienced during the day? Is the problem time or activity dependent?

Special questions
This category is important, to exclude any contraindications and highlight any precautions to treatment. Do any of the following conditions apply to the patient?

General
- Major operations.
- Serious illness.
- Diabetes.
- Epilepsy.
- Weight loss.
- General health.
- Drugs.
- Steroids.
- X-rays.

Spinal
- Bladder and bowel problems.
- Dizziness.
- Gait disturbance.

Peripheral
- Injections into the joint.

Recent history

Often, if there has been a clear incident of trauma or a distinct recent onset, then it is easier to start from that point. The therapist must try to complete a detailed account of the onset and sequelae (for example, the effects of any previous treatment, like drug therapy, periods of immobilisation or enforced rest), noting the general trend of the condition, either to improve, worsen or remain static.

If the history is long and insidious, try to establish a time in the recent past where there was some significant change, and discuss the problem from that point to the present time.

Long-term history

Any previous problems with the affected or associated areas must then be noted and will give further information as to the nature of the condition. It is important to obtain a clear picture of the duration, frequency and intensity of the bouts, to see if there is a progression of symptoms.

Planning

It is important to interpret the information gained in the previous section to establish the severity, irritability and nature of the condition to be treated. This allows for a systematic assessment which is safe and considerate to the patient, so the objective examination does not just turn into a list of manoeuvres to be completed.

Social history

Note the patient's degree of physical effort required for his job or hobbies – the therapist should try to aim for full recovery, but compromises must sometimes be made.

Body chart

This indicates the severity and area of the problem. If severe, you must not provoke the full-blown symptoms on testing, to avoid distress, just take the patient to the beginning of his discomfort. If the condition is not severe then you may move beyond the onset of pain and study its behaviour through its range to its limit (*see also* the next section, Aggravating and Easing Factors).

Aggravating and easing factors

This section again highlights the severity and also the irritability of the condition. If the symptoms do seem very troublesome, then movements should be kept to a minimum to avoid exacerbation, and testing must be to the onset of pain only. If symptoms are not so irritable, the behaviour of pain can be assessed through the range until the limit of movement is reached.

24-hour cycle

Daily activity may require modification to ensure that the patient is not worsening the condition unknowingly. This section also indicates the effect of rest *versus* activity, and the effect of weight-bearing *versus* non-weight-bearing. Try to assess the patient's ability to perform his daily tasks.

Special questions

Major operations   Has the patient suffered any malignancy in the past? Gastric surgery can lead to osteoporosis as there is a reduced area for absorption.

Serious illness   Is there any history of TB, Paget's disease, rheumatoid arthritis, ankylosing spondylitis, etc.?

Diabetes   Is it controlled by diet or insulin? Complications include peripheral vascular disease, neuropathy and delayed healing.

Epilepsy   Is it controlled? Remember the safety of the patient regarding electrical treatments.

Weight loss   May indicate malignancy if recent and rapid.

General health   Does the patient see his doctor on a regular basis for any other conditions? For example, increased blood pressure or hiatus hernia, which may affect the patient's ability to adopt certain positions.

Drugs   Relate these to the level of pain control and degree of severity of the pain and note any drugs related to other conditions.

Steroids   Prolonged steroid treatment leads to osteoporosis and impaired healing. If there has been a recent steroid injection, the behaviour of signs and symptoms will be altered.

X-rays   These exclude congenital abnormalities, serious pathology fractures, etc.

Cervical spine   Dizziness − the patient will need to undergo dizziness tests. Certain techniques may compromise the circulation and will therefore be contraindicated, others may require careful monitoring. Sometimes dizziness may be associated with ear disturbance, loss of normal proprioception or other factors.

Gait disturbance – this is present when there is compression of the spinal cord causing 'long tract' signs. This is usually described as loss of balance or tripping-up regularly. The therapist should test for increased tone.

Lumbar spine Bladder and bowel disturbance – cauda equina compression manifests itself as impairment of bladder or bowel control, or as loss of sensation in the saddle area. This may require surgical intervention.

History of present condition

The nature of the condition can be completely variable. There may, for instance, be a history of recent fracture or dislocation. Alternatively, the condition may be chronic, as in osteoarthrosis. It is important to remember, in cases of recent trauma, a need for caution in testing, to avoid further tissue damage.

Problems of insidious onset may be related to a type of activity the patient is performing on a regular basis, for which ergonomic advice may be needed, whereas chronic arthritic conditions may suffer periods of more acute exacerbation which require care on testing.

History

This indicates likely prognosis, which will be poor if there have been previous episodes and especially if there is increased frequency, duration and severity. Prognosis is good if there is no previous history of trauma or disease.

Important questions to ask yourself before the objective examination are:

- Which joints must I check? (Those underlying the symptoms, or possible sources of referred symptoms.)
- Which muscles must I check? (Those underlying the symptoms.)
- Is there any need for a neurological examination?
- Have I checked the joints above and below the lesion?
- Is the condition severe?
- Is the condition irritable?
- What is the exact nature of the condition?

Objective examination

The important rule to remember in the objective examination is: ensure the safety and care of the patient. The examination has to be formal, to allow standard testing between therapists, and thorough enough to ensure a complete understanding of signs and symptoms.

It is vital that by the end of the session the patient has confidence in the therapist. The following outline provides a framework.

Spinal objective examination

Observation must be carried out with the patient adequately undressed to view the spine from all sides. All the while, the therapist notes the patient's willingness to perform various activities.

More specifically, notes should be made regarding posture. For example:

- Cervical spine − position of the head and shoulders, look for a poking chin, etc.
- Thoracic spine − note kyphosis, scoliosis, shoulder and hip position, etc.
- Lumbar spine − equality of weight-bearing, the level and set of the pelvis, spinal rotation, scoliosis, kyphosis, etc.

Ask the patient about the presence of any symptoms in this position; any obvious deformity can then be corrected and the pain pattern reassessed. This eliminates postural pain and high-lights antalgic positions.

Usually, where possible, the patient will be asked to return to a neutral position to allow uniform testing procedures and stan-dardisation of tests.

The patient performs physiological movements, often leaving the most provocative until last. Close questioning by the therapist is important to establish how symptoms alter with each movement, to ensure a full understanding of behaviour through the range. Ask the patient to move either to the onset of symptoms (when pain is severe and irritable) or through to the limit of the range (when neither of the above applies). One must look for any decrease in quality of movement, such as 'hinging' at one level or 'rigidity' through the range. If any movement is pain-free and full range, gentle over-pressure may be applied to ensure that the movement is free of problems. The quality of the end-feel and the patient's response are recorded.

A neurological examination is compulsory in any patient with referred symptoms, and it is often useful to practise on every patient for purposes of elimination. This consists of testing sen-sation, muscle power and reflexes. Sensation testing usually involves testing to light touch, and may include pin-prick or two-point discrimination (note dermatomal distribution). The power of muscles innervated by each root level must be checked, and reflexes should be assessed by eliciting the response six times to detect subtle decreases in conduction, though the usefulness of this is open to debate.

Further isometric muscle tests can be made to those groups underlying the painful area. Here the therapist is looking to elicit the pain response to see if there is a local musculotendinous lesion, though it must be realised that these tests are often positive in the presence of joint lesions.

Joints peripheral to the spine are then tested, if they underlie the symptoms, to check their relevance to the problem. Where possible, test to end of range with over-pressure, which then clears the joint of any involvement.

Tension tests must be applied for a thorough examination of the spine.

For the cervical region, the upper limb tension test applies stretch to the brachial plexus and can be modified to highlight different root levels (only as necessary).

The thoracic and lumbar regions can be tensioned in a variety of ways: the tests one may include are passive neck flexion, straight leg raise (and then a combination of the two), prone knee flexion and, as necessary, the slump test.

Full descriptions of these tests are beyond the scope of this chapter (for further discussion, see Butler, 1991).

If tests are positive, they may indicate impingement of the structures that constitute the nervous system, either by, for instance, adhesions (which would be chronic and stable) or by a recent prolapsed intervertebral disc (in a more acute and unstable state).

All the above must be recorded accurately regarding degrees of available range and reproduction of symptoms, and can be used as treatments in their own right or as test movements.

Special tests must be included to assess any complications highlighted by the subjective examination. Dizziness testing is performed by sustained cervical rotation to both sides, then sustained cervical extension; these positions are held for 10 seconds, followed by 10 seconds, rest, and the patient is asked about the onset of dizziness (Sheehy et al., 1991). The standard test for increased tone associated with long-tract involvement is the Babinski reflex.

Palpation of the spine gives the therapist the opportunity to tie together all these findings. This consists of general techniques to evaluate the condition of soft tissue, noting any sweating or temperature variation, and tethering or thickening of paravertebral regions. Then check the position of spinous processes to familiarise yourself with the patient's spine. Next comes a more detailed intervertebral movement examination performed at each spinal level. The aim is to detect either local or referred symptoms, resistance to friction-free movement or muscle spasm. The therapist must judge at which point in the range these occur and how they behave through the range to the limit, finally noting the end-feel. After this, the patient is taken through the most significant active movement again and any change is noted. Finally, the patient is warned of the possibility of exacerbation of symptoms and asked to report any such at the next session.

The sequence of events should be amended to reduce the patient's change of position to a minimum, so the following sequence is a useful guideline.

Cervical spine

Sitting
• Observation.
• Active physiological movements.
• Neurological tests (or in supine).
• Active peripheral joint checks (or in standing).
• Isometric muscle tests (or in supine).

Supine
• Dizziness testing.
• Babinski reflex.
• Tension tests (only when necessary).

Prone
• General palpation.
• Passive accessory intervertebral movements (PAIVMS).

Thoracic spine

Standing
• Observation.
• Active lumbar physiological movements (only as necessary).

Sitting
• Active physiological movements.
• Active peripheral joint checks (including cervical spine).
• Tension test − slump sitting (only as necessary).
• Deep breathing or coughing.

Supine
- Tension tests – passive neck flexion, straight leg raise.
- Peripheral joint check – including sacro-iliac joint.
- Neurological examination.

Prone
- Isometric muscle tests (for pain).
- Complete neurological examination.
- General palpation.
- PAIVMS.

Lumbar spine

Standing
- Observation.
- Active physiological movements.
- Neurological examination – gastrocnemius.

Supine
- Tension tests – passive neck flexion, straight leg raise.
- Peripheral joint check – including sacro-iliac joint.
- Neurological examination.
- Isometric muscle tests (for pain).

Prone
- Isometric muscle tests.
- Tension test – prone knee bend.
- Complete neurological examination.
- General palpation.
- PAIVMS.

Sitting
- Tension test – slump sitting (as necessary).

The hip joint

Observation
Initially, as the patient enters the department, you should quickly assess the patient's willingness to use the affected part. Once the patient is adequately undressed, the therapist observes from the front, side and rear for any bruising, swelling, wasting or deformity. Note the general posture, the degree of weight-bearing, and look particularly for any shortening – checking for levels of the iliac crests and spines.

Quick test

While the patient is standing, the therapist can ask him to perform a functional movement test (its degree of difficulty dictated by the subjective), such as hip flexion or squatting. This may be used as a means of assessing the patient's overall condition on arrival in the department, prior to more thorough investigations of joint range and pain.

Proximal joints

Checks of lumbar spine movements (both physiological and accessory) are always carried out for the reproduction of pain and other symptoms. If there are positive signs, they must be considered in relation to the following examination.

Affected joint

Active testing In supine lying, with a pillow under the knees, the patient is asked to attempt active movements of the hip. The therapist can assist by describing and demonstrating with the unaffected side (note the patient's normal available range at this point). Localise the movement by fixing the iliac spines to provide accurate measurement and creating a repeatable test. All ranges should be measured to pain or the limit.

The Thomas test may be used to assess for fixed flexion deformity, where (in supine) the unaffected hip is fully flexed and held to the patient's chest. If the affected leg rises from the plinth, the test is positive, and the range can be measured for future reference.

When a movement is apparently full range and pain-free, overpressure is applied to exclude this from further unnecessary testing. Note that medial and lateral rotation can be measured in neutral or at 90° hip and knee flexion, if there is sufficient range, which gives greater accuracy.

Passive physiological testing Passive movement is then compared to active in relation to onset of pain, etc., and its quality through the range and end-feel can be gauged.

Resisted testing Static muscle tests are performed to check musculotendinous involvement; if pain is present the test may be positive, though a small amount of joint movement or compression cannot be ruled out, which can also produce a positive result. If there is no pain, then the muscle may be tested to assess strength.

Hip abduction weakness can be demonstrated by Trendelenburg's test. The patient is asked to bear weight through the affected limb — if the test is positive, the opposite side of the pelvis will tilt down (so the gluteal fold drops below the level of the weight-bearing side). The patient will usually compensate by side flexing the trunk to counterbalance the loss of normal muscle activity.

Distal joints

Those joints immediately distal to the hip (and possibly underlying the patient's symptoms) must be checked through to full range and overpressure applied. If positive, these will warrant further investigation at a later stage.

Palpation

It is important to be completely familiar with the surface anatomy of the joint, so that accurate palpation can be performed. Any area that gives rise to pain should be noted, and the structures likely to be involved can then be identified.

Shortening at the hip can be measured in two ways − to assess real shortening, from the anterior superior iliac spines to the medial malleoli, and from the umbilicus to the same point for apparent shortening.

In prone, one can look at hip extension (active and passive), check it with resistance and complete palpation.

Accessory movements

If you wish to treat the patient using passive accessory movements, this section will need to be included in the initial assessment; a full description is beyond the scope of this chapter (*see* Maitland, 1991).

Gait

Walking patterns should be assessed by asking the patient to walk at normal speed, so that he may be observed from in front, behind and from the side. It is best to adopt a systematic approach to observation and check movements at each joint in turn. Remember to ask the patient to walk forward, backwards and sideways, and note any variations.

Instructions to the patient

After the examination, the patient is warned of the possibility of exacerbation of symptoms and to report any at the next session.

Observation

Finally, as the patient dresses and leaves the department, remember to assess overall functional ability to see if this ties in with your previous findings, which should then confirm your initial impression.

The knee joint

For discussion of observation, quick test, palpation, gait, and instructions to the patient, see The hip joint, pp. 114–116.

Proximal joints

If the subjective examination suggests the possibility of proximal joint involvement, then each source of referral should be checked by active testing. Here, this includes the lumbar spine (both physiological and accessory ranges).

The hip should be cleared routinely, as it is the joint adjacent to the affected area. In a reclined position, the hip can be checked easily by movement into a combined position of flexion/adduction, and cleared with overpressure.

If there are positive signs these must be considered in relation to the rest of the examination.

Affected joint

Active testing   First, in long sitting, look at bilateral active ranges of flexion, extension and rotation, noting range, quality of movement, and the behaviour of symptoms.

Passive physiological testing   Passive movement is then compared to active, regarding onset of symptoms, etc., its quality through the range and the end-feel.

Resisted testing   Isometric tests are performed to check musculotendinous involvement. If pain is present the test may be positive though a small amount of joint movement or compression, which can also reproduce symptoms, cannot be ruled out. If there is no pain, then the muscles may be tested to assess strength. This is done for quadriceps, hamstrings and gastrocnemius.

Stability tests

The knee examination should also include special tests to stress the main ligaments.

First, look for excessive extension (recurvatum), which indicates general joint laxity.

Valgus stress test   This is performed with the joint in a few degrees of flexion. The therapist places his proximal hand on the lateral aspect of the joint, and applies an abduction force to the tibia with his distal hand. If the test is positive, there will be excessive movement at the joint line. (*Figure 6.2(a).*)

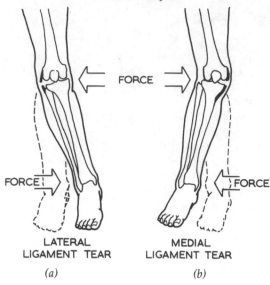

LATERAL   MEDIAL
LIGAMENT TEAR   LIGAMENT TEAR
(a)   (b)

Figure 6.2. Tears of the collateral ligament of the knee joint.

Varus stress test The starting position is similar, though the proximal hand is placed over the medial joint line. An adduction force is applied in the same way, and a positive test will demonstrate increased mobility. (*Figure 6.2(b)*.)

Lachmann's test This demonstrates damage to the anterior cruciate ligament. The knee is held in a few degrees of flexion, with the proximal hand fixing immediately above the joint on the lateral aspect. The distal hand holds the medial tibial condyle, so the therapist can move the tibia forwards and back. A positive result is shown by increased mobility.

Anterior drawer test If there is sufficient range available, the knee is positioned at 80°, the therapist anchors the foot with his leg. The tibia is held with both hands, close to the joint. An anterior drawer movement is then applied. When positive, excess movement can be seen and palpated at the anterior joint line. *Note* You must make sure that the hamstrings are relaxed as tension here will give a false negative result. (*Figure 6.3(a)*.)

Posterior drawer test The starting position is the same as in the previous test, though both legs must be positioned together. In this case, the therapist looks at the knees in profile, to compare the relative positions of the lower leg. A disrupted posterior cruciate will allow the tibia to slide backwards. (*Figure 6.3(b)*.)

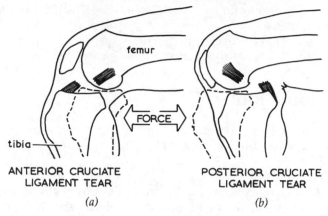

ANTERIOR CRUCIATE
LIGAMENT TEAR

POSTERIOR CRUCIATE
LIGAMENT TEAR

(a)   (b)

Figure 6.3. Tears of the cruciate ligaments of the knee joint.

It must be stressed that all the above tests are first performed on the unaffected side to allow for comparison, as everyone will present with variations in mobility. Results can be grossly positive, which would indicate rupture, and probable involvement of other structures. At other times, laxity may be only minimal and its detection improves with experience.

Meniscal test (McMurray's)

With the patient in supine, the therapist takes the knee into full flexion. Lateral rotation of the lower leg is added to squeeze the medial meniscus (this happens because the femur and tibia are pulled together as the medial collateral ligament is tightened). The knee is extended while the therapist palpates the medial joint line. There will be a click, which is usually painful, if the test is positive.

The same movements are repeated with medial rotation of the tibia, to detect lateral compartment problems.

It is difficult to assess meniscal problems clinically, and even when combined with an appropriate history, diagnosis cannot be conclusive without arthroscopy.

Distal joints

The joints immediately distal to the knee should be cleared. This includes testing the superior tibiofibular joint with passive antero-posterior glide, and full-range ankle movements with overpressure.

Accessory movements

If you wish to treat the patient using passive accessory movements, then this section will need to be included in the initial assessment; a full description is beyond the scope of this chapter (*see* Maitland, 1991).

In prone lying, check the posterior aspect of the joint and palpate for the hamstring tendons and gastrocnemius.

The hind foot

For discussion of observation, quick test, and instructions to patient, see The hip joint, pp. 114–116.

Proximal joints

If the subjective examination suggests the possibility of proximal joint involvement, then each source of referral should be checked by active testing. This includes the lumbar spine and the hip. The knee should be cleared routinely, as it is the joint adjacent to the affected area. The knee can be checked easily by thorough full active movement cleared with overpressure.

If there are positive signs these must be considered in relation to the rest of the examination.

Affected joint

Active testing   Look at active movements, bilaterally, to assess range, quality of movement, and the behaviour of symptoms. The movements available are dorsiflexion and plantarflexion, inversion and eversion, abduction and adduction, and rotation both medially and laterally.

Check for compensation which can occur at the mid-tarsal joint or further distally. If possible, overpress the movement to clear the joints, remembering to fixate immediately above and below, and note the end-feel.

Passive physiological testing   Passive tests are carried out and comparisons are made regarding symptom reproduction and range of movement.

Resisted testing   Isometric tests are performed to check musculo-tendinous involvement. If pain is present the test may be positive, though a small amount of joint movement or compression cannot be ruled out, which can also reproduce symptoms. If there is no pain, then the muscles may be tested to assess strength.

Stability tests

By applying stress tests at the ankle/subtalar complex the therapist can check for antero-posterior and lateral instability. It is important to check the unaffected limb to assess for individual variance. A positive result indicates the increased possibility of recurrent injury.

Distal joints

In prone, with the patient's knee flexed to 90°, the therapist can check the mid-tarsal joint by passive physiological and accessory movements. Be certain to locate the bony points accurately, and fix immediately proximal and distal to the joint line. Further testing of the forefoot also requires the use of accessory techniques.

Palpation

Place the patient in prone to look at and palpate the posterior aspect of the ankle, and the tendo Achilles. Also, see this heading under The hip joint (p. 116).

Accessory movements

If you wish to treat the patient using passive accessory movements, then this section will need to be included in the initial assessment; a full description is beyond the scope of this chapter (*see* Maitland, 1991).

Gait

For details, see this heading under The hip joint (p. 116), but add in toe and heel walking.

The shoulder joint

Observation

Initially, on entering the department, you should quickly assess the patient's willingness to use the affected part. Once the patient is adequately undressed, the therapist observes him from the front, side and rear for any bruising, swelling, wasting or deformity.

Quick test

The patient may then be asked to perform a quick test to give the therapist an idea of the functional level (its degree of difficulty is dictated by the subjective examination). This may be used as a means of assessing the patient's overall condition on arrival in the department, prior to more thorough investigations of joint range and pain.

Proximal joint

The cervical spine should always be checked by asking the patient to perform active movements in all planes and cleared with overpressure where applicable; accessory ranges must also be cleared. If there are positive signs, these must be considered in relation to the rest of the examination.

The shoulder girdle movements of elevation, depression, protraction and retraction must be checked, and cleared with overpressure where possible.

Affected joint

Active testing With the patient standing, look from behind him at active movements (bilaterally) to assess range, quality of movement, and the behaviour of symptoms.

Remember to observe the whole time for any alteration in scapular movement and scapulohumeral rhythm, which must be noted on the assessment form.

Passive physiological testing Ask the patient to lie down close to the side of the plinth, then check all available passive movements, and compare the range and severity of symptoms.

Resisted testing Static muscle tests are performed to check musculotendinous involvement and, if painful, may indicate a positive result. (Remember that some joint movement occurs and can also reproduce pain.) If there is no pain, then the muscle may be tested to assess strength.

Remember to include static resisted flexion and extension of the elbow − the 'long head' tendons of biceps and triceps may also be involved.

Distal joints
Check the elbow to full range with overpressure to eliminate any co-existing problem; also check any other joint underlying the symptoms.

Palpation
It is important to be completely familiar with the surface anatomy of all the joints, so that accurate palpation can be performed. Any area that gives rise to symptoms should be noted, and the structures likely to be involved can then be identified.

Accessory movements
If you wish to treat the patient using passive accessory movements, then this section will need to be included in the initial assessment; a full description is beyond the scope of this chapter (*see* Maitland, 1991).

Instructions to the patient
After the examination, the patient is warned of the possibility of exacerbation of symptoms and to report any at the next session.

Observation
Finally, as the patient dresses and leaves the department, remember to assess overall functional ability to see if this ties in with your previous findings, which should then confirm your initial impression.

The elbow joint

For discussion of observation, quick test, and instructions to the patient, see these headings under The shoulder joint, pp. 121 and 122.

Proximal joints
If the subjective examination suggests the possibility of proximal joint involvement, then each source of referral should be checked by testing active movement. This would always include the cervical spine, using both physiological and accessory ranges, and the shoulder. The latter is tested by asking the patient to take the limb into full elevation and, if symptom free, the therapist applies overpressure, noting any restriction. (Care must be taken to avoid the elbow at this stage.)

If there are positive signs, these must be considered in relation to the rest of the examination.

Affected joint

Active testing Examination of the affected joints may be carried out in supine. Examine elbow flexion and extension from its mid-position, as this is likely to be the patient's position of comfort. Ensure that the forearm position is consistent, as any change at the radioulnar joints will affect the range available at the elbow. Ideally, keep the forearm in mid-prone. Note the available range, pain and quality of movement.

Always remember to compare both sides, as the degree of extension available is subject to variation.

Measurement of active pronation and supination then follows with the elbow at 90°. The therapist must ensure that movement occurs at the radioulnar joints and be aware of the possibility of substitution at the shoulder or wrist.

Passive physiological testing Assess all the available passive movements, and compare the range and severity of symptoms with the above.

To test the radioulnar joints fix the elbow and grasp the inferior radioulnar joint to perform the movement, to make sure that the wrist is excluded.

Resisted testing Static muscle tests are performed to check musculotendinous involvement and, if painful, may indicate a positive result. (Remember that some joint movement occurs and can also reproduce pain.) If there is no pain, then the muscle may be tested to assess strength.

Distal joints

The wrist should be checked through all movements — to over-pressure where possible — to exclude the area from further investigation. Care of the elbow is important during these tests.

Accessory movements

If you wish to treat the patient using passive accessory movements, then this section will need to be included in the initial assessment; a full description is beyond the scope of this chapter (see Maitland, 1991).

The wrist and hand

For discussion of observation, quick test, palpation, and instructions to the patient, see these headings under The shoulder joint, pp. 121–123.

Proximal joints

If the subjective examination suggests the possibility of proximal joint involvement, then each source of referral should be checked by testing active movement. This would include the cervical spine, the shoulder, and the elbow. The latter should be cleared routinely, as it is the joint adjacent to the affected area.

If there are positive signs, these must be considered in relation to the rest of the examination.

Affected joint

Active testing The patient is asked to move the wrist through flexion, extension, and radial and ulnar deviation. The range and symptom response is assessed and recorded and, if symptom-free, the joints are cleared with overpressure. It is easiest to assess forearm pronation and supination routinely, as these joints are likely to be involved in any injury at the wrist. Measurement of active pronation and supination is performed with the elbow at 90°. The therapist must ensure that movement occurs at the radioulnar joints and be aware of the possibility of substitution at the wrist.

Passive physiological testing Assess all the available passive movements, and compare the range and severity of symptoms with the above, noting the end-feel at each range.

Resisted testing Static muscle tests are performed to check musculotendinous involvement and, if painful, may indicate a positive result. (Remember that some joint movement occurs and can also reproduce pain.) If there is no pain, then the muscle may be tested to assess strength.

Distal joints

Active testing of the joints below the wrist includes the carpo-metacarpal joint of the thumb and the metacarpophalangeal joints of the fingers (along with movements at the interphalangeal joints). The base of the thumb is tested actively to full range and over-pressure through flexion/extension, abduction/adduction, and opposition. Full finger flexion and extension should be carried out in the same way, and any associated problem highlighted.

Accessory movements

If you wish to treat the patient using passive accessory movements, then this section will need to be included in the initial assessment; a full description is beyond the scope of this chapter (*see* Maitland, 1991).

Finger and thumb assessment

This is largely similar to the above, but each individual joint of the affected digit must be measured for flexion and extension to make sure of accurate reassessment, remembering to differentiate between soft tissue tension and joint restriction. The adjacent fingers are then taken through the range to overpressure, clearing them where possible. Assessment of the base of the thumb is slightly more involved as there are five movements to consider, as mentioned above, but the important thing to remember is to fix the joint immediately above and below the joint line to ensure minimal movement at the carpus.

Conclusion

At the end of any joint examination, the therapist should be able to make a working clinical diagnosis of the condition, and have a good idea of the structures involved. This will complement the diagnosis of the referring doctor who will also have excluded any serious pathology.

The importance of a thorough examination cannot be over-stressed, because this gives the therapist precise information as to the present state of the tissues, thus helping her to select the type of treatment required at any one time, and the likely outcome. This information is then discussed with the patient, and realistic aims and objectives can be set.

References

Butler, D.S. (1991). *Mobilisation of the Nervous System*. Churchill Livingstone, Melbourne.

Maitland, G.D. (1991). *Peripheral Manipulation*, 3rd edition. Butterworths, London.

Sheehy, K., Middleditch, A. and Wickham, S. (1991). Vertebral Artery Testing in the Cervical Spine. *Manipulative Physiotherapist*, **22**(2), 15–18.

Bibliography

Bullock, M.I. (1990). *Ergonomics: The Physiotherapist in the Work Place*. Churchill Livingstone, London.

Butler, D.S. (1991). *Mobilisation of the Nervous System*. Churchill Livingstone, Melbourne.

Cailliet, R. (1980). *Low Back Pain Syndrome*, 3rd edition. F.A. Davis, Philadelphia.

Cailliet, R. (1981). *Neck and Arm Pain*, 2nd edition. F.A. Davis, Philadelphia.

Corrigan, B. and Maitland, G.D. (1983). *Practical Orthopaedic Medicine*. Butterworths, London.

Evans, P. (1980). The Healing Process at Cellular Level: A Review. *Physiotherapy*, **66**, 8.

Evans, P. (1986). *The Knee Joint: A Clinical Guide*. Churchill Livingstone, London.

Farragher, D. and Kidd, G.L. (1987). Eutrophic electrical stimulation for Bell's Palsy. *Clin. Rehab.*, **1**, 265–271.

Forster, A. and Palastanga, N. (1985). *Clayton's Electrotherapy*, 9th edition. Baillière Tindall, London.

Grieve, G.P. (1988). *Common Vertebral Joint Problems*, 2nd edition. Churchill Livingstone, London.

Grieve, G.P. (1991). *Mobilisation of the Spine*, 5th edition. Churchill Livingstone, London.

Hayne, C. (1984). Pulsed high frequency energy — its place in physiotherapy. *Physiotherapy*, **70**, 12.

Kidd, G.L. and Oldham, J.A. (1988). Motor unit action potential (MUAP) sequence and electrotherapy. *Clin. Rehab.*, **2**, 23–33.

Maitland, G.D. (1985). *Vertebral Manipulation*, 5th edition. Butterworths, London.

Maitland, G.D. (1991). *Peripheral Manipulation*, 3rd edition. Butterworths, London.

Melzack, R. and Wall, P. (1988). *The Challenge of Pain*, 3rd edition. Penguin Education, London.

Pheasant, S. (1991). *Ergonomics, Work and Health*. MacMillan, London.

Savage, B. (1984). *Interferential Therapy*. Faber and Faber, London.

Sheehy, K., Middleditch, A. and Wickham, S. (1991). Vertebral artery testing in the cervical spine. *Manipulative Physiotherapist*, **22**(2), 15–18.

Taylor, S. and Cotton, L. (1982). *A Short Textbook Of Surgery*, 5th edition. Hodder and Stoughton, London.

Thompson, J.W. (1988). Pharmacology of transcutaneous electrical nerve stimulation. *Intractable Pain Society*, **7**, 1.

7 Principles of Treatment Following Joint Examination and Assessment

K. Major

Although the therapist has many methods of treatment to choose from when confronted by a patient for the first time, the primary task is always to identify the problems accurately. Classify them under the following headings:

- Pain.
- Muscle weakness.
- Joint stiffness.
- Loss of function.

Following this, a series of short-term goals or objectives can be set, the overall aim of which is the restoration of full function.

The patient will usually have sought treatment because the pain of the condition has become a problem in normal daily life, so he will most appreciate some reduction in pain as a first aim. Once this is under control, the patient may then either improve spontaneously in all ways, or be able to co-operate with other techniques aimed at improving other aspects of the problem, for example strengthening exercises, gait re-education and proprioceptive retraining.

Whatever method is used the outcome is most likely to be successful when there is good communication between the patient and the therapist, enabling problems to be discussed objectively as well as ensuring that the plan of treatment is jointly agreed. It is the role of the therapist to encourage and educate the patient to participate fully.

This chapter contains a brief description of the methods currently available, an outline of their physiological effects and an idea of their use. Contraindications are not listed and must be checked elsewhere (*see* Bibliography to Chapter 6). The purpose is to provide a summary only of the details that will ensure that the method chosen is the most suitable for a particular patient.

Heat therapy

Heat may be applied in a variety of ways. The superficial tissues are most affected by the use of infra-red irradiation, electric heat pads, moist hot packs and paraffin wax. 'Deeper heating' is obtained by using short-wave diathermy.

The physiological effects of the above are broadly similar in that they increase blood flow, and therefore metabolic activity, as well as stimulate nerve endings to produce a sedative effect. The end results are erythema, muscle relaxation, a fall in blood pressure and an increase in the activity of the sweat glands.

This method is used to aid resolution of inflammation and so promote healing, relieve pain and decrease muscle spasm. The method of choice is dictated by the area of the body to be treated – whether deep or superficial, central or peripheral.

Some methods allow patients to continue their therapy at home between out-patient appointments. This is allowed only when the therapist has complete confidence that the patient has understood and can carry out the instructions necessary for a safe and proper treatment.

Each method carries its own particular precautions and contraindications, but in each case there is a legal requirement to test for normal thermal sensation at and around the area to be treated.

Other major contraindications common to all heat therapy methods include the presence of arterial disease (heat could precipitate gangrene), venous thrombosis or phlebitis, and recent haemorrhage.

Cold therapy

This can be applied in a variety of ways:

- Ice packs.
- Ice cube massage.
- Cold towels.
- Ice brushing.
- Cold sprays.
- Gel packs.

Physiologically the effect is to reduce temperature (skin temperature can fall to 10°C), which leads to stimulation of circulation to maintain homeostasis. Initially, there is vasoconstriction followed by vasodilation; these two states then continue to alternate (Lewis's hunting reaction), while the body attempts to find an even temperature.

Nerve conduction is slowed by cooling, and pain relief is achieved via the 'pain-gate' mechanism. Muscle spasm and spasticity may be reduced using the reflex inhibition of the anterior horn cells, though, alternatively, ice can have an excitatory effect with ice brushing over the appropriate dermatome.

Consequently, the indications for use of ice are twofold:

- Immediately post injury, vasoconstriction is elicited by short-term ice treatments of a few minutes' duration to reduce haemorrhage and excessive oedema.
- In the subacute condition, longer treatments of up to 20 minutes are needed to produce repeated constriction and dilation, so increasing circulation, reducing oedema, pain and muscle spasm.

Following this, movement and activity are made easier.

Major contraindications again involve vascular problems, including Reynaud's, and any patient with a recent history of cardiac disease (where ice can produce a sudden drop in blood pressure). Also contraindicated are those who have diminished sensation (where there is a risk of ice 'burn'), and others who are particularly sensitive can suffer an 'allergic' reaction, while some patients can be very reluctant to try the treatment.

Pulsed electromagnetic energy

Equipment used for this produces an electromagnetic field operating at a frequency of 27MHz. Two distinct fields of activity are produced during treatment, one electrical and the other magnetic, and most units at present work using these fields simultaneously.

The documented effects are an increase in the number of white cells, histiocytes and fibroblasts in a wound, and the reduction of inflammation, via an increase in the dispersal of oedema and absorption of haematoma. This treatment also speeds up the rate of collagen deposition and layering. Other effects include improved healing of the nervous system and stimulation of osteogenesis.

It is suggested that these changes are brought about by the action of the pulsed magnetic field on cells affected by the inflammatory process.

During inflammation, cell potential is reduced and the permeability of the cell to sodium ions increases. This produces local changes in osmotic pressure, therefore increasing extra-cellular fluid.

Restoration of the normal electrical potential is achieved by altering the throughput of ions at the cellular membrane.

This method is indicated for use immediately post injury or surgery to promote all of the above, and gain pain relief. This type of therapy is also useful in the treatment of open wounds.

Pulsed electromagnetic energy is not generally used for its thermal element, though at high-pulse frequency and high-peak power, heat can be generated. In these circumstances, skin testing is required.

The main contraindication to treatment is the patient who is fitted with a pacemaker. Those wearing hearing aids should be requested to 'switch off' before the machine is used, to avoid interference.

Interferential therapy

This is a means of applying electrical stimulation to the tissues, avoiding the discomfort associated with Faradic or galvanic currents. Two medium-frequency currents are used, one at about 4000Hz, and another operating in the range of 4000–4200Hz. Each current is applied using a pair of electrodes, placed so that the two currents intersect. Where this occurs, the resulting output is one of low frequency, operating in the range of 1–200Hz.

This allows the therapist to stimulate all types of nervous tissue – motor, sensory, sympathetic and parasympathetic. Each has a particular frequency at which there will be most response and, as a rule of thumb, the following settings may prove useful:

- At about 100Hz or higher, pain relief is achieved. The most effective setting is 130Hz. In the presence of acute pain, accommodation of sensory nerve endings is desirable, so the treatment is administered at a constant frequency. Treatment at around 5Hz can have a similar pain-relieving effect in chronic pain states.
- Re-education of muscle can be facilitated when stimulated by frequencies in the range of 10–50Hz.
- Interferential therapy also has a place in reducing oedema by stimulation of the parasympathetic nervous system, which increases blood flow, at 10–150Hz (Savage, 1984).

Treatment may be applied as either static or sweeping from one setting to the other, this being predetermined by the therapist, depending on the effect required. You may wish to avoid accommodation, in which case a small sweep can be introduced around the desired frequency. Alternatively, it may be necessary to achieve many effects simultaneously (e.g., pain relief and oedema reduction), which requires a larger sweep.

Therefore, interferential therapy is useful in a wide variety of conditions and has a place in the treatment of both acute and chronic problems.

Contraindications to this method include the presence of deep-vein thrombosis, the patient with a pacemaker, or any cardiac condition. It is also best to avoid malignancy (though there is no proven detrimental effect), and bacterial infections.

Ultrasound

When a quartz crystal is subjected to a piezo-electric effect, it will change shape. This phenomenon is used to deform the metal plate of the treatment head at frequencies of 1MHz and 3MHz, producing sound waves that penetrate the tissues to a depth of 4cm and 2.5cm, respectively. This brings about compression and rarefaction of the cells being treated. Ultrasound is subject to the laws of refraction, so it is important to place the treatment head perpendicular to the skin surface. Its physiological effects can be subdivided into mechanical, chemical and biological, and thermal.

Mechanical effects
Ultrasound creates a micromassage effect which can help to reduce oedema.

Bubbles of gas may be produced in the tissues as a result of treatment; this is known as cavitation. Stable cavitation is harmless as the bubbles remain intact, whereas in the unstable state bubbles expand and then collapse rapidly, causing an increase in temperature. Standing waves can produce inhibition of blood flow which results in the aggregation of blood cells. Both can be minimised by movement of the treatment head and a pulsed output (Dyson et al., 1968).

Chemical and biological effects
Where acoustic streaming (unidirectional flow of tissue components; Dyson and Suckling, 1978) is thought to have a beneficial effect in tissue repair, and pain is reduced by stimulation of mechanoreceptors, this is 'closing the pain gate'.

Thermal effects
These are produced by continuous ultrasound (see Heat therapy, p. 129).

Ultrasound is indicated in the treatment of recent injuries to reduce oedema, relieve pain and promote repair. Here, a typical starting dose may be pulsed $0.25-0.5w/cm^2$ for $2-3$ minutes (Forster and Palastanga, 1985). In chronic conditions, ultrasound can be used to break down organised oedema and adhesions, thus making scar tissue more pliable. In this situation, the dose may be continuous, and start at $0.8w/cm^2$ for 4 minutes (Forster and Palastanga, 1985).

Treatment is best applied by direct contact with a gel specifically manufactured for the purpose, which allows maximum transmission of energy. If the patient is very tender to the touch, treatment may be administered through water, but efficiency is reduced.

The dangers of ultrasound include burning the patient if the treatment head remains static, and damage to the head of the machine will result if the unit is operated in air.

Main contraindications are tumours, deep X-ray therapy in the previous 6 months, the presence of acute infection and thrombophlebitis. Patients who have a pacemaker can be treated in areas other than the chest wall.

Combined therapy

This is a treatment developed by applying ultrasound and interferential therapy simultaneously. The two machines are linked, and bipolar treatment is administered using the ultrasound head and an indifferent interferential electrode. The former is placed over the site of injury and the latter is positioned at some convenient point, depending on the position of the lesion.

With the machines working simultaneously, the affected area receives the benefits of both methods of treatment, but it should be remembered that, as the ultrasound prevents the body accommodating itself to the interferential therapy, treatment intensity for the latter is lower.

The primary physiological effect is the production of analgesia, which can last for 30 minutes post treatment or longer. For this reason, combined therapy should not be used on acute lesions, unless very minor, as injudicious pain-free movement may result in further damage.

Indications for use include conditions where ultrasound would aid the resolution of inflammation, and interferential therapy would provide pain relief; for example, in tennis elbow and tenosynovitis. For information on contraindications see the previous sections in this chapter.

Electrical muscle stimulation

This has been used for many years for a variety of purposes. Surged Faradism, i.e. short duration, interrupted, direct current, is used to facilitate muscle contraction or to re-educate muscle after injury and immobilisation. It can also be used to re-educate a new muscle action in cases of tendon transplant.

In the past, direct current was used to slow down the degeneration of muscle following denervation. This has now been abandoned as it was seen to be unrealistic and now it is known that tissue damage can result from inappropriate stimulation. This idea of treatment has now been evolved into a portable system. The electrical stimulus produced mimics the nervous system's own natural stimulatory codes and signals, resulting in a more beneficial effect than the older methods. This idea is known as Trophic Stimulation.

Treatment is administered on a daily basis. So the unit is supplied to the patient for home use, with strict instructions as to the placement of electrodes, and the intensity and duration of each session. For example, to prevent muscle atrophy the unit may be programmed to increase circulation and fatigue resistance of the muscle, resulting in hypertrophy of its slow oxidative fibres. In this case, treatment is given daily for 1 hour.

Protocols have been formulated for use of this treatment, primarily in cases of peripheral nerve lesion, in disuse atrophy due to pain or immobilisation, or for the support of muscle following nerve transplant.

Its use is contraindicated in patients who use demand-type pacemakers. It is advisable to avoid treatment in the vicinity of the carotid sinus, and not to treat during pregnancy.

Any muscle can be checked and measured by the use of strength duration curves.

Transcutaneous nerve stimulation

Transcutaneous nerve stimulation (TNS) is a method of achieving pain relief that can be delivered by hand-held portable units. This enables the patient to be ambulant while administering self-treatment. As this method allows much greater freedom over other types of therapy, the patient can choose the time at which the machine is used and, by monitoring the outcome of each session, the intensity, frequency and duration can be altered by the patient for the best effect.

The electrodes must be placed over the involved dermatome to be effective, but failing this the adjacent one may be used. The unit works by stimulating large-diameter sensory nerve fibres (beta fibres), which raise the threshold of pain perception in the segmentally related area, by pre-synaptic inhibition of the endings of the nociceptive (C) fibres. Therefore, the painful input is prevented from exciting the substantia gelatinosa in the dorsal horn, and transmission of impulses via the spino-reticular tract to the brain is prevented. This describes the gate control theory of pain (Melzack and Wall, 1965) in extremely simplistic terms; for further information refer to the Bibliography of Chapter 6.

The use of TNS is indicated in chronic pain states, as a means of long-term pain management, where other methods have failed to alleviate the patient's problem.

There are no side-effects to treatment other than that certain individuals become sensitive to the contact medium. Treatment is contraindicated for those patients with pacemakers. This therapy is always best avoided at the base of the neck, and at the lumbar spine in the early stages of pregnancy, though TNS is widely used as a method of pain control at birth.

Laser

The word laser is an acronym for Light Amplification by Stimulated Emission of Radiation. Lasers work by releasing light energy as photons. These are emitted when the energy source of the laser is stimulated. The usual medium used in physiotherapy is gallium arsenide aluminium which is located in the probe. This produces coherent, monochromatic, unidirectional light, the wavelength of which is in the order of 780–830nm. At this wavelength, body tissues absorb the maximum amount of energy.

The photons produced interact with structures in the tissues to bring about various physiological effects. Cell function is improved due to increased production of ATP in the mitochondria, so stimulating cell growth and regeneration. Pain relief is often noted shortly after treatment, as well as a decrease in oedema. This is thought to be due to the improvement in microcirculation.

Laser penetration is about 6–8mm, but the effects can penetrate more deeply as treatment creates a chain reaction from cell to cell which can reach depths of 4–5cm.

The energy levels required to produce effective treatment are usually between 0.5–10 joules per session, compared to ultrasound, which produces 240 joules for an average treatment.

Indications for treatment include acute problems, such as sports injuries, and chronic problems, such as tendonitis, bursitis and degenerative joint changes. Lasers are also useful in the treatment of ulcers and open wounds.

The type of laser used in physiotherapy is low level and non-thermal. The main danger of treatment is direct irradiation of the eye, as irreversible damage can occur. Other contraindications include tumour, DXT in the previous 6 months, epilepsy and pregnancy.

Rest postures

Immediately after injury or during an acute exacerbation of an inflammatory condition, the patient needs to rest the affected part to minimise further inflammation. While this can be combined with other forms of treatment already discussed, the essential aspect of this procedure is that joints should always be placed in a neutral position in order to reduce the stress on damaged ligaments, the capsule and other structures surrounding the joint.

Advice to the patient should emphasise the necessity of alternating gentle activity with rest, and the importance of periods of non-weight-bearing. For example, prone or supine lying in spinal disorders, and elevation when the lower limbs are involved.

In some cases, it may be prudent to avoid certain movements and in these situations it might be appropriate to splint the affected part, e.g. knee braces can be used during rehabilitation following ligamentous injury, thus preventing unwanted rotary, or valgus/varus stresses.

In spinal problems, the use of a temporary collar may be needed for a short period, usually up to 3 weeks. Prolonged use will compromise the cervical spine musculature and lead to more problems than it alleviates. Normal proprioception and confidence will be restored by a gradual weaning-off process which depends for its success on the patient's understanding and co-operation. Corsets achieve the same results and should be used in a similar way.

Mobilisation techniques

Broadly speaking, mobilisation techniques cover the use of rhythmic passive movements of a joint or joints, which are performed in either the accessory or physiological ranges. Each movement is performed within a range, and at a speed which ultimately can be controlled by the patient. High-velocity thrust techniques are not included in this description.

The foundation of mobilisation techniques, which are graded through the range, used to effect pain relief and increase joint motion, have been described by Maitland (1985, 1991). Many concepts have been described by other authorities and each has developed its own particular techniques which are of value to the therapist.

The concept peculiar to Maitland (1985, 1991) is to treat pain by mobilising within the pain-free range of joint motion, the theory being that mechanoreceptor stimulation activates the 'pain-gate' mechanism (Melzack and Wall, 1988). The same technique may be performed at the end of the range to decrease joint stiffness and stretch scar tissue.

Maitland (1985, 1991) emphasises that the techniques must be variable, the choice being determined by the presenting problem. Constant assessment and consequent modification are central to this concept if maximum benefit is to be achieved. Techniques may be performed at any point in a joint range, in any combination, the choice depending entirely on the patient's signs and symptoms, plus a careful consideration of the information gleaned during the pretreatment examination (see Chapter 6). It is absolutely essential that the therapist learns to sense movement at a joint.

Detailed knowledge of these techniques can be gained only by referring to specialist texts (see the Bibliography to Chapter 6).

Traction

This form of treatment may be regarded as a passive mobilising technique for the spinal column. It can be administered in one of three ways:

- Constant traction in hospital, on complete bed rest, for severe nerve-root pain.
- Intermittent traction administered once or twice a day for less severe nerve-root pain, usually on an outpatient basis.
- Intermittent variable traction used to mobilise joints and increase movements.

Traction does not necessarily bring about intervertebral separation. Even at $300lb/in^2$ pressure this is disputed. Traction is always applied with the affected joint in mid-position, which will be specific to each patient at each treatment session. The amount of force used is dependent on the patient's response to treatment. Ideally, this is the minimum necessary to effect an improvement in symptoms.

This method can be used to treat all areas of the spine, though care must be taken to avoid exacerbation of symptoms in areas other than that being treated.

Exercise

The use of exercise is the mainstay of physiotherapy, its aim being to ensure a fast and, it is hoped, permanent alteration in the patient's condition. Care should be taken when selecting movement regimes to see that they most precisely match the

1. Stand and walk tall and slim.

2. Always make sure your back is fully supported when sitting.

3. Use your whole body when bending and make sure that your hips and knees do the heavy part of lifting, keeping your back comfortably still and the weight close to your body.

4. Make sure your mattress is firm; if your back troubles you at night, even try putting boards between the mattress and the bed base.

CORRECT USE OF YOUR BACK — OF LIFELONG VALUE :-

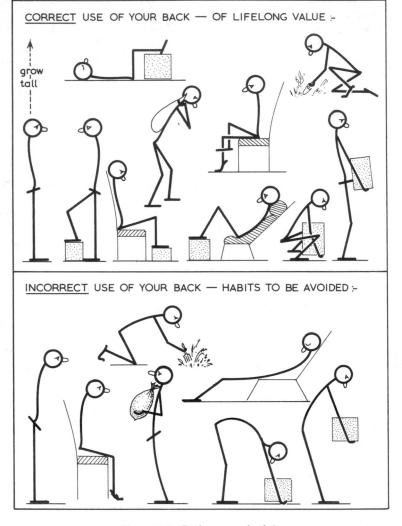

grow
tall

INCORRECT USE OF YOUR BACK — HABITS TO BE AVOIDED :-

Figure 7.1. Back care and advice.

needs called for by a particular problem. The broad categories are as follows:

- Small-range pendular movements within pain-free range, alleviating symptoms by direct stimulation of mechanoreceptors and by 'pumping the joint' to reduce oedema.
- Free exercise that mobilises joints to gain range; that is, moving to the onset of pain and applying stretch.
- Strengthening exercises tailored to the Oxford scale. This involves a progressive programme that at the earliest stage uses facilitatory techniques, sling suspension or a re-education board. The patient progresses to auto/active assisted exercises; then to free work in a variety of starting positions that can use or modify the effects of gravity. Finally, normal function is achieved by the use of resisted exercises with progressively heavier loads.
- Stabilising exercises work the affected muscle isometrically in various starting positions.

Once the exercise has been chosen, the number of repetitions at each session and the number of sessions per day must be understood and adhered to by the patient. Exercise is beneficial when carried out correctly, but irritability levels must be considered when deciding on the parameters for use.

Ergonomic advice

This involves a careful assessment of the patient's problems followed by an explicit programme of 'dos and don'ts' to be followed so that symptoms are alleviated and the possibility of exacerbation is minimised. As it may not always be obvious to the patient that some activities are liable to lead to an increase in pain, discomfort, etc., especially when there is a degree of latency in the pain pattern, activities of daily living need to be analysed and discussed in detail. Re-education is a major component of this therapy; its aim is to relieve the patient of his problems and ensure that future activities maintain that better state. (See *Figure 7.1.*)

References

Dyson, M., Pond, J., Joseph, J. and Warick, R. (1968). Stimulation of tissue regeneration by ultrasound. *Journal of Chemical Science*, **35**, 273–285.

Dyson, M. and Suckling, J. (1978). Stimulation of tissue repair by ultrasound. *Physiotherapy*, **64**(4), 105.

Forster, A. and Palastanga, N. (1985). *Clayton's Electrotherapy*, 9th edition. Baillière Tindall, London.

Maitland, G.D. (1985). *Vertebral Manipulation*, 5th edition. Butterworths, London.

Maitland, G.D. (1991). *Peripheral Manipulation*, 3rd edition. Butterworths, London.

Melzack, R. and Wall, P. (1965). Pain mechanisms, a new theory. *American Association for the Advancement of Science*, **50**(3699), 971–979.

Melzack, R. and Wall, P. (1988). *The Challenge of Pain*, 3rd edition. Penguin Education, London.

Savage, B. (1984). *Interferential Therapy*. Faber and Faber, London.

8 Osteoarthritis of Facet Joints and Lumbar Intervertebral Disc Disease

D. Jaffray

Introduction

Seldom is a patient with chronic back pain given a specific anatomical and pathological diagnosis. If we applied such behaviour to the hip joint or knee joint then we should be condemned. Why does non-specific backache remain non-specific? The answer is specific: it is a difficult diagnosis to make and very tiring to the clinician's brain and body. Much better and easier to diagnose is an osteoarthritic big toe, even though the metatarsophalangeal joint of the big toe is probably smaller than the L5/S1 facet. The important thing is that it is superficial and specific. Too bad if you have a facet problem which is deep and non-specific.

Degenerate disc disease also suffers from this problem. The disc, in some ways, resembles a knee meniscus, but the meniscus is superficial and specific. The examination and diagnosis of a torn meniscus are thus much easier than the diagnosis of a posterior annular tear; and yet both deserve attention.

Laziness is no excuse for failure to make a specific diagnosis. I hope to convince you in this chapter that the effort required to make the diagnosis is worthwhile. We will deal with the facet arthrosis and disc degeneration, but you must remember that there are many other pain sources in the spine. Diagnosis is first dependent on a history and examination. Everything else should be used to support this. X-rays, scans, etc., come after a full clinical history, examination and diagnosis.

History of a primary facet arthrosis

By definition the history will cover a long period of time. There is unlikely to be a history of a specific traumatic episode, but one of a more gradual slow onset and increase of symptoms. The pain will be in the low back and is commonly referred to the legs but usually not below the knees. It has no periodicity, but it is often worse at night. It is a deep dull pain and is not a toothache-like pain. Rest makes it worse, especially at night, and sitting is uncomfortable.

Ask your patients how long they can drive a car. They often avoid motorways because they have to stop frequently to walk, which allows − within limits − the pain to diminish. Bouts of severe pain are due to locking of the facets because of synovial damage and/or haemarthrosis. Usually, such episodes resolve as the effusion and/or haemarthrosis resolves within 3−4 weeks. The patient will often have received manipulation for such episodes. While taking the history, observe the patient's position in the chair and how he continually has to change position. The nature of his previous treatments will often support your diagnosis. I know of nothing better to make a facet arthrosis worse than a plaster jacket or a well-fitting corset. If you do not believe this, try putting a patient with osteoarthritis of the hip in a plaster spica and see if he tolerates it.

Your patient will have had physiotherapy. Exercises will have made him worse, just as active quadriceps exercises for an arthritic knee are not rewarding. Heat would have made it temporarily better and so too would have traction. The temporary benefit that many patients gain from their chiropractors describes facet arthrosis and patients' attitudes to it. They, unlike their chiropractors, get annoyed when it keeps coming back, and they resent the passage of time and its failure to resolve their condition.

Examination
This, by definition, must be secondary. Unlike osteoarthritic knee, which is large and superficial, a facet is small and deep. A skilled chiropractor, perhaps, can discern between facets, but mere clinicians have little chance. What signs there are may be non-specific to facet arthrosis, but they are worth mentioning.

Deformity can be symmetrical and take the form of a lost lumbar lordosis. A unifacet problem can give a scoliosis with a protective spasm. The degree of movement at any one level can be appreciated by placing the fingers over the spinous processes and using the patient's legs to lever the spine (this manoeuvre is just as painful to the examiner's back). Hyperextension is invariably very painful. Tenderness is frequently felt over the posterior superior iliac spines. The pain referral is most often into the buttocks and thighs, though it can be virtually anywhere in the lower limbs. Neurological examination will be negative, although referred pain can give false sensory loss, and pain naturally can restrict the power of muscles in the legs. Straight leg raising always causes pain in the back. Never confuse this with nerve-root irritation.

Investigations

These support or refute your clinical diagnosis based on a history and examination.

Plain X-rays   These may show obvious arthritic changes of the facet joints. Radiological changes, or the absence of them, in osteoarthritis of any joint do not correlate with the patient's symptoms. The asymmetry of the facet joints can be appreciated. Associated lesions that have caused the facet arthrosis, such as loss of disc height in disc resorption, may be obvious. Secondary effects of facet arthrosis, such as root canal stenosis, may be apparent.

CAT scans   These demonstrate facet joint arthropathy together with their secondary effects on root canals and the spinal canal (*Figure 8.1*).

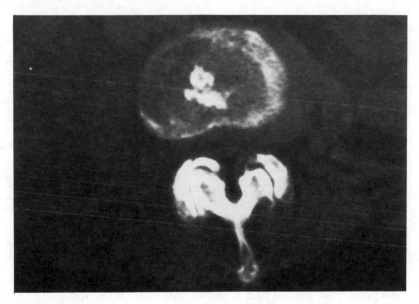

Figure 8.1. The facet joints are arthritic. The spinal canal is narrowed, but the root canals are wide. The intervertebral disc is calcified.

Pain reproduction   Facet arthrography can reproduce the patient's symptoms and subsequent marcaine injection can abolish them.

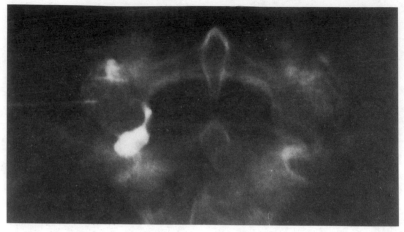

Figure 8.2. A facet arthrogram at L5/S1 with inferior capsular pooling of the dye.

This is the ideal, but it is accurate in only 40% of cases and requires high-class radiology (*Figures 8.2* and *8.3*).

Treatment

In theory the treatments to superficial osteoarthritic joints can be applied to a facet joint. Thus, heat and ultrasound, etc., to reduce inflammation, traction to stretch the capsule and manipulation to unlock a joint can all be tried. Whereas the results of a successful course of treatment for peripheral joints can be expected to last for a meaningful period of time, this is not to be expected with a facet joint (unless the therapist is dedicated to spinal work and is able to give time and patience). Even then, I seldom will waste the time of a therapist unless he thinks it is worthwhile to embark on a programme of treatment. It disappoints me to see hordes of patients with back pain referred for physiotherapy with no diagnosis and no proposed plan of treatment.

Lumbar supports, in my opinion, are a waste of time and money. In order to immobilise the lumbar spine a support has to incorporate the thighs. All a corset can do is keep the patient's back warm. If, by some remote chance, they are properly designed and fitted, then they are so uncomfortable that they force the patient to rest still. I have already explained that patients with a facet arthrosis cannot tolerate enforced immobilisation. A protuberant abdomen increases the lordosis and makes facet arthritis more painful.

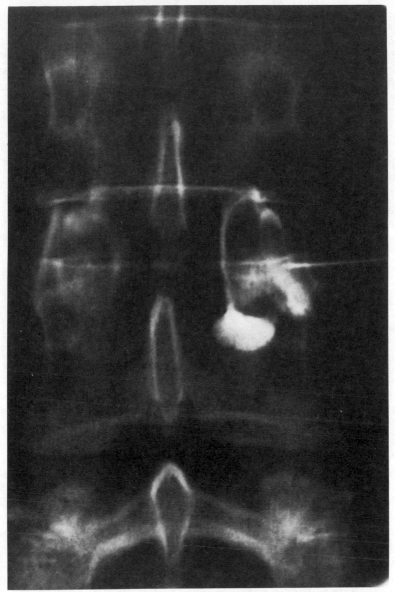

Figure 8.3. A facet arthrogram at L4/5, again with pooling of the dye.

Weight reduction is important. Corresponding strengthening of the abdominal muscles to compress the abdominal contents against the spine is also a good idea, but difficult in practice. I find swimming is likely to give the best chance.

Needless to say, NSAID (non-steroidal anti-inflammatory) drugs dampen the pain. Whether they cause more morbidity than they relieve is open to question. Do not dismiss injection of the facet joints with local anaesthetic or, better still, cryotherapy. Not only can these techniques be very useful in diagnosis, but they can be therapeutic. The relief that they can afford lasts, surprisingly, for many months and for the patient who is unfit for surgery or who prefers to avoid it, injection therapy can be a godsend. Surgery is dealt with in Chapter 9.

Of the three things that theoretically can be done to a facet joint, namely excision, replacement and fusion, only the last is appropriate at the moment.

In summary, the clinician can make a diagnosis of facet arthrosis and can explain it to the patient. This is seldom done for the reasons I have given above. However, when a diagnosis is made, a rational plan of treatment can be developed.

Lumbar disc disease

Traumatic

The force necessary to rupture the posterior annulus is surprisingly small. The protective mechanisms of the body, such as the proprioceptive and protective lumbar musculature, make this an uncommon injury, but any sudden unprotected or unexpected injury of surprisingly small dimensions can produce it.

History   There will have been a definite and sudden injury which the patient will describe if asked. Severe pain will be felt in the back alone. So severe will be the pain that the patient has to take periods of rest, usually on the floor, often for several weeks following the injury. During this time, referral pain patterns develop, which will involve one or other of the legs, but usually not below the knees. When the legs are involved, this can signal a sequestered disc through the rent in the posterior annulus. The patient will complain of pain made worse by movement and relieved by rest. This is in sharp contrast to a facet arthrosis. The sleep pattern will not be disturbed unless the patient has made sudden and gross movements in bed. Standing is uncomfortable, but sitting is acceptable. The patient has a longing desire to lie flat. Again, the various treatments described previously can aid the diagnosis. Corsets may have been appreciated.

Manipulations would certainly have made him worse. Traction, probably as an anchor to the bed, would have helped temporarily.

On examination The patient walks with a slow deliberate gait, avoiding sudden movements. Seldom is there any visible deformity and the back is held rigid. Movements of the spine are resisted and deep palpation over the spinous process is tender. Examination of the legs neurologically is normal. Straight leg raising will certainly be painful in the back, as the legs act as a lever on the back.

X-rays For a long time after the injury, X-rays will be normal, apart perhaps from the loss of lordosis. Eventually, there will be a loss of disc height with sclerosis of the vertebral end plates. Secondary facet arthritis, with possible root canal and spinal canal stenosis, occurs later.

Discography This will confirm the diagnosis (*Figures 8.4–8.7*).

Treatment Whether nature ever heals a posterior annular tear is unknown; I doubt it. Conservative treatment has unfortunately little to offer and surgery has to be considered if the symptoms warrant it.

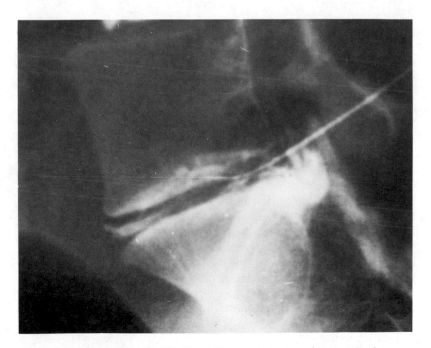

Figure 8.4. A narrow L5/S1 disc with a posterior annular contained tear.

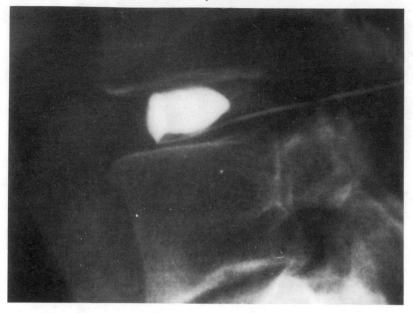

Figure 8.5. The L4/5 disc is normal.

Atraumatic

Isolated disc resorption   Why a disc in a young patient should rapidly lose its height and internal architecture is not known. Perhaps it is repeated micro-trauma, although some authorities believe it is an auto-immune phenomenon. It remains an enigma. It is a different process from degeneration of the disc in later life, although the end stages may be similar radiologically.

History   The patient is usually under 40 years of age. A gradual onset of back pain is the normal pattern. Its characteristics will be that of mechanical back pain, in many ways like that of the annular tear. Systemic symptoms are common. Lassitude, weight loss, depression, flushes, and headaches are the norm. Some authorities attribute such features to the inflammatory reaction of the anterior annulus and the adjacent sympathetic chain. On examination, the features are similar to that of an annular tear. X-rays show a dramatic reduction in disc height, with sclerosis of the vertebral end plates. Knuttson's sign is often present. Discography confirms the diagnosis (*Figure 8.8*).

Treatment   Initially, the treatment is that for mechanical back pain. As the disc height reduces, secondary facet arthrosis de-

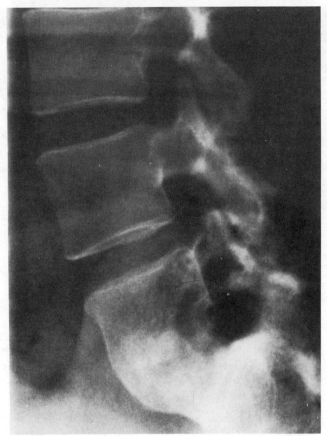

Figure 8.6. After interbody fusion the root canal is restored.

velops, the patient cannot rest and movement makes him just as uncomfortable. Surgery is the only chance of respite.

'Mixed' lesions

Seldom does a facet arthrosis or a disc resorption, etc., remain 'pure'. For example, a disc resorption leads to loss of disc height and a subsequent facet arthrosis. This gives a mixed picture, which makes evaluating a history even more difficult, but not impossible. Such patients will, of course, have pain at rest and on walking. The clinician should be aware of this and not become confused when the patient does not fit into 'pure' categories.

Prolapsed lumbar disc

So much has been written about this condition, I feel it is impertinent to add more. I know of no other diagnosis that has the

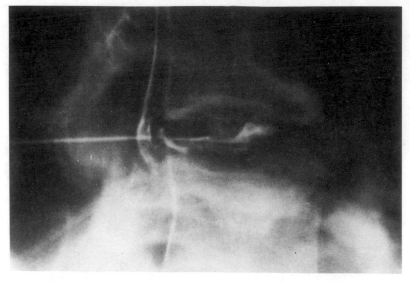

Figure 8.7. L4/5 annular tear with dye escaping into the epidural space.

potential to ruin poeple's lives. One wonders what happened before Mixter and Barr's classic paper describing this condition appeared in 1934. Certainly, Mixter and Barr may have had some regrets, once they had published their paper.

'The diagnosis of a herniated lumbar disc started all the damn trouble'
W.J. Mixter

'I am sorry that the discovery of herniation of the disc has led to so high an incidence of back cripples'
J.S. Barr

'They are more common and more severely impaired after surgery than they would have been had no surgical treatment been pursued'
J.S. Barr

At first glance one would expect the diagnosis to be easy. It is not. Unless one has a deep understanding of the nature of referred pain to the leg, described by Kellgren (1939), one will be confused. Unfortunately, there is not a back pain condition that straight leg raising does not make worse. True disc prolapse with nerve root irritation is uncommon; it is characterised by leg pain with a minimum of back pain and the motor sensory and bladder symptoms and signs are well described. The main sign I rely on is that of the popliteal nerve test (like a Tinel sign on the popliteal nerve), which I have seldom known to be false and is reliable. Prolapsed disc requires a clinical diagnosis. If you cannot make a

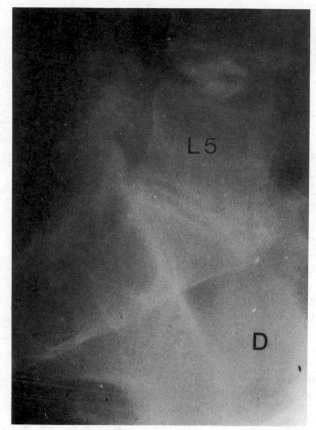

Figure 8.8. Resorption of the L5/S1 disc with a normal L4/5 disc.

clinical diagnosis, do not rely on myelograms or scans, which will always show bulges, etc. (*Figure 8.9*). Be accurate in your diagnosis. Most prolapses will cure themselves.

Whatever is done, the therapist can help nature shrink a prolapse by traction or, indeed, manipulation. The quicker the disc prolapse decreases in size, the less likely that surgery, percutaneous discectomy, etc., will be needed. Although the disc will never be normal again, it is better than no disc. In many ways it is like a knee meniscus – when the disc ruptures and the disc sequestrates then the situation is irretrievable. This does not mean that surgery is mandatory, but the disc has little chance of reasonable function, unlike a contained or prolapsed disc.

The surgical treatment of prolapsed discs is described in Chapter 9.

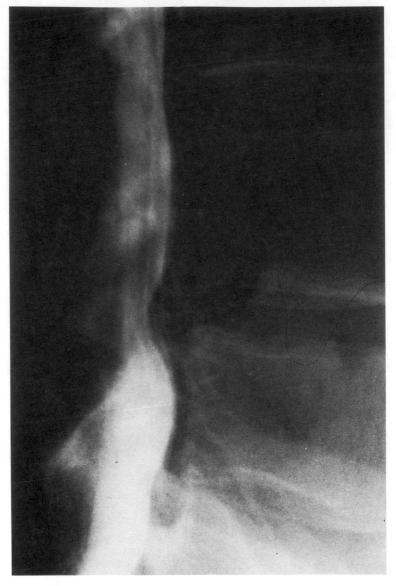

Figure 8.9. A central disc prolapse.

References

Kellgren, J.H. (1939). On the distribution of pain arising from deep somatic structures with charts of segmental pain areas. *Clinical Science*, **4**, 35–46.

Mixter, W.J. and Barr, J.S. (1934). Rupture of the intervertebral disc with involvement of the spinal cord. *New England Journal of Medicine*, **211**(5), 210–215.

Bibliography

Bough, B., Thakore, J., Davies, M. and Dowling, F. (1990). Degeneration of the lumbar facet joints arthrography and pathology. *Journal of Bone and Joint Surgery*, **72B**, 275–276.

Campbell, D., Goss, E. and Eisenstein, S.M. (1989). The natural history of low back pain. *Neuro-Orthopaedics*, **7**, 32–35.

Colhoun, E., McCall, I.W., Williams, L. and Pullicino, V.N.C. (1988). Provocative discography as a guide to planning operations on the spine. *Journal of Bone and Joint Surgery*, **70B**, 267–271.

Eisenstein, S.M. and Parry, C.R. (1987). The lumbar facet arthrosis syndrome. *Journal of Bone and Joint Surgery*, **69B**, 3–7.

9 Surgery for Spinal Disorders — Clinical

S. Eisenstein

Introduction

Reduced to its essentials, surgery for spinal disorders consists of two operations: stiffening the spine (arthrodesis); and clearing out the spinal canal to make more room for the neural tissue (decompression). Frequently, both types of surgery need to be done on the same patient under one anaesthetic. Traditionally, but quite incorrectly, the various types of stiffening or arthrodesis operations are called 'spinal fusions'. In these 'fusion' (arthrodesis) operations, surgeons place bone graft on the spine, but a natural biological process achieves the fusion. Equally incorrectly, the clearing or decompression operations are called 'laminectomies'. There is usually much more involved in spinal canal decompression operations than mere 'laminectomy'. Customary usage has, however, conferred a form of validity on these terms, and we all continue to use them.

In surgery for deformity of the spine, especially for the curvature called scoliosis, various techniques are used to straighten the spine, in combination with the spinal arthrodesis surgery which must always be done. The operations for deformity are described in more detail in Chapter 11.

The role of the physiotherapist in the surgery for spinal disorders may be negligible or critical, depending on the type of surgery, and the particular circumstances surrounding the surgery (Chapter 10). Where spinal surgery is performed on a regular basis, a physiotherapist should be allocated to join the surgical team as an indispensable member of that team. The major contribution of enthusiastic physiotherapy to the success of surgical treatment is too often taken for granted.

Spinal disorders and their operations

Below are described some of the more common spinal disorders, in approximate descending order of frequency; the operations which may need to be performed for them are given in brackets.

Mechanical pain (arthrodesis)

The pain may develop with age-related degeneration of the discs, or as a result of sprain and/or strain injuries of the spine. The most common spinal disorder, by far, is low back pain of this 'mechanical' type. Pain in the neck (cervical spine) of similar origin is the next most common disorder.

In the great majority of cases, there is no obvious cause for the mechanical pain, either in the history or in the plain X-rays. Occasionally, however, one may find on X-ray an ununited fracture of part of the lamina of a lower lumbar vertebra (spondylolysis). This is a fracture which will have occurred in childhood,

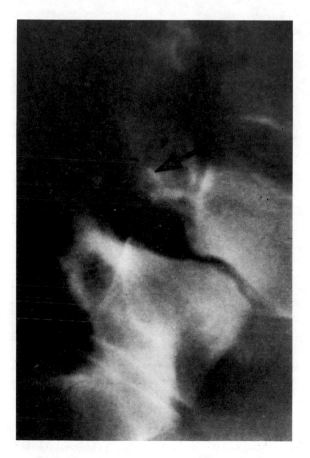

Figure 9.1. Spondylolisthesis causing backache. Arrows show ununited fracture.

usually quite forgotten or not even known of at the time of occurrence, and presenting with pain in adult life. It is never a congenital defect. If the gap has opened significantly, the whole spine above the gap will have shifted forward on the vertebra below (spondylolisthesis) (*Figure 9.1*).

Disc prolapse (decompression)

The bulging or frank rupture of a disc anulus, posteriorly at the lower two lumbar segments, is quite common in physically active young or middle-aged adults. The condition comes to light only because irritation, by the disc, of a root of the sciatic nerve causes intense pain and paraesthesiae ('sciatica') down one lower limb (*Figure 9.2*). Surgical decompression of the nerve becomes neces-

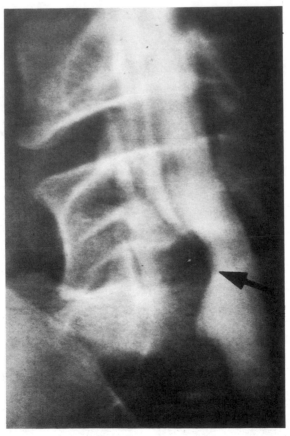

Figure 9.2. Disc prolapse has compressed the nerve root, causing an indentation in myelogram contrast.

sary to relieve severe pain if non-surgical methods have been unsuccessful for about 10 days. When a large midline bulge of the disc causes paralysis of the bladder, then this must be considered a surgical emergency.

The problem occurs also in the cervical spine, causing intense pain down one arm, but this is rare.

Deformity (arthrodesis)

Scoliosis (side-to-side curvature with a twist, *Figure 9.3*) and kyphosis (forward tilt) may be progressive in a youngster, and unresponsive to brace treatment. Spinal arthrodesis, with various forms of metal internal fixation, will then be necessary to prevent further deformity and to improve the appearance (*see* Chapter 11). Physiotherapy has no role to play in the prevention of these deformities in young people, except in respect of management of a bracing programme.

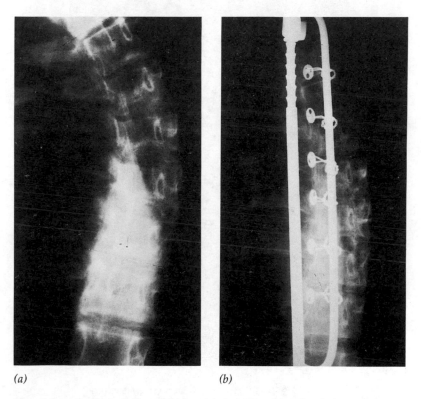

(a)   (b)

Figure 9.3. Scoliosis deformity before (a) and after (b) arthrodesis surgery.

Spinal stenosis (decompression, sometimes with arthrodesis)

This is a generalised narrowing of the spinal canal (*Figure 9.4*), usually in the elderly, and the result of age-related bony overgrowth and buckling ligaments crowding into the canal. Patients complain of weakness, numbness, tingling, and pain in the lower limbs, aggravated by walking, and in spite of a good peripheral circulation. When these symptoms force a patient to stop walking after a certain distance, the condition is called spinal claudication.

Spinal stenosis is also associated with achondroplastic dwarfism, and may be developmental in origin, but these are rare causes.

Again, physiotherapy has no role in prevention or treatment, except in conjunction with surgical decompression.

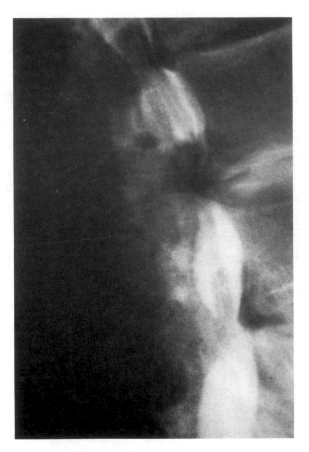

Figure 9.4. Spinal stenosis 'beaded' appearance on myelogram.

Spinal injury (decompression and arthrodesis)

Where major violence has caused a spinal fracture (*Figure 9.5*), with or without dislocation, the unfortunate result frequently is paralysis of the lower limbs and of bladder and bowel control (paraplegia). The management philosophy differs markedly between hospitals and nations. In many institutions it is considered important to operate on these patients to decompress the spinal cord and nerves in the faint hope of restoring some neural function, and to arthrodese the spine for early rehabilitation to mobility.

Where the injury is to the cervical spine, the patient may be paralysed in all four limbs and in some of the muscles of respiration (quadriplegia or tetraplegia).

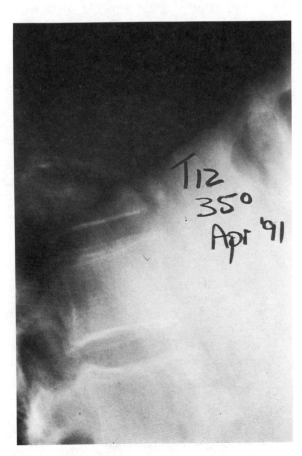

Figure 9.5. Crushed T12 vertebra after a fall from a horse.

Infection (decompression with or without arthrodesis)

Almost every infecting bacterium and fungus has at some time infected the spine, causing varying degrees of destruction of the vertebral body and disc (*Figure 9.6*). Paralysis is a possible tragic outcome if the resulting kyphosis deformity and abscess formation produce pressure on the spinal cord or spinal nerves. The two most common infecting organisms are pyogenic (staphylococcus) and mycobacterial (tuberculosis). Decompression may be sufficient in early cases, but it is more usual to have to add a supporting bone graft.

Inflammatory diseases (arthrodesis: occasional decompression, or osteotomy)

Rheumatoid arthritis uncommonly causes such destruction of disc and vertebra that a kyphosis deformity will endanger the spinal

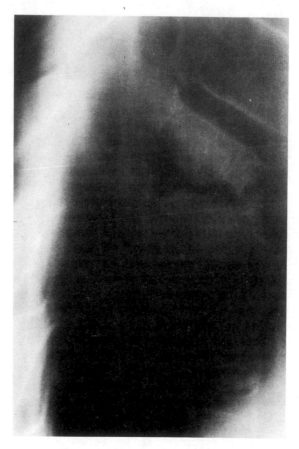

Figure 9.6. Two vertebrae destroyed by infection.

cord. More common is the destruction of ligaments that secure the odontoid peg in the upper cervical spine, creating a danger of tetraplegia or sudden death. Arthrodesis is a remarkably successful solution in both circumstances.

Ankylosing spondylitis produces a spontaneous fusion of the spine (*Figure 9.7*), of varying extent, but often in a kyphosis deformity of the whole spine. These patients are young and middle-aged adults (usually male), so bent over that they cannot see more than a few feet of ground ahead. In this situation, the vertebral column must be cut across in the lumbar area (osteotomy) to improve the deformity. An arthrodesis must be added to secure the correction. It may be necessary to perform similar surgery at the cervico-thoracic junction if the deformity is extensive and severe.

Cancer (decompression and arthrodesis)   Cancer originating in the spine (*Figure 9.8*) is rare. The vertebral column is usually

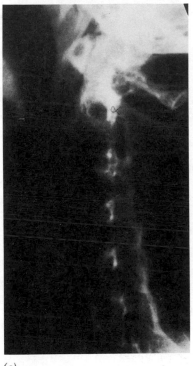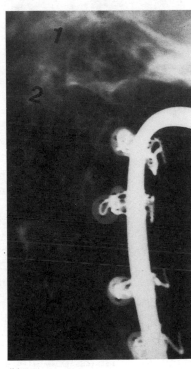

(a)   (b)

Figure 9.7. Spontaneous fusion of the spine in ankylosing spondylitis (a), and after correction by osteotomy and fixation (b).

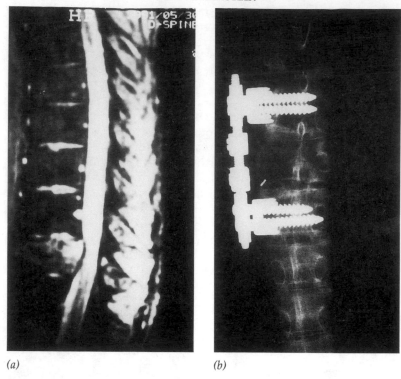

(a)   *(b)*

Figure 9.8. Cancer of the vertebrae (a) and appearance after decompression and fusion (b).

involved by spread of cancer from breast, kidney, lung, bowel, and prostate. The patient presents with great pain and established or impending paralysis from the destruction of one or more vertebral bodies. Decompression and arthrodesis can prevent paralysis (or occasionally improve it), and reduce the pain sufficiently to provide an acceptable quality of life remaining.

The 'salvage' situation (decompression and/or arthrodesis)

The best efforts of spinal surgeons occasionally result in failure through a conspiracy of circumstances, or for reasons which cannot be established. It is then too easy to point a finger and pontificate that the patient should not have had the surgery in the first place. Spinal surgeons are all too aware that many consider their practice esoteric and of doubtful need, so that decisions for surgical treatment are seldom lightly made. A decompression may need to be repeated, for instance, where a further fragment of disc tissue has emerged to press on a spinal nerve. A spinal arthrodesis may have failed to produce a complete fusion and additional bone grafting will be necessary. Internal fixation may have to be removed or replaced because of displacement or breakage. Infection is an ever-present danger. 'Salvage' or 'revision' surgery is never easy, never as successful as primary surgery can be, and is cursed with a high complication rate.

Indications for spinal surgery

Much of this subject has been covered in the text above. It remains true, *in general*, that spinal surgery is contemplated only when all non-surgical treatments have been tried without success. This is true especially for chronic low back and neck pain, where the non-surgical treatments available are many and varied. The condition does not, in any event, affect life expectancy; and the results of surgery for spinal pain are unpredictable.

On the other hand, there are important exceptions to the generalisation made above: the pain of nerve compression (e.g., in lumbar disc prolapse) becomes more difficult to treat successfully the longer the delay in applying surgical decompression; loss of bladder control is a surgical emergency; certain spine deformities (e.g., congenital scoliosis) are known to be quite unresponsive to non-surgical treatments; a spinal abscess needs urgent surgical drainage; spinal cancer may be slowed by radiotherapy, but only arthrodesis will provide the stability required to mobilise the patient; and a few spinal injury patients may be more easily rehabilitated after arthrodesis.

The exceptions described above are relatively clear-cut: there is little controversy surrounding the decision for surgical treatment. *The great dilemma is the matter of deciding for surgical treatment in the most common spinal disorder, chronic mechanical low back pain.* Here it is certainly the case that surgery should be held back as 'a last resort'.

While spinal arthrodesis is the only surgical treatment known to have any chance of providing some degree of pain relief when all else, including physiotherapy, has failed, the results of surgery are notoriously unpredictable from patient to patient, even assuming technically successful operations with complete consolidation of the bone graft. As far as the physiotherapist is concerned, there is a danger that every patient finally selected for surgery is seen by the therapist to represent a personal failure. It is closer to the reality of the matter to regard physiotherapy as a stage in the selection process leading to surgery.

Selecting the patient for surgery

There is no difficulty in selecting patients for spinal surgery when they are afflicted with serious spinal disease, deformity, or injury: relatively simple rules govern the situation as it presents itself. On the other hand, the vast majority of patients attending a spinal clinic have no serious spinal disease: they have 'mechanical' pain, which may have originated in a sprain or strain, or in some degenerative process common to all humans. This 'mechanical' pain will not affect life expectancy, nor will it produce paralysis, but it may cause such a disruption of the normal conduct of daily life as to constitute a disability nearly equivalent to paralysis. These patients present the greatest challenge in the matter of selection for surgery and therefore deserve a little more discussion, given here under the headings of Disability, Personality, and Special Investigations.

It is important to remember that the vast majority of back pain patients are satisfactorily treated without surgery. The discussion that follows applies to those few unfortunate patients whose symptoms are refractory to all non-surgical treatments.

Disability

Disability is the cornerstone of patient selection for spinal arthrodesis in mechanical back pain. Pain at any level produces some degree of disability, most of which the majority of people can cope with sufficiently well to continue their daily lives more or less uninterrupted. Pain is a matter of perception, and perception is 'in the eye of the beholder'. It follows that the disability which flows from the pain is also a matter of perception and differs markedly from one personality to the next. Even so, we must all complete certain tasks in our daily living to be able to continue a reasonable existence. Once it is no longer possible to conduct a reasonable semblance of a daily life routine, then it can be said that disability is of sufficient degree to justify an attempt at surgical treatment. It is possible to measure disability for a particular patient by means of a questionnaire that covers all aspects of daily living activities. For that particular patient, the resulting disability 'index' is real and valid. The Oswestry Disability Index (ODI; *see* Appendix) is usefully comprehensive without being burdensome. This index is now widely used internationally.

Personality

Pain perception, apart from being dependent on neurological physiology, is also a function of mental attitude or *personality*. Experience over the years has produced a wariness in spinal surgeons of the back pain patient who does not respond adequately to conservative treatments and who begs that 'something more' be done. Spinal arthrodesis is the only 'something more' that remains to be tried, but all too often patients have declared that the operation has made them 'much worse', even when it can be shown that the operation has been technically successful. Surgeons then begin to question the patient's motivation and sincerity, and their own ability to judge personality traits. Cynicism and suspicion come to poison the relationship between surgeons and prospective surgical patients. In seeking to resolve this situation, surgeons have employed a variety of questionnaires designed to assess patients' personalities, in the hope of weeding out those patients who will complain of continuing pain, however successful the surgery. The best known of these tests is the Minnesota Multiphasic Personality Inventory (MMPI). Eysenck, Millon, and Beck are names associated with others: there are many more. Unfortunately, none of these tests is wholly reliable and failed expectations have produced more disillusionment.

In the end, the surgeon's own judgement of the patient's personality may remain the best guide to patient selection, accepting that this judgement will be fallible and incorrect in a number of instances.

Special investigations

Special investigations in the context of spinal pain are almost always radiological. Various blood tests are useful to eliminate nagging doubts raised by the possibility of infection, inflammation, or cancer being the cause of pain. Special X-ray tests are required to locate a source of pain or to eliminate some spinal structure as a source of pain. Plain X-rays show only the bones of the spine and none of the soft tissues. The bones (vertebrae) are very rarely the source of pain. The discs are the major soft-tissue connections in the spine and therefore the most likely to be painful. Discography involves injecting into a series of discs, usually lumbar, using some contrast medium which will show up internal disc abnormalities on X-ray (Figure 9.9), and noting the patient's reaction as to the type and distribution of pain experienced. Facet arthrography is a similar technique (Figure 9.10) for proving or eliminating the facet joints as a source of pain.

If it is not certain whether some lower limb pain is being caused by a disc prolapsing on to a spinal nerve, then myelography (see Figure 9.11; also called radiculography) will help to decide the matter. Contrast medium is injected into the spinal canal: where a disc presses on a nerve, no contrast medium will be seen. Computerised tomography produces excellent cross-section views of the spine (see Figure 9.12), usually without the need for any

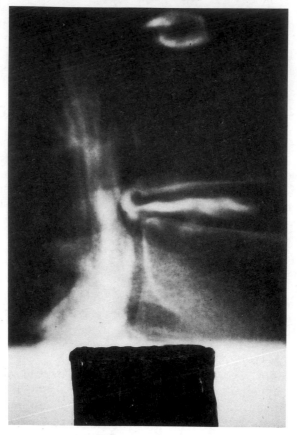

Figure 9.9. Discography showing normal disc above and abnormal below.

injection into the spine, and is frequently used instead of myelography.

Magnetic resonance imaging (MRI) does not use X-rays at all, but records the tissue images produced when very high magnetic forces are sent through the body to stimulate the tissue ions (see *Figure 9.13*). These images are useful for detecting the extent of various diseases in both the spine *and* soft tissues, but they are of no assistance in detecting the sources of pain in 'mechanical' back pain. *Radio-isotope bone scan* (see *Figure 9.14*) records the concentration of radio-activity in the bone, after the injection of radio-active technetium[99]. It is useful for locating cancer, infection, and inflammation, but is of little help in 'mechanical' back pain. Wherever there is a suspicion of cancer or infection of the spine, a *biopsy* of bone or disc tissue will help to make a certain

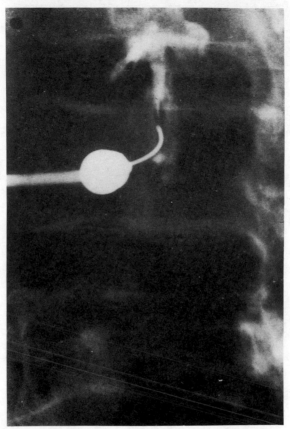

Figure 9.10. Facet arthrography.

diagnosis. A special wide-bore needle is directed to the diseased area: fragments are extracted for microscopy and bacterial culture.

For all the sophistication of modern investigations, there is still no satisfactory method of imaging or locating those sources of pain that must arise in the vast mass of muscle and ligamentous tissue which extends from the back of the vertebral column to the subcutaneous fat.

The operations

Arthrodesis
Arthrodesis (or 'fusion') can be performed at the anterior or posterior aspect of the spine, depending largely on the preference

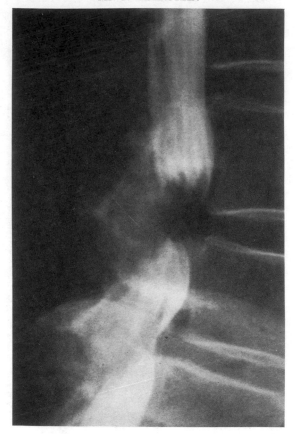

Figure 9.11. Gap in contrast shows where the disc compresses the nerve.

of the individual surgeon, but also on the need for associated decompression surgery.

A *posterior fusion* anywhere in the spine involves splitting the soft tissues that cover the spine, usually from a midline incision, and shifting the tissues laterally to expose the bone surfaces of the laminae right out to the tips of the transverse processes. The bone is scraped until a bleeding surface is produced. Slices of bone graft are taken from the patient's own pelvis and placed over the scraped surfaces. Further procedures to keep the spine still and stable while the bone graft consolidates are becoming increasingly popular.

These *internal fixation* procedures consist of a variety of screws, bars, wires, and plates of stainless steel or other surgical metal, fixed to the spine over the length of the fusion to be desired. At

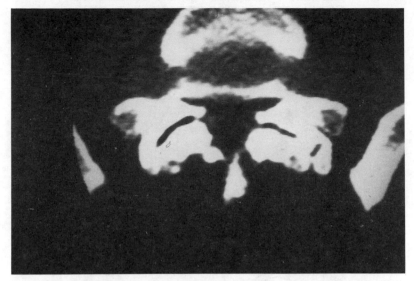

Figure 9.12. Computerised tomography scan of an arthritic spine.

the time of writing, the strongest fixation results from screws inserted into the pedicles of the vertebrae and connected to each other by longitudinal rods (Oswestry pedicle screw system; Cotrel–Dubousset system; *Figure 9.15*) or plates (Steffee system; Luque system).

An *anterior fusion* can also be performed at any level of the spine but complex anatomy at the junctions (cervico-thoracic and thoraco-lumbar) makes for complex surgery at these levels. Once the spine is exposed, whether through the neck, the chest, or the abdomen, the relevant disc segments are excised, the adjacent vertebral body surfaces scraped till bleeding, and pelvic bone graft blocks hammered into position. Where the vertebrae have been crushed or split by injury, it may be desirable to add extra stability by inserting metal screws and connections into the vertebral bodies above and below the injured vertebrae. Whether or not internal fixation is used, it is probably best to protect the grafted area postoperatively by some sort of external support for a period of weeks or months. A firm collar will do for the cervical spine, for 6–8 weeks. For the thoracic spine and lumbar spine, a custom-fitted polyethylene brace is used for 3–6 months.

Decompression
Decompression is performed most frequently for a prolapsed disc in the lumbar spine. It is obvious that the least damaging surgical

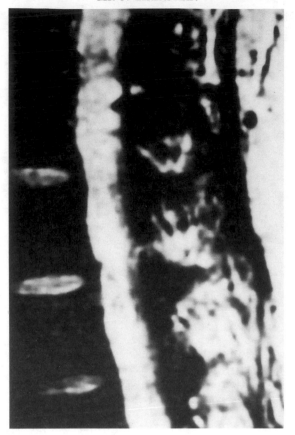

Figure 9.13. MRI, showing normal discs (white) and degenerative discs (grey).

dissection will be the approach of choice. Sometimes it is possible to perform a discectomy through a *fenestration* approach, i.e. by cutting a window in the ligamentum flavum only and on the affected side only. Where this approach does not give sufficient access to the disc, some bone must be nibbled away from the adjacent laminar edges on the affected side – a *laminotomy*. If, rarely, greater exposure is needed, a whole lamina on one side must be removed – a *hemi-laminectomy*.

The principle of minimal exposure has led to the increasing use of percutaneous techniques for decompressing the disc. *Chemonucleolysis*, now less favoured than it was, requires an injection into the disc of an enzyme (chymopapain) derived from the skins

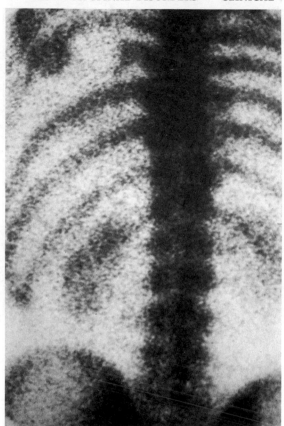

Figure 9.14. Radioisotope scan showing spine infection (dark areas).

of unripe paw-paws. *Nucleotomy* involves disc removal through an automated biopsy needle connected to a suction device.

Percutaneous discectomy is simply the removal of disc material via a wide-bore tube inserted through the skin and tissues, and using long nibblers. A compromise between formal fenestration or laminotomy, and these percutaneous techniques, is *microdiscectomy* (*Figure 9.16*), where a small incision (2−3cm) is nevertheless large enough to permit a formal discectomy, because a surgical microscope is used by the surgeon to achieve excellent visualisation of the surgical field.

The advantage of all these 'minimal' approaches is in increased patient comfort and early mobilisation: the postoperative task of

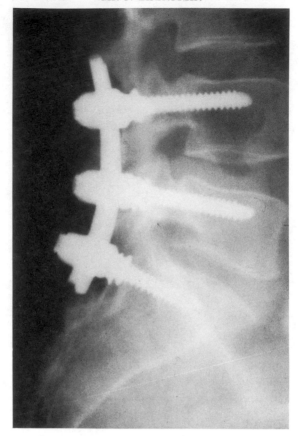

Figure 9.15. Oswestry pedicle screw fixation for lumbar spine fusion.

the physiotherapist is much reduced, and the mechanical stability of the spine is better preserved.

In degenerative lumbar spinal stenosis, it is usually necessary to excise the whole lamina on both sides and at several levels, followed by widening of the nerve root canals − *multilevel laminectomy and under-cutting facetectomy.*

In major spinal diseases, such as cancer and tuberculosis, it may be necessary to decompress the spinal cord from the front, by *vertebrectomy,* i.e. removal of one or more whole vertebrae. This is always followed by a bone graft to fill the gap, and anterior internal fixation may be added. If this operation has to be done in the thoracic spine, as is so often the case with tuberculosis, then access through the chest wall is by *thoracotomy,* and involves the removal of a rib.

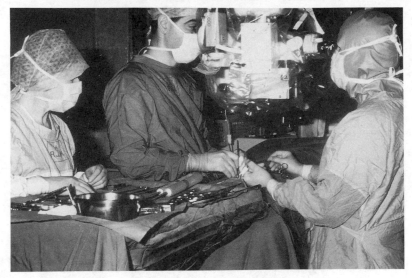

Figure 9.16. Microdiscectomy.

The rehabilitation of the patient after major spinal surgery, from recumbency to independent walking, requires dedication, care, and persistence on the part of the physiotherapist. Where a thoracotomy has been necessary, the physiotherapist is crucial in helping the patient regain full respiratory function while still in great pain and subject to the inconvenience of a chest drain.

Appendix

The *Oswestry Disability Index* was developed in 1976, and has provided a useful measure of disability, through spinal pain, for the more severely disabled. It has been validated by a number of separate studies conducted elsewhere and is in daily use in many countries.

Each section is scored from 0–5, there being six levels of disability in each section. The figures for all sections are added together and multiplied by two to give a score out of 100. This final score does not in any sense represent a percentage disability, but is merely a score against which to measure disability on subsequent occasions in the same patient. In no way is the score intended to be compared to those of other patients.

MR S. EISENSTEIN

Confidential

Score:

THE OSWESTRY DISABILITY INDEX FOR LOW BACK PAIN

THE ROBERT JONES AND AGNES HUNT ORTHOPAEDIC HOSPITAL, OSWESTRY, SHROPSHIRE DEPARTMENT FOR SPINAL DISORDERS

NAME: ....DATE OF BIRTH: ....
ADDRESS: ....DATE: ....
.................................AGE: ....
OCCUPATION: ....
How long·have you had back pain? ......Years ......Months .... Weeks
How long have you had leg pain? ....Years ......Months .... Weeks

PLEASE READ:

This questionnaire has been designed to give the doctor information as to how your back pain has affected your ability to manage in everyday life. Please answer every section, and mark in each section only **ONE BOX** which applies to you. We realise you may consider that two of the statements in any one section relate to you, but please just **mark the box which most closely describes your problem.**

SECTION 1 – PAIN INTENSITY
0 ☐ My pain is mild to moderate: I do not need pain killers.
1 ☐ The pain is bad, but I manage without taking pain killers.
2 ☐ Pain killers give complete relief from pain.
3 ☐ Pain killers give moderate relief from pain.
4 ☐ Pain killers give very little relief from pain.
5 ☐ Pain killers have **no** effect on the pain.

SECTION 2 – PERSONAL CARE
(Washing, Dressing, etc.)
0 ☐ I can look after myself normally without causing extra pain.
1 ☐ I can look after myself normally, but it causes extra pain.
2 ☐ It is painful to look after myself and I am slow and careful.
3 ☐ I need some help, but manage most of my personal care.
4 ☐ I need help everyday in most aspects of self care.
5 ☐ I do not get dressed; wash with difficulty; and stay in bed.

SECTION 3 – LIFTING
0 ☐ I can lift heavy weights without extra pain.
1 ☐ I can lift heavy weights, but it gives extra pain.
2 ☐ Pain prevents me from lifting heavy weights off the floor, but I can manage if they are conveniently positioned, e.g., on a table.
3 ☐ Pain prevents me from lifting heavy weights, but I can manage light weights if they are conveniently positioned.
4 ☐ I can lift only very light weights.
5 ☐ I cannot lift or carry anything at all.

SECTION 4 – WALKING
0 ☐ I can walk as far as I wish.
1 ☐ Pain prevents me walking for more than 1 mile.
2 ☐ Pain prevents me walking for more than ½ mile.
3 ☐ Pain prevents me walking for more than ¼ mile.
4 ☐ I can walk only if I use a stick or crutches.
5 ☐ I am in bed or in a chair for most of every day.

SECTION 5 – SITTING

0 ☐ I can sit in any chair as long as I like.
1 ☐ I can sit in my favourite chair only, but for as long as I like.
2 ☐ Pain prevents me from sitting for more than 1 hour.
3 ☐ Pain prevents me from sitting for more than ½ hour.
4 ☐ Pain prevents me from sitting for more than 10 minutes.
5 ☐ Pain prevents me from sitting at all.

SECTION 6 – STANDING

0 ☐ I can stand as long as I want without extra pain.
1 ☐ I can stand as long as I want, but it gives me extra pain.
2 ☐ Pain prevents me from standing for more than 1 hour.
3 ☐ Pain prevents me from standing for more than 30 minutes.
4 ☐ Pain prevents me from standing for more than 10 minutes.
5 ☐ Pain prevents me from standing at all.

SECTION 7 – SLEEPING

0 ☐ Pain does not prevent me from sleeping well.
1 ☐ I sleep well, but only by using tablets.
2 ☐ Even when I take tablets, I have less than 6 hours' sleep.
3 ☐ Even when I take tablets, I have less than 4 hours' sleep.
4 ☐ Even when I take tablets, I have less than 2 hours' sleep.
5 ☐ Pain prevents me from sleeping at all.

SECTION 8 – SEX LIFE

0 ☐ My sex life is normal and causes no extra pain.
1 ☐ My sex life is normal, but causes some extra pain.
2 ☐ My sex life is nearly normal, but is very painful.
3 ☐ My sex life is severely restricted by pain.
4 ☐ My sex life is nearly absent because of pain.
5 ☐ Pain prevents any sex life at all.

SECTION 9 – SOCIAL LIFE

0 ☐ My social life is normal and causes me no extra pain.
1 ☐ My social life is normal, but increases the degree of pain.
2 ☐ Pain affects my social life by limiting my more energetic interests only (dancing, etc.).
3 ☐ Pain has restricted my social life and I do not go out as often.
4 ☐ Pain has restricted my social life to my home.
5 ☐ I have no social life because of pain.

SECTION 10 – TRAVELLING

0 ☐ I can travel anywhere without extra pain.
1 ☐ I can travel anywhere, but it gives me extra pain.
2 ☐ Pain is bad, but I manage journeys of over 2 hours.
3 ☐ Pain restricts me to journeys of less than 1 hour.
4 ☐ Pain restricts me to short necessary journeys of less than 30 minutes.
5 ☐ Pain prevents me travelling except to the Doctor or Hospital.

COMMENTS:

....
....
....
....
....
....
....
....
....
....
....
....
....
....
....

COUPER, EISENSTEIN, FAIRBANK, O'BRIEN

10 Surgery for Spinal Disorders — Physiotherapy

E. Goss

The types of patient found in an orthopaedic spinal disorders unit are varied. Many will have had previous surgery, for example a laminectomy, or perhaps a laminectomy followed by an exploration, and still be in their teens. Approximately nine-tenths of the patients will have low back pain and the rest some degree of spinal deformity.

The causes of back pain may be:

- Congenital, e.g. hemivertebra producing a kyphotic deformity, or spina bifida producing a scoliosis deformity associated with low back pain.
- Acquired, e.g. infective tuberculosis or poliomyelitis producing both low back pain and deformity, or as a result of heavy work producing degenerative changes resulting in low back pain.
- Due to trauma, e.g. fracture of the spine, or spondylolisthesis.

The lumbar, thoracic and cervical spine may be affected individually or as a whole.

Physiotherapy aims to prevent postoperative complications and to help the patient regain independence and safe gross motor function, including transfers from bed to standing and to toilet, and gait training. Advice in back care and safe lifting is also important.

The philosophy underlying the physiotherapist's role is basically:

- To reassure the patient.
- To give the patient a general understanding of his back problem.
- To give the patient confidence in himself and enable him to manage his back problem.
- To give the patient and his family any advice which will enable them together to reduce the overall effect that the condition may have on lifestyle, including marriage, family and work.

MacNab (1979) wrote ' . . . Treat a patient — not a spine. Find out about the patient who has backache as well as finding out as much as you can about the back pain that the patient has.'

Assessment

A full assessment should always be carried out on every new patient, even though it may take up a lot of the physiotherapist's time. The history, as accurate as possible, of the patient's back pain is very relevant. A thorough examination of posture, gait, pain patterns, disability, range of movement, neurology and muscle power should all be recorded. The patient's height and weight are also important.

Pain patterns can either be recorded on a form or be photographed. Photography will also show the back contours, e.g. sway back or round shoulders, and will be useful for comparison — pre- and post-operation — of antero-posterior and lateral views. A scoliosis series — pictures to show the curve in all dimensions — will show the deformity and any pain.

If the photographic method of recording pain is to be used, the physiotherapist should start her palpation for pain and/or tenderness from the cervical spine and work distally. She should mark the pain patterns on the skin using mercurochrome for red and gentian violet for blue; bony, muscle trigger points or nerve pressure points are marked in red. The patient is then asked to indicate the pattern of referred pain, which is marked in blue. The patient will usually outline the painful area quite accurately; if he cannot it may be easier to note where the finger passes over the skin and ask the patient to state if and when the sensation changes. Areas of sensitivity can then be marked as indicated above. This change in sensation will be a dermatome-type representation of the painful area referred from the 'red' tender spots already drawn. *Figures 10.1* and *10.2* show pain patterns from cervical and lumbar lesions, respectively.

Disability forms which are filled in by the patient can give good insight into his problems (Fairbank et al., 1980).

Range of movement is relevant depending on the painful episodes experienced by the patient. One method of measuring this is to palpate the posterior superior iliac spines, i.e. the dimples; mark this line, and extend it laterally to the left and right hip, respectively. Place the tape measure with the 10cm mark on the line and your thumb on the 15cm mark; as the patient bends backwards the measurement will be between the 15 and 10cm mark. Side flexion is measured in the same way using the lateral

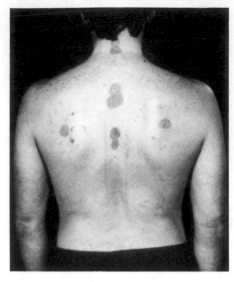

Figure 10.1. Pain pattern from a cervical lesion.

marks: to measure left side flexion the tape is held on the right side as the patient bends towards the left; this is then repeated for the other side. This way of measuring is a modification of the Schober method (Schober, 1937).

Muscle power should be tested using the Medical Research Council (MRC) scale of grading muscle power (Oxford scale) to define associated limb weakness. If the patient has been bedbound or disabled for a long time, disuse atrophy is quite common. A myometer reading of muscle groups is interesting to have, but not essential.

Neurological examination may consist of testing reflexes, sensory changes, femoral and sciatic stretches, positive bowstring, and Babinski test.

Femoral nerve stretching is done with the patient prone and lifting the affected leg into extension. The knee may be flexed. If there is a positive femoral stretch, pain will be experienced indicating femoral nerve irritation.

Sciatic nerve stretching is done in the supine position by lifting the affected leg with the knee fully extended into flexion, and then dorsiflexing the ankle and forefoot. Note whether there is

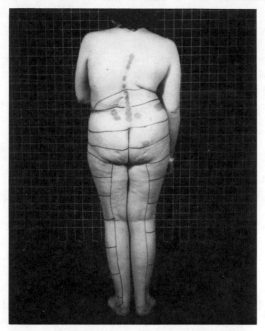

Figure 10.2. Pain pattern from a lumbar lesion.

back or leg pain on straight leg raising (SLR). If the hip flexes to
90° and the leg is pain-free, it is a negative SLR. A crossed SLR
may also be present — when the unaffected leg is raised, pain is
felt on the affected side of the back. If there is any doubt about
the reaction of the patient to SLR, testing should additionally be
undertaken in a different position, for example in sitting.

To test for a positive bowstring, the patient is in supine lying
with the affected leg flexed to 90° at the hip and the knee; the
ankle is supported by the examiner. Pressure is applied to the
popliteal fossa and pain is felt over the sciatic nerve, again
indicating nerve root irritation. Dural stretching can also be tested
by fixing the sternum with the palm of one hand, patient supine,
and passively flexing the cervical spine with the other hand,
approximating the chin to the chest. This may produce the
patient's low back pain. Likewise, SLR can be combined with
neck flexion as an initial test, and on re-examination to show
progress of treatment and less dural tethering.

Anterior tenderness of the lumbar spine can be palpated and will indicate disc inflammation. This may be quite acute and produce back and leg pain. To test for anterior tenderness the patient should be in relaxed crook lying. The examiner places the fingers at a perpendicular angle 2.5cm below the umbilicus and applies pressure gently to the lumbar spine. This will be approximately the lumbar 5–sacral 1 area. Pain may be experienced slightly higher or to the left or right of the lumbar spine. If the patient is not relaxed, ask him to breathe out deeply. While performing this examination watch for a full bladder, or tenderness due to abdominal symptoms or scars.

The social worker may be involved with some patients to assess whether their lifestyle is compatible with surgery and its effect postoperatively during their rehabilitation.

The ward nursing staff can provide valuable help in the assessment of the patient's disability. The following should be noted on the ward: walking time, sitting time, bed-rest positions, posture and pelvic tilt, exercise tolerance, pain tolerance and what tablets are needed during the day and at night, and the amount of sleep that the patient requires. A general opinion can be given as to the relationship between patient and staff, as well as patient to patient.

After the initial assessment of his pain and disability the patient may be put through a physiotherapy programme to see what improvement can be gained. Hydrotherapy is one of the easiest and most enjoyable forms of treatment; patients become more relaxed and confident, and exercise is easier due to the bouyancy, warmth and good feeling of the water.

Pre-operative physiotherapy

The aim of physiotherapy is to ensure that the patient is as fit as possible. This includes improving the chest expansion and vital capacity (which should be recorded in the notes), muscle power and general tone, circulation and endurance. Depending on the surgery, a brace or corset may be needed postoperatively. This can be measured and fitted initially and be ready to use when the patient is able to begin mobilising.

An explanation of the operation will be given by the doctor, and the physiotherapist will teach the necessary breathing and leg exercises to be done immediately postoperatively.

Following surgery, and once the patient is fully awake, chest expansion and foot and ankle movement are checked.

The postoperative management will differ according to the type of surgery

General aims of postoperative physiotherapy

The general aims of treatment are:

- To keep the chest clear and expanding fully.
- Maintenance of muscular power of the upper and lower limbs (but not pushing hip flexion if the patient has had a spinal fusion).
- Relief of pressure.
- Orientation, i.e. preparing for change of position from lying to sitting to standing by elevating the head end of the bed.

Preparation of the patient for getting out of bed includes strengthening exercises for the arms if crutches or sticks are to be required. A corset may be recommended and will be fitted by the physiotherapist who will ensure that the 'bones' are bent to the patient's lumbar spine. To put the corset on in bed the patient may bridge or roll.

There are two methods used for getting the patient out of bed:

- The patient is turned into a prone position and gets out of bed feet first, with the hips supported on the bed. He keeps a straight back and comes upright using his hip and back extensor muscles with arm support. The bed height is important with this method.
- The patient is turned onto the pain-free side; he slides his legs over the side of the bed and comes to sitting, pushing up with both arms, while the legs go down with gravity. The arms are then supporting the back in the sitting position. The patient moves forward, perching on the bed with his feet firmly on the floor. This method helps to overcome initial dizziness while the patient is still supported.

On the first time out of bed, re-education of balance with weight transference using arm support should be practised. If the patient is not dizzy a short walk helps regain confidence. The patient then progresses until he is independent with the help of one stick, out of doors if necessary. Depending on the surgery, sutures are removed 10–14 days after surgery, and metal clips after 5–7 days (occasionally alternate clips on consecutive days); steristrips may be left *in situ* at discharge. The patient is then discharged in a plaster-of-Paris jacket, plaster-of-Paris spica, polythene brace, corset, or with no support.

Depending on the type of operation, the immobilisation period and the following mobilising will vary. The end goal is a return to work *and* relief of pain. Building-up of confidence and reassurance is essential to achieve independence for the patient.

Patients should be advised on activities of daily living by the occupational therapist and the physiotherapist. Each patient is given a progressive exercise programme, which will include mostly isometric and relaxation exercises. A general advice form may be given. A follow-up appointment will be given to each patient at which time the spinal support — jacket or spica — may be removed and a mobilising programme started. Follow-up treatment will depend on the sugeon's wishes.

Specific physiotherapy

One-level anterior spinal fusion

Pre-operative Before a spinal fusion, the height, weight and vital capacity of the patient are recorded. He should be taught breathing exercises, general maintenance exercises for his arms, legs and trunk muscles and how to get out of bed following surgery. The orthotist will measure the patient for an anterior fastening polythene brace.

Postoperative

- Days 1—5: Breathing exercises and general maintenance exercises. Do not flex the legs beyond 90°.
- Day 5: Patient allowed up with brace to stand and sit for a short time, 30—60 minutes.
- Days 5—10: The patient starts to mobilise with the brace, plus walking aids, i.e. crutches or sticks, if necessary. The aids will be determined by muscle weakness of the arms and legs, e.g. a patient with a leg affected by poliomyelitis may require a caliper on the affected leg, and elbow crutches. (A good rule for the average patient without previous muscle weakness is to get up with two helpers supporting his arms on the first postoperative day, one helper and a stick the second day, then one stick, and thus the patient is independent on the third.) Ambulation is gradually progressed with gait re-education, relaxation, posture correction and starting to use stairs.
- Day 10 or after: The sutures are removed (clips will already have been removed) and the patient is discharged, in a brace, worn for approximately 6 months while up and about, but not while in bed.

The general aim is for the patient to be discharged without aids and to be completely independent. He should be able to manage stairs, walk 100 yards and be able to sit comfortably for an hour. A stick may be given for use outdoors. If he goes home in a jacket, it should be kept on for a minimum of 3 months, but often 6 months, and it may then be changed to a corset. Special out-patient physiotherapy is *not* needed — only arm and leg strengthening exercises and *no* back exercises (other than isometric contractions). At the clinic follow-up, 3 months after surgery, the patient will be advised to start swimming and do simple exercises, depending on the consolidation of the fusion.

Two-level anterior spinal fusion

Pre-operative This is the same as for the one-level fusion (*see* above).

Postoperative The patient is mobilised and allowed out of bed, wearing a brace, following a period of slightly longer bed rest, perhaps up to 2 weeks. The brace should be worn for 3—6 months.

Posterior fusion with bone graft only; posterior fusion with bone graft and metal instrumentation

Pre-operative As previously described; in addition 'log rolling' is taught, as follows. The patient must *never* move the shoulders first and hips later, thereby rotating the trunk. Head, shoulders, hips and legs, flexed to a comfortable position, should turn all in one easy movement. The position of crook lying makes the movement easier. If log rolling is to be done with straight legs, then on rolling to the right the left ankle should be crossed over the right ankle to facilitate rolling without trunk rotation.

Postoperative

- Days 1—5: General maintenance exercises are carried out in bed as previously described.
- Day 5: Up with brace to stand and sit well-supported for a short time; continue mobilising as for anterior surgery.

If the patient is kept in bed for 1—2 weeks, it is useful to use a tilt table; this will help with circulation, chest expansion, head control and arm and leg movement using gravity. The patient may be transferred to the tilt table either by lifting, via a sliding board, or by rolling from bed to table.

Anterior and posterior fusion 2−3 weeks
apart or simultaneous

Pre- and immediately postoperative regimes are as previously described. Strong analgesics, e.g. papaveretum (Omnopon) or morphine, are necessary for the first 3 days; they are given intramuscularly to facilitate movement and relaxation, thereby reducing chest and urinary complications. The drugs are then changed to mefenamic acid (Ponstan), or to what the patient was taking preoperatively, and gradually reduced. While the patient is being nursed in bed, urinals are used for both men and women: bedpans are *never* used, to prevent the back being strained; incontinence pads are used for bowel care.

Bed rest is maintained until the brace is fitted after the desired immobilisation. If the patient is kept in bed for a longer period, it is useful to use a tilt table; this will help with circulation, chest expansion, head control and arm and leg movement using gravity. The patient may be transferred to the tilt table by lifting, via a sliding board, or by rolling from bed to table.

Once the patient is allowed to mobilise on land, the routine is again the same as for anterior surgery. Walking, after having an anterior approach compared with a posterior approach, may be slower because of the pain felt at the donor site from which the iliac bone is taken.

If the patient is stiff, or has had a long period of bed rest preoperatively, hydrotherapy may be very beneficial. This would encourage free arm and leg movement and a more relaxed gait. Otherwise, the patient tends to develop a stiff walk, which in turn leads to a stiff, painful thoracic and cervical spine with limitation of movement at the neck and the shoulders.

He will be supplied with aids by the occupational therapist. These may include dressing aids, e.g. a long shoehorn, gadgets for pulling-up stockings or socks, or elasticated shoelaces; personal toilet aids, such as a long back scrubber for reaching down to the feet; and alterations in the house, including grab rails in the toilet, raised toilet seats or the installation of showers. Provision of walking aids and wheelchairs may be arranged by different members of the team, according to the procedure of the individual unit.

With the above procedure the patient may become depressed due to the wait between operations; the stress and longer stay in hospital seem to slow down rehabilitation. The combined procedure appears to have quicker results in pain-free mobility when compared with the staged operations.

Laminectomy; discectomy

Once any infusion lines and drains have been removed the patient may be mobilised. A corset may be fitted if ordered by the surgeon. Strong isometric exercises and active back extension and abdominal exercises should be taught. Initially, sciatic stretch can be done in side lying and then in supine. The patient is discharged when the sutures, clips or steristrips have been removed, and he often continues as an out-patient.

If the decompression is done with metal fixation, i.e. for spinal stenosis, especially in the younger patient, isometric exercises only are taught. The patient is discharged in a jacket or a corset.

Microdiscectomy

Pre-operative and immediate postoperative routines are as previously described:

- Day 1: The patient is up and mobilising in an elasticated corset, with or without a stick, as needed.
- Day 2 onward: Hip and knee flexion exercises are carried out standing, alternating sides, using a conveniently high chair. The patient is discharged in a corset, to be worn for 6 weeks while he is up and about. When clips or steristrips are removed and the skin is healed, the patient may begin hydrotherapy. Gradual weight-lifting is then added to the programme, and he can return to work in 6 weeks.

Percutaneous discectomy/Chymopapain injection

- Day 1: The patient is up in a corset and mobilising with a stick if needed.
- Day 2 onward: Hydrotherapy, which aims to reduce any muscle spasm in the spinal muscles following the procedure, reduces stiffness and any soreness. Leg pain should be minimal. Walking is encouraged with limited sitting, gradually progressing to weight lifting and return to light work at 6 weeks. Driving should be limited for the first 4 weeks. Discharge from day 2 onward, but hydrotherapy is beneficial as an inpatient if he does not have this facility at home.

Lifting and bending

Correct lifting should be taught to all back patients during their time in hospital, before and after surgery. Prior to surgery, patients will have managed at home, perhaps by making beds while kneeling or ironing for short periods seated. They will already have adapted to their activities of daily living. They would tend to leave lifting to other people in the household or move objects one by one instead. Low cupboards and high shelves have probably been avoided as much as possible.

After admission patients find they have a locker in which to put their possessions. Usually, the largest space for clothes is at the bottom, so they must bend to get at slippers for everyday use. Correct lifting is taught by putting the strongest leg behind the other leg and bending the knees as if genuflecting. The back remains straight. The knee of the back leg then rests on the floor so that the position is stable. The patient can then safely use his arms.

When lifting an object off the ground, the weight should be clasped tight to the chest. The stronger back leg then pushes up while the front leg controls the movement, the back remaining straight. If the legs are together, then bending down and rising is unstable and the patient is likely to wobble. If the object being lifted is an awkward shape or heavy, it should be lifted in stages. First from the floor to a table or chair placed directly in front of the object, and then carried away. Do not turn or twist while lifting.

Therefore, to bend the knees and keep the back straight is the ideal way to lift, but not all people have strong quadriceps or pain-free knees. In some cases, it may be easier to bend forwards from the hips on the stronger leg and counterbalance with the other leg extended. This is the way a patient in a single-hip spica would have to bend. If the arms are free they can be used for support.

When lifting light objects, such as clothing, it is much easier to use a 'helping-hand' aid with perhaps just a slight bend of the knees. Most of these aids have a magnet on them, so are useful for moving things like pins and other objects out of the way.

Complications following spinal surgery

Complications that may follow surgery include deep vein thrombosis, pulmonary embolus, paralytic ileus (this is most likely to occur immediately postoperatively when an abdominal approach has been used), associated stiffness of the thoracic spine, neck and shoulders, wound infection, neuralgia and graft site pain. If a plaster-of-Paris support is worn then particular care must be taken of the skin.

Fitting corsets, plaster jackets and hip spicas

Corsets

Corsets are used for supporting the abdominal and back muscles in patients with low back pain, e.g. the overweight patient with poor abdominal musculature; a patient who has been recumbent and is to be mobilised; or a person whose work demands lifting and where the extra support of a corset would be beneficial. They may also provide the support needed following some spinal surgery (*Figure 10.3*).

Corsets can be obtained 'ready-made' either by hip or waist measurement. They vary in type of material, depth, amount of support, e.g. bones or metal struts, and types of fastening. A corset, which is mostly made of elasticated fabric, can be pulled

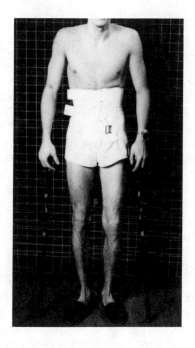

Figure 10.3. A well-fitting corset.

tight and thus give a very firm support. Some suppliers make male and female corsets which vary in hip measurement and so give a better fit. If the patient is not suitable for a ready-made corset, he will require one made to measure. This may be for coccygeal pain, when the corset needs extending to the gluteal fold; or after thoracic surgery, when the corset should be extended to the shoulders with shoulder straps.

The measurements required to make a corset are: waist; hips at the widest region; xiphisternal notch to groin anteriorly; and the lower border of the scapula to mid-buttock posteriorly, with arms by the side. The metal struts used in the corset should be exactly moulded to the contours of the patient and inserted. After a spinal fusion the back contour will very likely alter and should be checked if the corset was fitted prior to surgery. After spinal surgery, especially with posterior instrumentation, the lumbar curve flattens and so lengthens the spine; there is a similar effect on the thoracic curve. Some corsets have pads inserted for extra lumbar support and warmth.

Applying a spinal jacket (plaster-of-Paris or other material)

Jackets may be applied for patients with low back pain and /or following surgery. For a patient with stability of the spine post-operatively, the jacket can be applied with the patient standing; if necessary, traction may be given by application of a head-halter apparatus. This ensures a comfortable jacket with good correction.

If the spine is unstable in standing or following Harrington rod instrumentation for scoliosis, the patient must have a jacket applied before weight-bearing. It is then applied with the patient supported, in lying, on a special frame, such as the Abbot frame.

A three-point pressure for a plaster-of-Paris or other material jacket is required: anteriorly at the sternum or below the nipple curve; at the symphysis pubis; and posteriorly in the lumbar area. The plaster should be trimmed so that there is no pressure while sitting, arm movement is full and the patient independent for toilet purposes. Skin care is very important; cream and powders soften the skin and should not be used, instead, surgical spirit or soap and water should be used to clean and toughen the skin.

Depending on the material used, the plaster may be waterproof or not. Plaster-of-Paris is still the most useful because it conforms to the body shape, but it is not waterproof. Elasticated plaster-of-Paris (Orthoflex) used with Soroc is very durable and gives a good tight fit. Hexalite, Baycast and Scotch cast are other materials

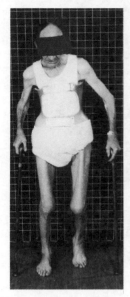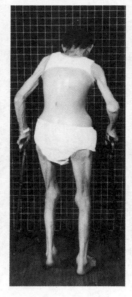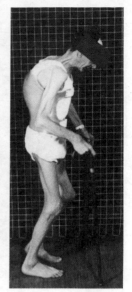

Figure 10.4. An adapted Boston brace: anterior, posterior and lateral views.

used; they are not so easy to mould or apply, but they are waterproof.

Braces made from polythene are very acceptable cosmetically and for comfort, as they can be tailor-made from a plaster-of-Paris cast. A cotton vest, preferably without side seams, should be worn between the brace and skin to add to the general comfort and for skin care.

Other orthoses may be used and/or adapted for the following conditions:

- *The Boston brace* is made of polythene for patients with scoliosis or low back pain. It is more convenient as the brace may be removed for toilet purposes and is made to measure from a plaster-of-Paris cast (*Figure 10.4*).
- *The Jewitt brace* is made of metal alloy and leather and is used for thoracic support, perhaps following surgery to stabilise the thoracic spine after removal of a hemivertebra.
- *The Milwaukee brace* is also made of metal alloy and leather and is used to support scoliosis patients with a curve suitable for splinting (*Figure 10.5*).

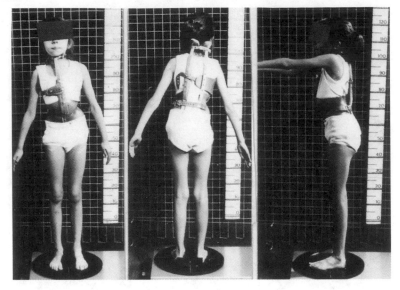

Figure 10.5. The Milwaukee brace: anterior, posterior and lateral views.

Braces may be specially lined with sheepskin as an extra safeguard if the skin is sensitive, as with a spina bifida patient who has undergone posterior spinal surgery.

References

Fairbank, J.C.T., Couper, J., Davies, J.B. and O'Brien, J.P. (1980). The Oswestry low back pain disability questionnaire. *Physiotherapy*, **66**, 271–273.
MacNab, I. (1979). *Backache*. Williams and Wilkins Co, Baltimore.
Schober, P. (1937). Lendenwirbelsäule und Kreuzschemeren. (The lumbar vertebral column and backache). *Müenchener Medizinische Wochenschrift*, **84**, 336.

Bibliography

Cailliet, R. (1981). *Low Back Pain Syndrome*, 3rd edition. F.A. Davis Co, Philadelphia.
Keim, H.A. and Kirkaly-Willis, W.H. (1980). *Clinical Symposia*, **32**, 6.
MacNab, I. (1979). *Backache*. Williams and Wilkins Co, Baltimore.
Maurice-Williams, R.S. (1981). *Spinal Degenerative Disease*. John Wright and Sons Limited, Bristol.

Moll, J. and Wright, V. (1980). Measurement of Spine Movement. In *The Lumbar Spine and Back Pain*, 2nd edition (Jayson, M. (ed.)). Pitman Books Ltd, London.

Onik, G. and Helms, C.A. (1988). *Automated Percutaneous Lumbar Discectomy*. Radiology Research and Education Foundation, University of California Printing Department.

White, A.A. and Panjabi, M.M. (1978). *Clinical Biomechanics of the Spine*. J.B. Lippincott Co, Philadelphia.

11 Spinal Deformities

S. Eisenstein and V. Draycott

Introduction

The management of spinal deformity is a means of returning to the origin of orthopaedic philosophy and the earliest traditions of orthopaedic practice, when the aim was simply the achievement of 'straight children'. In those early days almost all of orthopaedics was conducted by external splintage rather than by surgery, and exemplified by the many representations of Andry's crooked sapling lashed to a stake (*Figure 11.1*). The badges of orthopaedic professional associations around the world proudly display this emblem, which is the crest of the British Orthopaedic Association.

For the newcomer to spinal deformity practice, there is a new language to learn. This should not be regarded as a deterrence to novices, but as a challenge when joining a fascinating and rewarding clinical endeavour.

The deformities

Scoliosis

Scoliosis is a side-to-side 'S' bend in the spine, or part of an 'S' bend, produced by something more than just wilfully incorrect posture (*Figure 11.2*). The term implies an element of permanence because of some structural abnormality inherent in the spine.

In addition, there is almost always some degree of 'twist' in the spine (rotation), where several vertebrae are permanently turned about their vertical axis so that the spinous processes point into the concavity of a bend. This rotation can be the most important feature in a scoliotic spine, because it is the *rotation* of thoracic vertebrae which causes the unattractive rib hump. It is the *rib hump* (*Figure 11.3*) that we usually see as the obvious deformity in the patient, and not the curved spine. The ribs are attached to the sides of the vertebrae: as the vertebrae rotate, the ribs rise up on one side to form the hump (*Figure 11.4*).

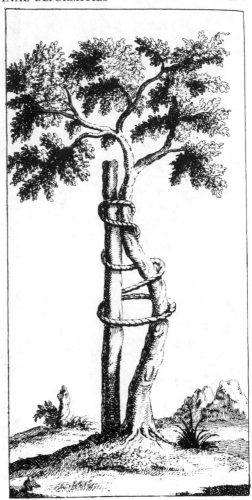

Figure 11.1. Andry's crooked sapling.

Kyphosis

Kyphosis is a smooth forward bend of the spine. The thoracic spine has a normal forward bend of up to 40°, so that in this instance the kyphosis is normal or physiological. In practice, the term implies an excessive forward bend (*Figure 11.5*), and may be found together with scoliosis, i.e. kyphoscoliosis.

Kyphos or gibbus

Kyphos (or gibbus) is a sharp forward bend (more like a kink than a bend in the spine) traditionally, but not exclusively, associated with the destruction caused by tuberculosis (*Figure 11.6*).

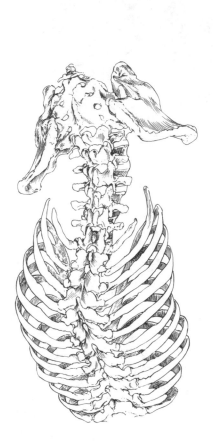

Figure 11.2. Scoliosis.

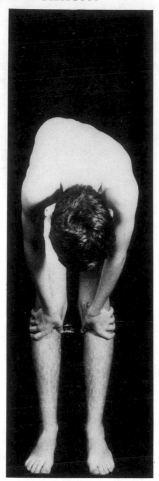

Figure 11.3. Rib hump of scoliosis.

Lordosis

The opposite of kyphosis, lordosis is a smooth backward bend of the spine, found as normal posture in the cervical and lumbar spines to balance the thoracic kyphosis, but again usually indicating an excessive or pathological condition. It may be found in the lumbar spine as compensation for a pathological kyphosis in the thoracic spine.

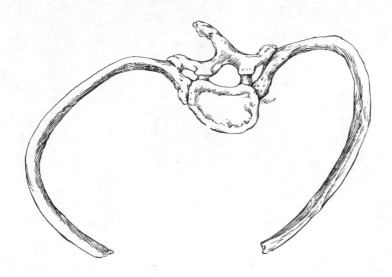

Figure 11.4. The ribs rise up on one side to form the hump.

Spondylolisthesis

Spondylolisthesis is a horizontal shift of one vertebra in relation to another, as if a vertebra slides along the one below it, in any direction, to take up a new abnormal, but permanent, position (*Figure 11.7*). As it happens, the direction of shift is usually forward. (Spondylolisthesis must not be confused with similar-sounding words, such as spondylosis – degenerative changes in the spine – and spondylolysis – an ununited fracture of the lamina of a vertebra.)

Nature of the deformity

It is sometimes held that spine deformities are 'only cosmetic', as if they did not matter much because they are usually painless and no longer associated with a diminished life expectancy. The point not to be missed is that there is a degree of cosmetic deformity which is so pervasive as to go well beyond a question of mere

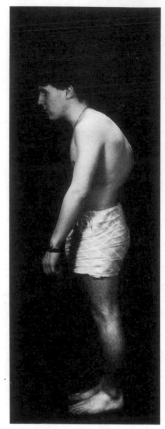

Figure 11.5. Kyphosis thoracic spine: an excessive forward bend.

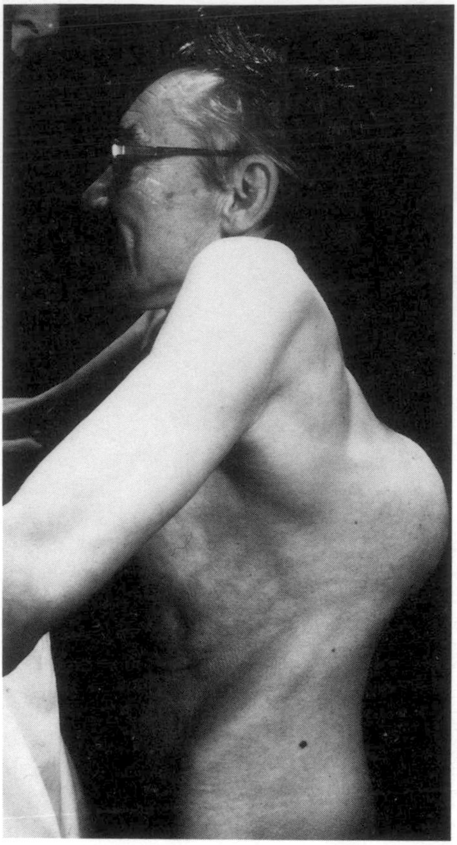

Figure 11.6. Gibbus in spine tuberculosis.

vanity, such as may be posed by a small mole on the face. Scoliosis is just such a deformity. The whole body shape may be altered to a degree which is simply unacceptable to the patient and which materially affects patients' perception of their place in society. Moreover, the deformity is very likely to be progressive and may indeed cause disabling pain later in adult life.

The causes

Scoliosis
By far the most common deformity that requires treatment is

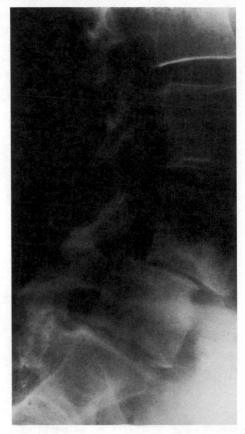

Figure 11.7. Spondylolisthesis.

scoliosis. There are several types of scoliosis, classified according their origin, and each type needs a different therapeutic programme.

Idiopathic (or 'cause not known') This is the most common diagnosis in scoliosis, affecting adolescent girls and producing a thoracic curve with a right-sided rib hump. The spine is normal at birth but deforms with rapid growth for reasons not yet understood. Because the curve is associated with a loss of the normal thoracic kyphosis, the deformity is more correctly termed 'lordoscoliosis'. Despite the term 'idiopathic', we know that there is frequently some genetic influence, so this type of scoliosis tends to run in families.

Idiopathic scoliosis can appear also in infants and juveniles, less commonly, but when it does it presents major problems in management because the deformity starts so early in life.

Congenital The spine is deformed from the start of its development in the foetus, either through failure of the vertebrae to form symmetrically, or through failure of the vertebrae to separate completely from each other (*Figure 11.8*). The worst of these deformities are found when the two types of failure occur together. This type of scoliosis presents the greatest treatment challenge of all scoliosis.

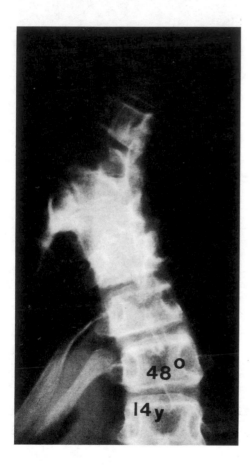

Figure 11.8. Congenital scoliosis: note the wedge shape at the apex of the curve.

Neuromuscular (or 'paralytic') The spinal column may be normal at birth, but one of many paralysing conditions will affect the stabilising muscles of the spine, and scoliosis develops. These paralysing conditions are spinal injury, cerebral palsy, poliomyelitis, and the muscular dystrophies (especially Duchenne muscular dystrophy in boys, *Figure 11.9*). The paralysis of myelo-

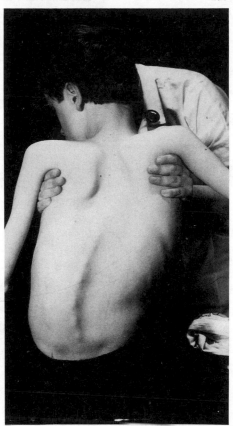

*Figure 11.9. Paralytic
scoliosis of muscular
dystrophy.*

dysplasia will be present from birth and may be compounded by
the presence of congenital abnormalities, as described above.

Other causes This is a disparate group of rarer causes, such as
the scoliosis secondary to spinal tumours, acute back strains, disc
prolapse, and hysteria.

Kyphosis
Kyphosis is far less common than scoliosis, and successful treatment can be more difficult to achieve.

Juvenile osteochondrosis (Scheurmann's disease) is a mysterious
condition and probably the most common cause of mild-to-
moderate kyphosis. The end-plates of the thoracic vertebrae of
teenage boys are damaged in some way that produces anterior
wedging of the vertebral bodies and results in the 'round shoulders'

despised by parents. Patients often complain of low back pain in a compensatory lumbar lordosis.

Infection, in the form of tubercular destruction of one or more adjacent thoracic vertebrae, is probably the most common cause of a pathological kyphosis in Third World countries. The deformity is more likely to be a gibbus, which can be so acutely angled to the spinal cord that it produces paralysis (*Figure 11.10*).

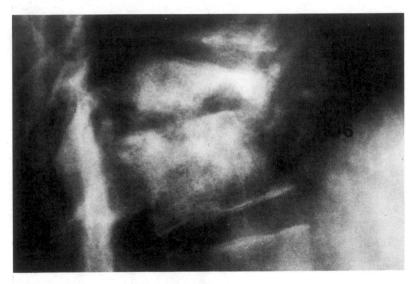

Figure 11.10. Tuberculosis kyphosis (gibbus): lateral X-ray.

Spinal injury is a potent cause of kyphosis, following a crush of one or more vertebral bodies, and frequently associated with paralysis through direct damage to the spinal cord at the level of the crush (*Figure 11.11*).

Biochemical changes in the bone (osteoporosis), associated with the menopause, dietary inadequacy, and alcoholism, are the most important cause of kyphosis in adults. The bone of the vertebral body collapses under the normal loads of daily living. The pain produced in this condition is severe and almost incurable.

Congenital abnormalities occur less frequently in the sagittal plane, but they can cause a severe and progressive kyphosis with a likelihood of producing paralysis if untreated.

Rheumatoid disease of the spine, as exemplified in ankylosing spondylitis, can produce a kyphosis and devastating disability in young adults (*Figure 11.12*).

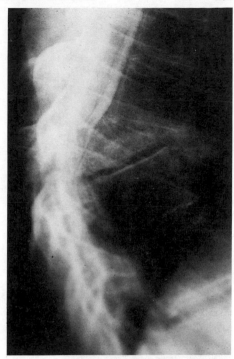

Figure 11.11. Spinal injury: A fall from scaffolding crushed one vertebra to form a sharp wedge.

Idiopathic kyphosis is rare and is probably the forward-deforming conterpart of idiopathic lordoscoliosis. The thoracic vertebrae are all very slightly wedged, as are the disc spaces between them.

Degenerative changes of ageing in the discs of the cervical and lumbar spine are frequently associated with a relative kyphosis (loss of lordosis) in these areas, producing the typical stoop of the elderly.

Lordosis

Lordosis is almost always a deformity to compensate for a primary deformity (usually kyphosis) elsewhere in the spine. It is also the logical response to fixed flexion deformities at the hip. On the other hand, lordosis in the thoracic spine is probably the primary cause of idiopathic scoliosis.

Spondylolisthesis

Spondylolisthesis may result from degenerative disc disease (spondylosis), especially at L4/5 in obese women in middle life; or from an ununited fracture of the lamina between the facet joints (pars interarticularis); or from a weakness in the bone of

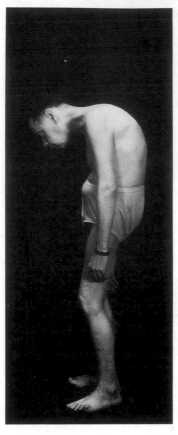

Figure 11.12. Ankylosing spondylitis.

the lamina (dysplasia) which allows the lamina to stretch as it grows so that the vertebral body slides forward; or from a violent spinal injury which may disrupt the neural arch so severely that the vertebral body is free to slide forward.

Degenerative disc disease may cause a vertebra to slide backward (retrolisthesis), and scoliosis in the lumbar spine of adults is sometimes associated with a rotation slide to one side.

Spondylolisthesis is almost always in the lower lumbar spine, but is not always painful: it may be discovered quite by chance during X-ray investigations for non-spinal problems.

Diagnosis and assessment

On the basis that scoliosis is by far the most common and most important deformity with which we deal, the remainder of this chapter is devoted largely to it.

Scoliosis is a problem not just because it exists, but also because it tends to be progressive. The greater problem is that advanced scoliosis is very much more difficult to treat well than is mild or moderate scoliosis, but we have no certain way of knowing which curve will progress nor how far it will progress. The partial solution to this problem is a combination of early diagnosis and continued vigilance. Once progression is confirmed, a scheme of treatment can be planned for the individual patient.

Early detection was only partially successful when left to parents and teachers, because it is difficult to notice subtle changes in posture in someone who is seen casually on a daily basis. A formal programme of clinical examination at school (school screening) was expected to solve this problem, but proved too expensive for the number of cases discovered.

The clinical examination is simple in the extreme and requires merely the inspection of the back of a child bending forward, looking for a rib hump and other asymmetries of the trunk. Greater general awareness of scoliosis has increased in recent years, but the problem of achieving early detection has not yet been solved.

X-ray examination of the spinal curvature is the next step, when surgical consultant staff are satisfied that the deformity warrants a more accurate assessment. On the erect (standing) antero-posterior (A-P) view, a standard method of measurement of the side-to-side bend (Cobb method) and the rotation (Pedriolle method) allows comparison with similar measurements made at intervals of months or years.

The Cobb method uses an ordinary protractor to measure, in degrees, from the top to the bottom of any one curve, for as many curves as necessary on one X-ray. The Pedriolle method uses a specially designed protractor to measure the rotation in degrees.

The erect A-P view allows an assessment of the extent to which the spine is out of balance, that is, by how many centimetres the cervicothoracic junction is shifted off to one side of the lumbo-sacral junction (*Figure 11.13*). This information is of particular importance when considering the possible need for surgery.

These X-rays should also show the iliac crests so that a rough assessment can be made of the patient's skeletal maturity according to the technique of Risser: in general, spinal curvatures will cease or slow in their progression as skeletal maturity is reached (*Figure 11.14*).

The lateral view is used to assess the extent of lordosis or kyphosis.

The rib hump

The rib hump is measured by one of a number of devices available for this purpose, either directly on the patient's back or by one of

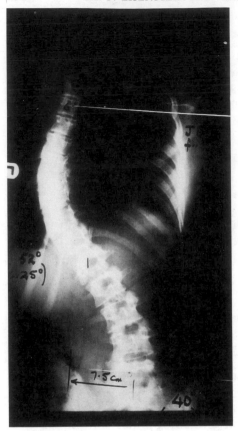

Figure 11.13. Scoliosis with out-of-balance curve in a 13-year-old girl.

the imaging techniques, such as Moire screen photography or computerised contour mapping (Isis). Clinical photography remains an important means of recording the cosmetic appearance of the whole spinal deformity.

Further examinations
Further examinations depend on circumstances: if the patient with idiopathic scoliosis is being considered for surgical treatment, antero-posterior X-rays will be needed, to show the spine bent as far as possible to left and right in order to assess curve stiffness. If congenital scoliosis is discovered, there is always the suspicion that there may be other abnormalities in the spinal canal (split cord or diastematomyelia), kidneys, and heart. Myelography, computerised tomography, intravenous pyelography, and cardiac

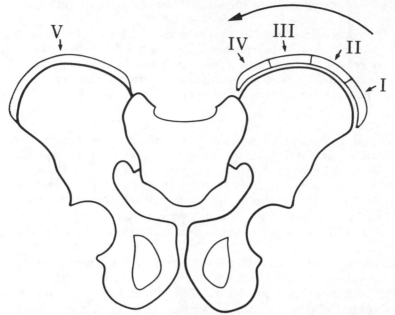

Figure 11.14. Risser measurement of skeletal maturity graded I–IV. When the iliac apophysis fuses with the iliac blade, this is called grade V.

function tests are necessary to assess patients with congenital scoliosis, especially if surgery is being planned.

Treatment

Conservative

For many years there was a rule of thumb whereby idiopathic scoliosis was left untreated if the Cobb measurement was less than 20°; treated conservatively in a Milwaukee brace if it was between 20°–40°; and treated by spinal fusion operation if it was beyond 40°.

This rule remains current in many centres, but variations to it are appearing in some places: bracing has been abandoned, not only because it is unacceptable to self-conscious teenagers, but also because recent studies have raised serious doubts as to its efficacy.

The non-bracing philosophy relies on the scoliosis to halt its progression spontaneously or to prove its need for surgical treatment by demonstrating progression beyond 35°–45°.

There was a time when it was thought that certain exercises had some influence on the deformity, but this has been disproved:

the only exercises now prescribed are as part of the bracing regimen.

Electrical stimulation of the muscles on the convexity of the curved spine, at night, has been used as a substitute for bracing mild curves because it is more acceptable to patients. There is evidence that electrical stimulation is as effective as bracing, but it remains a controversial treatment.

Surgical

The decision to opt for surgery is based on three factors: *curve dynamics*, *curve severity*, and the *skeletal maturity* of the patient.

Dynamics consist of curve progression, curve stiffness, and spinal balance. Severity relates to the degrees of bend and rotation. Skeletal maturity describes the level of development of the bony spine, irrespective of the patient's chronological age.

A decision in favour of surgical treatment is likely to be made:

- For a patient with a progressive curve which corrects but little on side-bending and shows a definite list to one side.
- Where the curve is greater than 35° with an unsightly rib hump.
- Where the patient has a Risser sign of III or less and has not yet reached the menarche (*Figure 11.15*).

The *purpose* of surgery is not only to halt progression of the curve, but to achieve some correction of the curve and its rib hump as well.

All the operations involve a spinal fusion (bone graft) of some sort, to slow the growth of the spine and to stabilise it in that position. All modern operations involve the insertion of some system of metal fixation to stabilise the spine until fusion is complete: all these systems provide some correction as well.

In *congenital* scoliosis the purpose of surgery is to set the stage for future growth to halt the progression of the deformity, and possibly to reverse it, but striving too much to achieve correction during the operation can be dangerous for the spinal cord.

The *operations* most commonly performed (together with bone grafting to the spine) are:

- *Harrington posterior instrumentation*: A rod supports hooks at either end so as to spread open the concavity of the curve (distraction); this is sometimes combined with a compression system on the convex side.
- *Harrington–Luque technique*: As above, but sublaminar wire loops along the concavity are used to help pull the curved spine towards the straight rod (thus most closely recreating the old orthopaedic symbol of Andry's deformed tree, *Figure 11.16*).

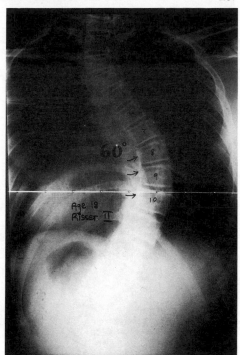

Figure 11.15. Severe and stiff scoliosis: here it is progressive and needing surgery.

- *Zielke method*: An anterior instrumentation through the chest (and through the diaphragm into the abdomen, if necessary) which places screws transversely through the vertebral bodies, supporting a rod passing through the screw heads. This technique is ideal for curves with an apex at the thoraco-lumbar junction. It is capable of an impressive degree of derotation of the spine. The Webb–Morley system is a British version of this German system.
- *Cotrel–Dubousset*: This technique is applied posteriorly and is a major advance on the Harrington system, using double rods and multiple hooks or screws; it is also capable of impressive derotation (*Figures 11.17(a)* and *11.17(b)*).
- *Luque segmental sublaminar system*: A posterior procedure, ideal for neuromuscular scoliosis, where most of the thoracic and lumbar spine has to be fused in one operation. Double rods are secured to the spine by wires looped around the laminae (*Figure 11.18*).

Two other procedures are frequently used in conjunction with the above operations, usually under the same anaesthetic: anterior

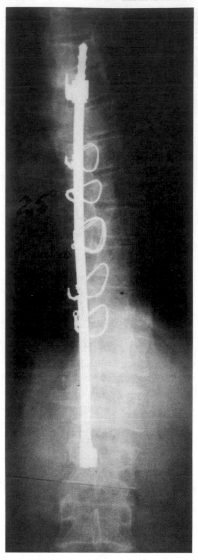

Figure 11.16. Harrington–Luque technique (same patient as in Figure 11.15*).*

discectomy, at several levels, most often through a thoracotomy, to loosen a particularly stiff curve; and excision of part of several ribs in the rib hump (costoplasty) to improve that factor of greatest importance to the patient, the cosmetic appearance.

In *congenital scoliosis* it is sometimes necessary to remove all of a 'wedge' vertebra, by a combined anterior and posterior approach.

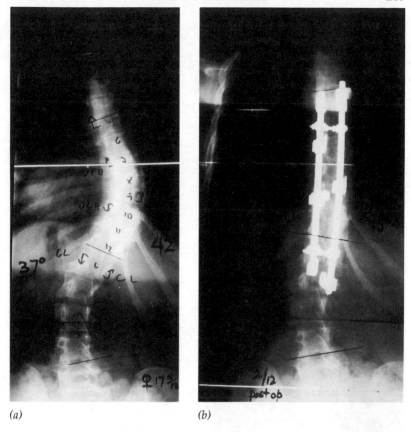

(a)   (b)

Figure 11.17. Scoliosis before surgery (a) and after surgery (b).

At other times, it is necessary to destroy the vertebral body end-plates along the convexity of a curve (epiphyseodesis), in order to slow down the deforming growth on that side.

In the presence of a stiff, severe, and disabling *kyphosis*, such as in juvenile osteochondrosis, it is necessary to perform major anterior and posterior surgery, strutting the spine front and back. The Gardner Distractor is useful here, inserted into the thoracic spine through the chest. In ankylosing spondylitis it is too dangerous to operate on the thoracic spine for fear of damage to the spinal cord. A combination of osteotomies (cutting across vertebrae) in the lumbar spine and cervico-thoracic junction will produce gratifying improvements in posture and the ability to see ahead again.

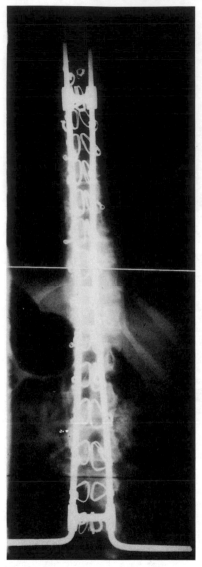

Figure 11.18. Luque technique for scoliosis with paralysis.

The role of the physiotherapist

Traditionally, physiotherapists have been intimately involved in scoliosis bracing programmes. With the reduction in bracing and the realisation that exercises alone could not alter the course of scoliosis, it was thought that there would be little part for physiotherapists to play in the management of this and other deformities.

The fact of the matter is that physiotherapists are *more* intensely involved than ever before, because of the greater complexity and hazard of the newer operations for deformity.

Since many of these operations require entry into the chest and through the diaphragm, the physiotherapist is required not only to prepare the patient for surgery with breathing exercises, but also to provide the basic lung function assessments (*Figure 11.19*). In this pre-operative phase, the physiotherapist has a further important role as confidant, giving reassurance and encouragement.

In the immediate postoperative period, the physiotherapist is of extreme importance in restoring a clear airway, encouraging breathing in spite of pain, supervising the chest drain care, and helping the return of joint movement in all limbs (*Figure 11.20*).

The role of the physiotherapist continues uninterrupted throughout the rest of the rehabilitation, encouraging an early resumption of sitting, standing, and walking. A cast is usually required prior to discharge, for protection of the whole operation in the critical early weeks of rehabilitation; in many centres the physiotherapist is the best-placed person to apply the cast (*Figure 11.21*).

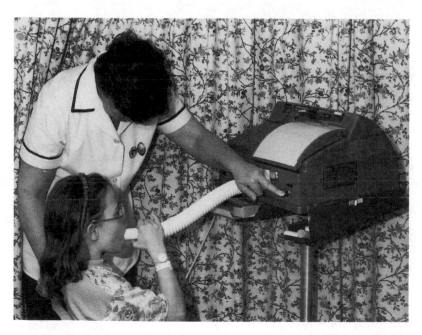

Figure 11.19. Physiotherapist conducting lung function assessments.

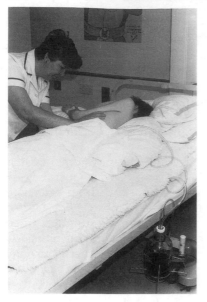
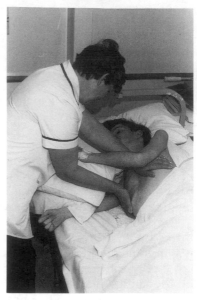

Figure 11.20. Physiotherapist with patient post-operatively.

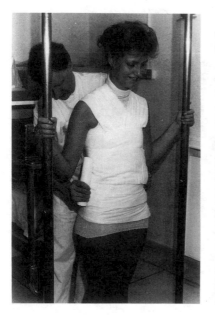
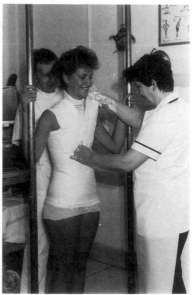

Figure 11.21. Physiotherapist applying post-operative cast.

The cast is usually removed after 6 weeks and a polythene brace applied. It is the physiotherapist who should assess the adequacy of the brace and the patient's function in it, over a period of days. Repeat rib-hump measurements are taken, as are clinical photography and X-rays, for comparison with the pre-operative situation.

12 Rheumatoid Arthritis and Juvenile Chronic Arthritis

R.C. Butler and M. Kerr

Rheumatoid arthritis

Rheumatoid arthritis (RA) is a common disease which affects some 2% of the population, i.e. more than one million people in the UK. Women are affected more frequently than men in a ratio of about 3:1. A high proportion of cases present between the ages of 25 and 55; it is very rare before the age of 5 years, but can present throughout life to extreme old age. It occurs worldwide, but some populations, e.g. Yakima Indians, appear to be particularly susceptible. The importance of environmental factors is illustrated by the observation that the prevalence of RA is more common in urban than rural South African blacks.

Diagnosis

The diagnosis is made on clinical grounds. RA is typically a symmetrical arthropathy with painful, tender and swollen joints, morning stiffness, erosive changes on X-ray and rheumatoid factor in the serum. Rheumatoid nodules and other extra-articular features may be present. The criteria of the American Rheumatism Association (Arnett *et al.*, 1988) are often used for clinical studies; four of the seven criteria have to be satisfied:

- Morning stiffness in and around joints for at least an hour.
- Soft tissue swelling, observed by physician, of at least 3/14 joint groups (right or left): metacarpophalangeal (MCP), proximal interphalangeal (PIP), wrist, elbow, knee, ankle, metatarsophalangeal (MTP).
- Soft tissue swelling in a hand joint (MCP, PIP or wrist).
- Symmetrical joint swelling in one joint area.
- Rheumatoid nodule.
- Rheumatoid factor in serum.
- X-ray changes in wrist and/or hand: erosions or juxta-articular osteoporosis.

Rheumatoid factor is an autoantibody directed against the immunoglobulin IgG. It is found in the serum of some 80% of patients with RA, but it is also found in some patients with systemic lupus erythematosus (SLE), Sjögren's syndrome, scleroderma and other rheumatic disorders so its presence cannot be regarded as a diagnostic test. In addition, it can be found in some healthy persons: fewer than 5% of young adults, but over 10% of the very elderly. Healthy people with a positive test for rheumatoid factor are at increased risk of developing RA subsequently; the higher the titre of rheumatoid factor, the greater the risk.

The earliest radiological features of RA are soft tissue swelling and peri-articular osteoporosis (*Figure 12.1*). Later, typical erosions develop at the margins of articular cartilage and diffuse destruction of cartilage leads to joint space narrowing. Later still, joints become subluxed and, in advanced disease, bony ankylosis may occur, especially in carpal bones (*Figure 12.1*).

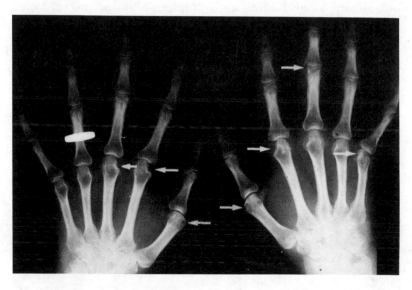

Figure 12.1. Radiograph showing erosive changes in the hands.

Aetiology

The cause of RA is not known. Genetic factors are important, since up to 10% of patients with RA report a first-degree relative with the condition. The tissue type HLA−DR4 is present in some 70% of patients with RA, in comparison with only 25% of the population at large. Recent work indicates that susceptibility is associated with a particular amino acid sequence shared by some sub-types of DR4 and other HLA molecules, including DR1, but current evidence suggests that additional genetic factors are involved. It seems likely that a variety of as yet unidentified viral and/or other micro-organisms may trigger the disease. In susceptible individuals these agents provoke a damaging immune reaction, which leads to synovial inflammation and joint damage. Sometimes RA develops after profound psychological or physical trauma, but psychological factors do not appear to be sufficient by themselves to account for the onset of disease.

Pathology

Normal synovium consists of loose connective tissue with a thin lining of synovial cells. In RA the blood vessels proliferate, dilate and become congested and the tissue oedematous; the lining layer is greatly increased in thickness and the surface may become necrotic. The synovium is infiltrated by large numbers of chronic inflammatory cells (lymphocytes, plasma cells and macrophages), which take part in a vigorous immune response. Other potentially noxious substances, including enzymes, immune complexes, free radicals, cytokines and complement are present in the rheumatoid joint (Harris, 1990). Numerous polymorphonuclear leucocytes accumulate in synovial fluid, which often contains fibrinous clots. At the interface between cartilage and synovium a mass of granulation tissue (new blood vessels and fibroblasts with an inflammatory cell infiltrate) forms: this is known as pannus. It gradually

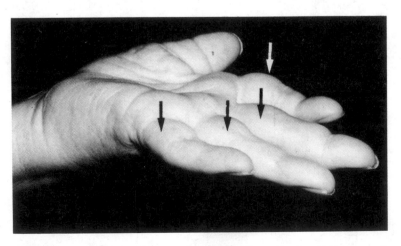

Figure 12.2. Flexor tendon sheath distension due to RA.

erodes the adjacent cartilage and subjacent bone and so gives rise to the joint-space narrowing and characteristic erosions seen on X-ray. The inflammatory process also damages ligaments around the joint, which leads to joint instability and deformity and may cause tendon rupture. Synovial tissue lines bursae and tendon sheaths and these may be similarly involved (*Figure 12.2*).

Rheumatoid nodules typically occur in fibrous connective tissue, such as that overlying the elbow. They consist of a central necrotic area (fibrinoid necrosis) with a rim of histiocytes arranged radially in palisades and a surrounding infiltrate of chronic inflammatory cells. Rheumatoid vasculitis may affect arteries and venules. The vessel walls are infiltrated by lymphocytes and polymorphonuclear leucocytes and may become necrotic, while the lumen is occluded by thickening of the intima and secondary thrombosis. The precise cause is uncertain, but immunoglobulin and/or complement can often be identified in the walls of affected vessels and immune complexes may well be responsible.

Clinical features

Onset is variable; it can develop overnight or over a few days or insidiously over several months. There may be polyarticular arthritis from the onset or increasing numbers of joints may be involved over a period of weeks or months. Some patients present with the syndrome of palindromic rheumatism, in which there is severe acute arthritis of one or two joints, such as the wrist or shoulder, which resolves completely in 24—48 hours. After recurrent attacks over a variable period of time the disease evolves in some patients into typical RA. The mode of onset appears to be a poor guide to long-term prognosis. Systemic features, such as malaise, fatigue, anorexia with some weight loss, a low-grade fever and mild depression, are all common.

Any synovial joint may be affected, but the pattern of involvement varies in individual patients. The hands (MCP and PIP joints), wrists and MTP joints are usually involved early and symmetrical involvement is typical. The knee, shoulder, hip and, less commonly, ankle and elbow may be involved later. The cervical spine is affected fairly frequently during the course of the disease, but other regions of the spine are usually spared. Affected joints are swollen due to a combination of synovial proliferation and joint effusion. They are painful, tender and stiff, with consequent impairment of function, and may be hot, but overlying erythema is uncommon. Morning stiffness is usual, but may occur in other forms of inflammatory arthritis. It is probably caused by accumulation of oedema in inflamed joints during sleep; this is gradually dispersed with movement. Wasting of muscles is often seen around affected joints. In advanced disease, damage to joints, ligaments and tendons may give rise to deformities, often fixed, or instability.

Course and prognosis

The course of RA is variable and difficult to predict at onset. Older patients tend to do worse than younger ones and women worse than men; patients from low socio-economic groups tend to do badly. Circulating rheumatoid factor, especially in high titre, persistently raised erythrocyte sedimentation rate (ESR), plasma viscosity or serum C-reactive protein (CRP) and the early appearance of erosive disease all tend to be associated with severe disease. Some patients (perhaps 10–20%) have an acute episode followed by prolonged remission. Others (some 30–40%) have an intermittent course with recurrent episodes of arthritis, but intervening periods free of active arthritis. The remainder have progressive disease and, although the majority of these will have periods of relatively quiescent disease between exacerbations, the general trend is of progressive disabling disease. Many patients with mild RA never attend hospital, but of those who do at least 50% end up with severe disability despite treatment after 20 years.

RA is not fatal but the average life expectancy is reduced somewhat: perhaps by five years. The cause of death is variable and resembles that in the general population, but infection is quite often involved. Treatment in the form of steroids and non-steroidal anti-inflammatory drugs (NSAID) undoubtedly contributes to death in some cases.

Individual joints

Cervical spine Compression of cervical roots may cause root symptoms and signs, including severe pain radiating up over the occiput. Kinking of the vertebral artery may give rise to symptoms of vertebrobasilar insufficiency. Rheumatoid involvement often leads to subluxation in an antero-posterior plane, most often at the atlanto-axial level, but sometimes subaxial (*Figure 12.3*). If lateral radiographs of the neck are not taken in both flexion and extension such instability may be missed. These problems can cause cervical myelopathy with pressure on the cervical cord causing pyramidal and/or posterior column signs and, in severe cases, tetraplegia. Occasionally, there is rostral migration of the odontoid peg through the foramen magnum with compression of the medulla and even greater risk of neurological damage. Fortunately, cervical myelopathy occurs in only some 1% of hospital patients with RA, even though atlanto-axial instability can be demonstrated in some 30%. Imaging of the cervical spine has

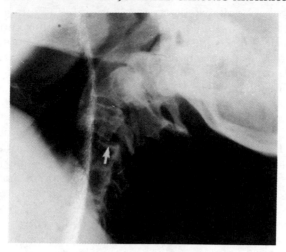

Figure 12.3. Radiograph showing subaxial subluxation in RA.

been greatly improved by CT scanning with cervical radiculography and the non-invasive technique of magnetic resonance imaging (MRI).

Patients are at particular risk during intubation for anaesthesia, if they suffer a whiplash injury or if subjected to manipulation of the neck. A collar will often help root symptoms, but decompression and cervical fusion will be required if there is evidence of cord compression.

Temporomandibular joint Apart from pain, difficulty in mouth opening can make it difficult for the patient to eat. Involvement of these joints is fairly common but tends to be episodic; a local steroid injection may help.

Cricoarytenoid joint Occasionally this joint is involved and hoarseness results. It is important to exclude alternative causes of hoarseness, such as laryngeal tumours. Stridor may develop and a tracheostomy be required, but this is extremely rare.

Shoulder and shoulder-girdle Involvement of the gleno-humeral joint is very common and rotator-cuff lesions are often superimposed. The acromio-clavicular and sterno-clavicular joints may also be affected. Shoulder–girdle dysfunction often leads to difficulties in self-care, including dressing, feeding and personal hygiene, especially if the elbows are also affected.

Elbow Lack of full extension is common, but minor degrees give rise to little disability, whereas inability to flex can make it very difficult for the patient to feed himself or comb his hair. Inability to rotate the elbow can also give rise to considerable functional impairment. Entrapment of the ulnar nerve at the elbow is not uncommon.

Wrists Pain in the wrist impairs function in the whole hand. Carpal tunnel syndrome is common and may be a presenting feature of RA; it can often be relieved by use of a splint and local steroid injection, but surgical decompression may be required. Dorsal subluxation of the ulnar styloid is painful and, when associated with synovial proliferation, often leads to rupture of the extensor tendons to the little, ring and sometimes middle fingers. Dorsal tenosynovitis overlying the carpus may also lead to tendon rupture. Surgical repair is required for tendon rupture; decompression and ulnar styloidectomy may prevent recurrence. In late or neglected disease there is often palmar subluxation of the wrist which adds to disability. Radial deformity of the wrist appears to contribute to the development of ulnar drift of the fingers (*Figure 12.4*).

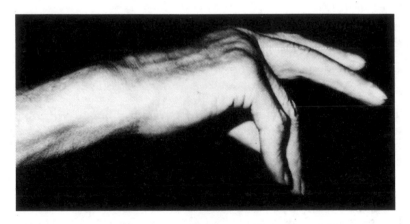

Figure 12.4. Ruptured extensor tendons to the fourth and fifth fingers related to the subluxed lower end of ulna.

Hands Arthritis of MCP and PIP joints (*Figure 12.5*) is usual and often a presenting feature, and is frequently accompanied by tenosynovitis of the long finger flexors (*Figure 12.2*). Involvement of distal interphalangeal (DIP) joints is relatively uncommon.

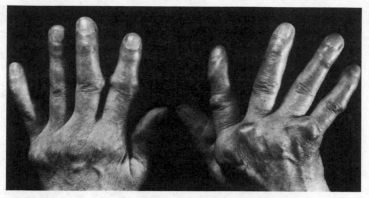

Figure 12.5. RA of the hands showing (a) ulnar deviation at the metacarpophalangeal level of the right hand; (b) soft tissue swelling of the metacarpophalangeal joints; (c) nodule formation; (d) vascular lesions of the nail beds.

Inability to close the fingers fully with weakness of grip leads to functional impairment; inability to undo buttons or jars and to turn taps are common complaints. Ulnar deviation of the fingers is a typical deformity but not invariable; preventive splints and joint protection advice are given with a view to lessening the risk of this deformity.

Finger deformities are common in RA. The swan-neck deformity (*Figure 12.6(b)*) consists of hyperextension at the PIP caused by shortening of the intrinsic muscles with compensatory flexion at the DIP joint. At first this can be overcome, but the deformity may become fixed with inability to close the fingers. A boutonnière (button-hole) deformity consists of flexion at the PIP and hyperextension at the DIP joint (*Figure 12.6(a)*); it results from damage to the central slip of the extensor hood over the PIP joint with lateral and forward slip of the lateral bands, so that they flex the PIP joint. A Z-shaped (Nalebuff) deformity of the thumb is characterised by flexion of the MCP joint and hyperextension of the interphalangeal joint of the thumb.

Hips   Hip involvement eventually occurs in some 40% of patients, but is rarely a presenting feature. It leads to difficulty in walking, climbing stairs, transfers, putting on shoes, etc. Sexual difficulties are also common but rarely vocalised. Pain from the hip is often referred to the thigh and knee and may be experienced solely in the knee.

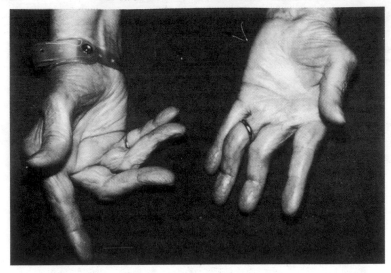

Figure 12.6. RA of the hands showing: right hand, *button-hole deformities (boutonnière's) and* left hand, *swan-neck deformities.*

Knees   Knee swelling due to effusion and synovial proliferation is common throughout the course of the disease and often leads to limitation of both flexion and extension. Later instability may result from damage to collateral ligaments, valgus deformity being more common than varus (*Figure 12.7*).

Popliteal (Baker's) cysts result from accumulation of fluid within a popliteal extension of the knee joint; the fluid tracks posteriorly, but cannot return due to a ball−valve type mechanism. The cysts can become large and tense (*Figure 12.8*), cause discomfort and difficulty in flexing the knee and may rupture. Release of synovial fluid into the calf causes acute pain and inflammation, with clinical features indistinguishable from those of a deep vein thrombosis. Only arthropraphy (*Figure 12.9*) and venography can clarify the clinical problem accurately.

Hindfeet   The subtalar joint is more often involved than the ankle itself and pain when walking on uneven ground is a common complaint. Damage to the ligaments which bind the tibia and fibula to the talus leads to instability of the hindfoot and a valgus deformity commonly results (*Figure 12.7*). Valgus deformities of the ankle and knee are often seen together and each will aggravate the other and lead to worsening problems. Surgical treatment of the hindfoot is much less satisfactory than for the hip or knee

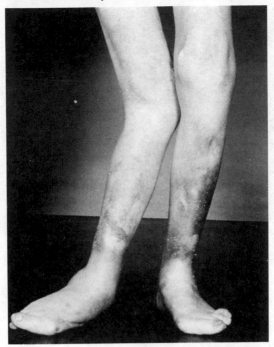

Figure 12.7. RA of the knees showing the wind-swept deformity. Note also the valgus position of the right foot. Skin changes on the shins are due to long-term corticosteroid therapy.

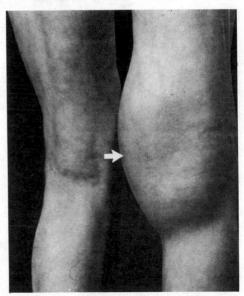

Figure 12.8. RA affecting the knee showing a Baker's cyst.

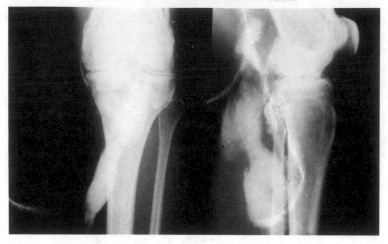

Figure 12.9. Arthrogram of the left knee joint showing a ruptured Baker's cyst (A-P and lateral views).

and early use of splints to stabilise the hindfoot may prevent subsequent problems.

Metatarsophalangeal joints   These joints are often involved early in the course of the disease and radiographs may show changes in the absence of forefoot symptoms. The patient typically complains of the sensation that they are walking on pebbles. Subluxation is common with hyperextension of the MTP joint and secondary flexion of the toes. This results in increased depth of the forefoot with difficulty in finding suitable shoes, callosities under the heads of the metatarsals and abrasion of the toes. Difficulties with footwear are compounded by an increased width of the forefoot and hallux valgus. Metatarsal insoles and/or special footwear can greatly improve walking capacity.

Assessment of disease activity
The activity of RA varies with time and is influenced by treatment. Decisions regarding changes to therapy can be made with more confidence if there are serial measurements of disease activity, and in many rheumatology units these are carried out by metrologists who may be trained physiotherapists, occupational therapists or nurses. The activity of RA can be assessed in a number of ways (*Table 12.1*). Changes in the various measures tend to occur in parallel, but none can be considered ideal and new methods are being developed (Scott *et al.*, 1989; Bellamy, 1988).

Table 12.1. Assessment of disease activity in rheumatoid arthritis.

Duration of morning stiffness
Visual analogue pain score
Number of swollen joints
Number of tender joints
Walking time
Grip strength
Functional class
Global score
Health assessment questionnaires
Laboratory measures, e.g. ESR and CRP
X-rays

Early morning stiffness   This varies according to the severity of the disease and patients can usually give a reasonable estimate of the duration of morning stiffness.

Pain   The visual analogue score (VAS) has proved to be practical and useful for pain assessment. It consists of a 10cm line, at one end of which is written 'no pain' and at the other 'worst possible pain' or a similar phrase. The patient makes a mark on the line which corresponds to his level of pain. Thus, a mark 7.5cm along the line would give a VAS pain score of 75%.

Number of swollen joints   A count of the number of swollen joints can be a useful guide to the extent and activity of RA. The size of individual joints can be measured, most often and conveniently the knee, although jewellers' rings can be used for PIP finger joint size.

Number of tender joints   The Ritchie articular index (Ritchie *et al.*, 1968) is widely used to assess activity of RA in rheumatology units. Individual joints or groups of joints are gently squeezed and the degree of tenderness judged according to response, i.e. 0 = no pain; 1 = patient reports pain; 2 = patient reports pain and winces; 3 = patient reports pain, winces and withdraws joint. The scores for individual joints or joint groups are summated. Clearly, the response will depend to some extent on the pain threshold of the patient and the pressure exerted by the examiner, but serial measurements in a given patient by the same examiner can give useful information.

Walking time   It is easy to measure the time taken by a patient to walk a given distance, conventionally 50ft. This reflects only lower limb function so is of limited value for overall disease assessment.

Grip strength Modified sphygmomanometers can be used to measure grip strength. This will vary according to disease activity, but the technique is of limited value in advanced disease, since fixed hand deformities will cause weakness of grip whether the disease is active or not.

Functional class The Steinbrocker functional index has four classes: 1 = complete functional capacity; 2 = functional capacity adequate to conduct normal activities despite handicap or discomfort or limited mobility of one or more joints; 3 = functional capacity adequate to perform only a few or none of the duties of usual occupation or of self-care; 4 = largely or wholly incapacitated with patient bedridden or confined to wheelchair permitting little or no self-care. The problem with this index is that it is insensitive, since most patients fall into classes 2 or 3.

Global scores These are simple, yet have proved fairly sensitive and valuable in clinical trials. The patient is asked to rate their arthritis on a five-point scale. This can take the form of 1 = asymptomatic; 2 = mild; 3 = moderate; 4 = severe; 5 = very severe, or 1 = much better; 2 = a little better; 3 = no change; 4 = a little worse; 5 = much worse.

Health assessment questionnaires Several questionnaires have been developed to assess the patient's ability to wash, dress, walk, undertake self-care, etc. These give information which is much more relevant to the patient's level of function than, say, measurement of knee or finger PIP circumference. The Stanford health assessment questionnaire (HAQ) is widely used in the UK and appears more sensitive and relevant than does the Steinbrocker functional class.

Laboratory measures and X-rays The ESR, plasma viscosity and CRP concentration are all used to monitor changes in disease activity in RA. All tend to be high during exacerbations of disease and they tend to be persistently high in patients with progressive disease. Widespread erosion of the bone is associated with progressive deforming arthritis and patients who develop numerous erosions early in the course of the disease are likely to do badly. A number of scoring systems have been devised to assess erosions and cartilage damage; most are time-consuming and so few units use them in routine clinical practice.

Extra-articular features

The arthritic manifestations of RA command attention, but systemic involvement is common (*Table 12.2*) and extra-articular features can be life-threatening. Extra-articular features tend to be seen in patients with long-standing and severe disease, although occasionally patients present with such features. The prognosis for both survival and degree of disability is significantly worse for patients with extra-articular disease than for those with arthritis alone. Almost all these patients have circulating rheumatoid factor, usually in high titre.

Table 12.2. Extra-articular involvement in rheumatoid arthritis.

	Percentage
Anaemia	50
Lymphadenopathy	30
Nodules	25
Pleurisy	40
Pericarditis	40
Sjögren's syndrome	20
Amyloid	5
Neuropathy	2
Vasculitis	2
Felty's syndrome	1
Pulmonary fibrosis	1
Scleritis	1

Haematological Anaemia is common and is typically of a secondary type, which reflects disease activity in RA. Deficiencies of iron, folate and B_{12} due to poor diet and, in the case of iron, gastrointestinal bleeding, may contribute, as may drug toxicity, e.g. to sulphasalazine. The platelet count tends to be high during phases of active disease, but thrombocytopenia may result from drug toxicity, e.g. to gold and penicillamine. The white cell count is usually normal, but it is reduced in Felty's syndrome and there is an increased susceptibility to infections which can be life-threatening. Thrombocytopenia is often seen in Felty's syndrome, as are splenomegaly and vasculitic leg ulcers.

Nodules The pathology of rheumatoid nodules is described above. They are most often seen over the olecranon or the extensor surface of the proximal ulna, but are also seen over the sacrum, Achilles tendon and occiput. Sometimes multiple nodules may be seen on the fingers. Nodules can be soft, mobile and rubbery, or hard and attached to the underlying periosteum. Vasculitic lesions may develop over them and they may ulcerate and discharge over long periods. Nodules may also occur in the lung or on the eye or vocal cords.

Vasculitis Necrotic nail-fold lesions (*Figure 12.5(d)*) are sometimes seen on the fingers and may be the first evidence of
vasculitis. Purpura, ischaemic leg ulcers or gangrenous digits are
more serious manifestations of the same process. A mixed motor
and sensory neuropathy and mononeuritis multiplex may result
from vasculitis of the vasa nervorum. Vasculitic infarction of the
gut is a life-threatening surgical emergency which is fortunately
rare.

Eye The most common problem is a sensation of dryness or
grittiness of the eye due to secondary Sjögren's syndrome (*see*
Chapter 14); dryness of the mouth may also occur. Scleritis is a
more serious problem which causes a red, painful eye and can
lead to corneal ulcers and thinning of the sclera and, ultimately,
to impaired vision. Prolonged steroid therapy may cause cataracts
and antimalarial drugs can accumulate in the retina and cause
blindness.

Lung Pleurisy is commonly found at post mortem (*Table 12.2*),
but is rarely a clinical problem in patients with RA. Rheumatoid
nodules can resemble primary and secondary intrathoracic
tumours and thoracotomy with histological examination may be
the only means by which to make the distinction. Fibrosing
alveolitis (interstitial fibrosis) can cause dyspnoea and cough, but
fortunately lung failure is uncommon in RA.

Gut By far the most common problem is irritation of the oesophagus, stomach and duodenum by NSAID. This may cause dyspepsia or contribute to iron-deficiency anaemia, but some patients
have an acute gastrointestinal haemorrhage with haematemesis
or malena due to bleeding from or perforation of a peptic ulcer.

Kidney Amyloid is a significant cause of nephrotic syndrome,
renal failure and death in patients with severe, long-standing RA.
Amyloid is a protein which accumulates in the kidney, gut and
heart as a result of prolonged inflammation or infection. It can be
diagnosed by biopsy of rectum or kidney. RA is now a more
common cause of amyloid than infections such as tuberculosis,
bronchiectasis and osteomyelitis. Some studies have suggested
that more than 5% of patients with RA develop amyloid deposits,
but fewer than this develop significant renal disease. NSAID may
cause renal impairment, but 'analgesic nephropathy' – papillary
necrosis and interstitial nephritis resulting from prolonged intake
of analgesics – appears to be less common now that phenacetin
has been withdrawn from sale. Gold and penicillamine can cause
a nephrotic syndrome.

Bone Peri-articular osteoporosis is commonly seen in radiographs of inflamed or relatively immobile joints. Patients with RA are also susceptible to generalised osteoporosis which can predispose to fractures of vertebrae (*Figure 12.10*), femur and other long bones and make joint replacement surgery difficult. Patients with severe, long-standing disease and limited mobility appear to be most at risk; poor nutrition and long-term steroid therapy also appear to be important risk factors.

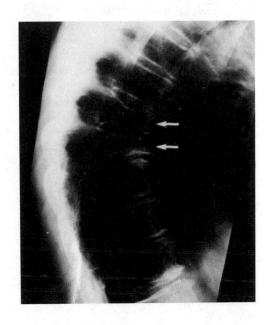

Figure 12.10. Radiograph showing vertebral collapse due to osteoporosis following corticosteroid therapy for RA.

Heart Pericarditis is also a common finding at post mortem but is rarely symptomatic. Very rarely a large pericardial effusion will accumulate and give rise to cardiac tamponade which requires urgent aspiration while chronic pericarditis may necessitate pericardectomy. Conduction defects, valvular disease and coronary vasculitis also occur occasionally.

Muscle Muscle wasting is a common problem in RA which can usually be attributed to reduced muscle use due to pain, joint swelling and immobility. High-dose steroid therapy may cause a proximal myopathy. Very occasionally, patients have tender muscles and a low-grade myositis.

Oedema Peripheral oedema is fairly common in patients with RA. In a few patients this results from poor cardiac, venous or renal function; in the remainder it seems to be due to extravascular pooling caused by the impaired muscle pump effect of reduced mobility, by low serum albumin secondary to active disease, by poor nutrition, and possibly by lymphatic dysfunction.

Psychology   Severe depression sometimes occurs in patients with RA, but is much less common than a mild reactive depression associated with frustration about disability and anxiety about the future. Many patients find that disability is much more difficult to come to terms with than pain. Severe RA will often make it difficult for the patient to continue to work, whether in employment or in the home. The patient has to face loss of employment and reduction in income as well as pain and disability, and these factors will affect the interpersonal relationships within a family and change the dynamics of a marriage. Patients respond in different ways; some have a determined attitude and may try to ignore or even deny their arthritis, whereas others adopt a very passive and dependent role from an early stage of their disease.

Sexual relationships are often adversely affected by arthritis as a result of pain, difficulties due to joint deformities, loss of libido, apprehension about pregnancy and fear of exacerbating the arthritis, either on the part of the patient or spouse. Although difficulties are common they are not often communicated to health workers; patients will often broach the subject hesitantly with the person with whom they feel most comfortable, which may be a doctor, physiotherapist or nurse, and it is important that the response is sympathetic. Advice on different positions and reassurance regarding misconceptions about possible adverse effects of sex on the patient's arthritis can help a sexual relationship to resume.

Management

Management consists of much more than changes to drug treatment. RA tends be a life-long complaint in those patients who attend hospital regularly, although there is always the hope that the disease will 'burn itself out'. The functional impairment which develops over the years demands regular reassessment and patients require different types of practical and psychological support at different stages of their illness. It is vital to know something of the patient's home environment, including family members and interpersonal relationships; type of dwelling; ability to negotiate stairs if not on one level; availability of downstairs toilet and washing facilities; ability to wash, dress, cook, do housework and get to shops; availability of home help, helpful friends or neighbours. Without such information one cannot target appropriate help to the individual patient.

The management of someone with RA is a multi-disciplinary task in which close collaboration between the different specialities and ease of communication is vital. Each member of the team has a special area of expertise and close liaison between for instance, the physiotherapist and orthotist or occupational therapist will achieve the best results. The scope of the task can be merely outlined here.

A programme of management for patients with rheumatoid arthritis includes:

- Regular assessment of measures of disease activity and disability.
- *Education.* Arthritis and Rheumatism Council (ARC) booklets can be useful. Advice regarding joint protection, pregnancy, footwear, etc., is valuable.
- *Physiotherapy.* A regular exercise programme is valuable, as well as measures directed at specific problem joints. Requirements will vary according to activity and stage of disease.
- *Splints.* Working and resting splints can be valuable, but need to be checked periodically.
- *Occupational therapy* (OT). Apart from assessment and provision of aids and appliances much education can take place in the OT unit. The occupational therapists can liaise with the social services' department about modifications to the home, such as the provision of ramps to permit wheelchair access, etc.
- *Nursing.* Apart from conventional nursing care, nurses tend to spend longer with patients than any other member of the team and so play a large role in education, especially regarding the disease and medication.
- *Social work.* Patients often experience financial difficulties and need advice about benefits and local facilities. Problems with housing are common and social workers are well placed to liaise with the local housing department and can help to organise home help, care assistants and meals on wheels. As well as providing advice and information, counselling is often helpful.
- *Orthotist.* The provision of suitable splints, footwear, etc., can improve the quality of the patient's life and may prevent deformities. The skills of the orthotist have been underused and undervalued in the past.
- *Employment.* The disablement resettlement officer (DRO) of the local employment centre will help to find suitable employment.
- *Voluntary organisations.* Patients often gain significant support from meeting fellow sufferers. Meetings of local branches of the ARC or of Arthritis Care can be enjoyable social functions, which can also be educational. The latter organisation runs several hotels which cater for patients with disability.

- *Drug treatment.* It is vital that there is effective communication between the rheumatology unit and the patient's general practitioner, since many of the drugs used in treatment are potentially toxic. Pharmacists are playing an increasing role in the education of the patient regarding how and when to take drugs, and the possible side-effects.
- *Surgery.* This is often required at different stages of the disease. Orthopaedic surgeons are tending to specialise in certain areas, e.g. the cervical spine or hand, so patients may see different surgeons for different problems.

Drug therapy

Four classes of drugs are commonly used in the treatment of RA. These are simple analgesics, non-steroidal anti-inflammatory drugs (NSAID), second-line drugs, and corticosteroids.

Analgesics These are rarely sufficient by themselves, but are often used by patients throughout the course of their illness for pain relief. The dose can be varied according to the severity of the arthritis and activities to be undertaken. Paracetamol is often used either by itself or in combination with dihydrocodeine (codydramol) or dextropropoxyphene (coproxamol). Codeine phosphate and dihydrocodeine can be used, but tend to constipate. Newer drugs include nefopam and meptazinol. Opiates are very rarely appropriate except in the peri-operative period.

Non-steroidal anti-inflammatory drugs (NSAIDs) These have an anti-inflammatory as well as an analgesic action. RA is an inflammatory condition and it is very difficult for patients with active arthritis to cope without NSAID. There are many NSAIDs (*Table 12.3*); all are effective, but all can cause of side-effects. Individual patients will usually find some more effective than others; often the choice of preparation is dictated by absence of side-effects. By far the commonest problem is irritation of the gastrointestinal tract. Dyspepsia is common and some patients have chronic low-grade blood loss, but a few suffer potentially

Table 12.3. Non-steroidal anti-inflammatory drugs.

Azapropazone	Benorylate	Diclofenac
Diflunisal	Etodolac	Fenbufen
Fenoprofen	Flurbiprofen	Ibuprofen
Indomethacin	Ketoprofen	Mefenamic acid
Nabumetone	Naproxen	Piroxicam
Sulindac	Tenoxicam	Tiaprofenic acid
Tolmetin		

life-threatening haematemesis or malena as a result of a bleeding or perforated peptic ulcer. The elderly appear to be particularly at risk of such serious toxicity. Occasional patients develop significant renal impairment and these drugs must be used with great care in anyone with any degree of renal insufficiency.

Second-line drugs These are also known as disease-modifying anti-rheumatic drugs (DMARDs); slow-acting anti-rheumatic drugs; remission-inducing drugs (RIDs) and specific anti-rheumatic drugs. The profusion of terms indicates that none is entirely satisfactory. Several drugs are available (*Table 12.4*) and share several features. First, they have no direct analgesic effect, so patients need to take an analgesic or NSAID in addition. Second, it takes a minimum of several weeks and sometimes some months before an effect is seen. Third, there is a high risk of side-effects, some of which are potentially serious. These drugs generally give best results when used early in the course of the disease, but can be useful in exacerbations of arthritis in patients with long-standing disease. They cannot be expected to achieve anything in patients with inactive disease and will not reverse fixed deformities.

Table 12.4. Second-line anti-rheumatic drugs.

Sulphasalazine
Hydroxychloroquine
Auranofin
Penicillamine
Sodium aurothiomalate
Methotrexate
Azathioprine
Cyclophosphamide

NSAIDs do not affect the long-term outcome of the disease, whereas second-line drugs can suppress the disease, at least in a proportion of patients. They are therefore used in the hope of bringing the arthritis under control and so improving the long-term outcome. Because of their potential toxicity, second-line drugs are rarely given in the first few days or weeks of RA; in any case, there is often some uncertainty regarding the diagnosis and a fairly high rate of spontaneous remission in the earliest stage of the disease. These drugs are commonly used in patients whose arthritis remains active despite treatment with NSAID, those with progressive disability or deformity, those who cannot tolerate NSAID, and those with radiographic evidence of active erosive disease. They are also commonly used in patients with extra-articular manifestations of rheumatoid disease and for a steroid-sparing effect. If one second-like drug does not work or causes side-effects then it is usual to try another. Patients who achieve remission on a second-line drug sometimes relapse if the drug is withdrawn and do not respond when it is re-introduced. There is, therefore, a tendency to continue second-line drugs even if the patient is in remission, or at least to tail them off very slowly.

Some typical drugs are:

- *Sulphasalazine*: This has been widely used for the treatment of RA and other forms of inflammatory arthritis in recent years. Benefit is often experienced after 1 month of treatment, which is faster than with some of the other second-line drugs. It is fairly well tolerated but nausea, abdominal discomfort, headaches and rashes are not uncommon. Blood dyscrasias are rare.
- *Hydroxychloroquine*: Antimalarials have been used in the treatment of RA since it was noted that patients with the disease improved while taking them for malaria prophylaxis. They have a modest effect, which usually takes some 2 months to become apparent, but some patients find them very useful. Side-effects other than mild nausea are uncommon, but there is a small risk of retinal toxicity which can cause blindness. The risk is greatest in patients who take high doses over long periods, especially if unsupervised, and in the elderly. Regular ophthalmological assessment is necessary so that the drug can be stopped at the first sign of problems developing.
- *Gold salts*: Injectable gold (sodium aurothiomalate) has been used for the treatment of RA for some 70 years. It is commonly regarded as one of the most effective second-line drugs, but side-effects are common, notably pruritic rash and mouth ulcers. Proteinuria is fairly common and can produce nephrotic syndrome, while thrombocytopenia and leucopenia also occur. These abnormalities resolve if the drug is stopped, but leucopenia can progress to aplastic anaemia if gold is continued. Regular blood counts and urine tests for protein are therefore mandatory. Recently, an oral preparation of gold (auranofin) has become available. This seems to be similar to injectable gold in efficacy and toxicity, although side-effects tend to be less common and less severe. One additional side-effects is diarrhoea, which is fairly common.
- *Penicillamine*: This is widely used and is similar in efficacy and toxicity to injectable gold, so careful checks on blood count and urine need to be undertaken.
- *Methotrexate*: This has been used with increasing frequency in recent years. It is given in oral form, with the advantage that it

only has to be taken once weekly and seems to have a fairly rapid onset of action. Nausea sometimes occurs, as can blood dyscrasias, so regular blood counts are necessary. The main concern is hepatic fibrosis, but this does not appear to progress to cirrhosis except in those with a high alcohol intake.

- *Azathioprine*: This is another valuable second-line drug, but it does sometimes cause nausea or blood dyscrasias.
- *Cyclophosphamide*: This is very rarely used for arthritis alone, but is valuable for the treatment of rheumatoid vasculitis. It can be given either in oral form or as a high-dose intravenous infusion.

Corticosteroids   These are the most effective agents we have for the treatment of active RA, but unfortunately long-term use is often associated with side-effects. They are often used for patients with active disease who have not responded to NSAIDs or second-line drugs and for those with profound disability; they are usually required for extra-articular manifestations of RA. Once patients have been started on steroids it is often difficult to discontinue them, since the disease flares as the drug is tailed off.

Side-effects are related to the dose used, but even if the daily dose does not exceed 10mg prednisolone or equivalent patients commonly develop thin skin, steroid purpura, osteoporosis and reduced resistance to infection after 10−20 years of treatment. In an attempt to reduce the risk of side-effects, pulsed intermittent intramuscular or intravenous steroid has been used rather than regular daily oral medication, especially during the first 2 months of second-line drug therapy.

Intra-articular steroids are widely used. They are particularly useful when one joint is very inflamed, but arthritis elsewhere is under reasonable control. The risk of infection is slight if sterile precautions are taken and, although there is a theoretical risk that intra-articular steroid may hasten destruction of the joint, this does not appear to happen in practice, at least if the injection of a single joint does not exceed about three per year.

Surgery

Extensive discussion of this subject is outside the scope of this chapter, but advances in orthopaedic surgery have undoubtedly improved the outlook for patients with RA. In the lower limbs, hip and knee replacements are very successful as can be forefoot arthroplasty; hindfoot fusion can be worthwhile in patients with intractable hindfoot problems. In the wrist, excision of the ulnar styloid and wrist fusion can be valuable and silastic implants for MCP joints can give good results in selected patients. Repair of ruptured tendons can restore hand function. Prostheses for elbow and shoulder have been developed but have not yet achieved the success rates for hip and knee replacement. Techniques for fusion of the cervical spine have improved considerably and this can be of major benefit for patients with neurological signs or symptoms.

Physiotherapy

As noted above, many professionals are involved in the care of a patient with RA, but the physiotherapist plays an important part in the management programme. The physiotherapist must assess the patient carefully, determine the physical problems, mental stresses, the patient's expectations, and establish a realistic plan of treatment. When the goals of treatment have been met, physio-therapy should be discontinued and the patient discharged with appropriate advice. This stimulates the patient to have a progressive and realistic attitude to the benefits of physiotherapy, knowing that further effective treatment can be provided in the future if necessary. (See *Figure 12.11* p. 242.)

Physiotherapy should not be used as a prop for the patient in the sense that a visit to the department or hydrotherapy pool becomes a weekly outing to prevent isolation or provide the opportunity for a good wash. When this happens it creates a situation in which there are no goals for the patient or physio-therapist and an impasse results. It is important for the physio-therapist to try to avoid this situation, but if it occurs treatment should be reduced and a social worker should become involved to try to improve the home environment and so make better use of resources.

Out-patient work   Ideally, a physiotherapist should be present at out-patient clinics to check splints, give advice about pain, troublesome joints or wasting muscles, to check footwear and walking aids and to give advice to new patients. Often staff shortage does not permit this and the physiotherapist has to rely upon the rheumatologist identifying a problem in the clinic and making the referral for appropriate help.

The majority of patients with RA never require more than this service. They may attend for local pain relief, splintage, muscle re-education, solving gait problems, dealing with stiffness in hands, hydrotherapy or other treatments. Patients should be treated in their nearest hospital wherever possible, since long journeys may cause such fatigue as to make the session worthless. Ideally, a physiotherapy department should have one physio-therapist to whom all rheumatology referrals are made. This will stimulate the physiotherapist's interest and expertise and will result in better treatment and advice for the patient.

Community physiotherapy For various reasons some patients cannot attend a hospital physiotherapy department and so community physiotherapy is requested. The community physiotherapist has relatively few resources and it is necessary for the hospital unit to support and liaise with her so as to provide optimal treatment.

In-patient treatment Hospital admission may occur for several reasons. These include an exacerbation of arthritis with marked disability; inability to cope at home; medical problems which require investigation and treatment; for mobilisation with intensive physiotherapy; and joint surgery.

Assessment The physiotherapist must make a thorough assessment, set goals, devise a treatment plan and implement it. A dated, written assessment will be useful for future reference. Several topics should be considered:

- *Social history and activities of daily living.* Since arthritis can create such severe problems it is necessary to know something of the patient's life: who lives at home? Is the patient employed and if not did arthritis force him to stop work? Are there stairs and if so can the patient manage these? Are the toilet and bathroom accessible? Who does the cooking, cleaning, washing and shopping? Is there a home help or meals on wheels? Are there any outings or visits to or from friends, relatives or neighbours? How does the patient manage everyday tasks, such as getting out of bed, washing, dressing, toileting, picking up things from the floor, rising from a chair, climbing stairs, eating, reading and writing. By asking such questions one gains considerable insight into the life of the patient and can determine priorities for treatment.

- *Medical history.* The duration of arthritis should be noted and the presence of any co-existent medical problems which may influence treatment, e.g. presence of a pacemaker. A note of medication may be useful.
- *Subjective problems.* The site(s), type and duration of pain should be determined, along with aggravating and relieving factors. Morning stiffness is characteristic during active disease and the duration and any relieving factors are worth noting. Difficulty in using certain joints due to limitation of movement should be noted.
- *Objective assessment.* Ranges of joint movement can be measured with a goniometer. Areas of muscle wasting should be noted and muscle power can be graded according to the MRC scale.

Grip strength can be measured with a modified sphygmomano-
meter. Joint swelling can be measured with a tape measure or
ring guage. Any inequality of leg length should be noted. It is
vital that gait is observed since it is difficult to predict from
examination on the couch; walking time can be recorded. Skin
should be observed and any abrasions or ulcers noted. If there
are pulmonary problems then spirometry is valuable. All
measurements should be recorded for future reference.

• Footwear should be inspected for suitability, pattern of wear
which will indicate style of gait, and any pressure areas. Walking
aids must be assessed for height, safety, suitability and mode
of use. All splints should also be checked.

When the assessment is complete the physiotherapist will have
a fair idea of the patient's current problems, although some patients
will of course reveal more of their private fears and difficulties
than others on initial assessment. Some treatment goals must
now be set.

Treatment   The aims of treatment are to:

• Relieve pain.
• Increase range of joint movement.
• Increase muscle power.
• Support and stabilise joints where necessary.

Pain relief   Physiotherapy involves an active approach to pain.
Various methods can be used, including heat, cold, rest, relaxation,
education, transcutaneous nerve stimulation and hydrotherapy.
During acute flares of arthritis, affected joints should be rested
and only isometric exercises given. Splints may make the joints
more comfortable and will prevent deformity but the joint should
be put gently through a range of passive movement daily to
prevent loss of movement.
    Heat can be applied in the form of heat packs, infra-red, wax or
as hydrotherapy. Other methods include ultrasound, pulsed short-
wave diathermy and interferential machines. All increase circulation and reduce muscle spasm and pain. Heat is usually helpful,
but some patients prefer ice. Following pain relief, exercise can
be carried out.
    Education may help pain control. The patient should be encour-
aged to consider if anything precipitated the pain – overuse or
inappropriate posture – and to note any aggravating or relieving
factors. Instruction in relaxation techniques may prove useful.
Prevention of pain or use of simple measures, such as a splint or
heat, is preferable to regular use of analgesics.

Transcutaneous nerve stimulation (TNS) is useful for the treatment of chronic pain. When applied to a painful area it causes sustained transmission of impulses in thick myelinated afferent nerve fibres, which reduces transmission of pain impulses from thin and unmyelinated fibres up the spinal cord and so reduces pain perception. It is possible that acupuncture works by a similar mechanism. If initially helpful it is reasonable to loan the patient a machine for 3–4 weeks, but then reassessment is necessary to ensure that it will be of value in the longer term.

Increase in range of movement   Loss of movement may result from protective muscle spasm, instability, tendon rupture, fibrosis or damage to articular surfaces. One must remember that joint tissues are inflamed and vulnerable in RA and stretching and mobilising techniques without voluntary control may lead to instability.

To increase the range of movement, heat should be applied first to reduce muscle spasm. Active exercises should follow and active assisted exercise can be introduced if the response is insufficient. Hold–relax and contract–relax techniques can also be used. Ideally, patients with RA should perform a routine daily exercise programme to encourage maximum joint mobility. The exercises should involve all major joint and muscle groups and be performed slowly with sustained stretch-and-hold in the optimum position.

Increase in muscle power   Muscle groups which act across an inflamed joint are likely to become weak and wasted in part due to disuse and in part as a result of reflex inhibition. Muscle power should be recorded according to the MRC scale and reviewed with treatment. In active disease, only isometric exercises should be used, but as the disease settles active exercises, active resisted exercises, and the use of weights and springs can be introduced progressively. The aim should be a return of grade 5 power although this will not always be possible.

Hydrotherapy   This is a much valued resource in the treatment of RA since it can be used to reduce pain and increase both range of movement and muscle power. The pool temperature should be close to body temperature (approximately 35°C). The hot water relaxes muscles and the water supports the body and reduces the need for antigravity muscular activity which greatly reduces the pain associated with movement. The water can be used to assist or resist movement and exercises can be active or passive depending on the needs of the patient. Swimming can be encouraged as a good form of active exercise. Floats, rings and collars can be used according to the patient's needs. Bad Ragaz techniques can be used and modified for the severely disabled or apprehensive patient. In patients with weak muscles, gait training and step practice can begin in water sooner than would be possible on dry land. This can encourage the patient and demonstrate to him the feasibility of rehabilitation. The underwater douche can be used to give a kneading massage which can reduce muscle spasm and pain.

A treatment session of 20−30 minutes is reasonable for someone with RA but the patient must never be overtired. After a shower and dressing the patient should have a drink, rest and cool down for some 30 minutes or so.

Support and stabilisation of joints   Rheumatoid joints often need some form of splint or support to reduce pain, stabilise the joint or prevent deformity. A wide variety of splinting materials is available (*Table 12.5*). The purpose of the splint should be determined and an appropriate material selected. Plaster of Paris is most suitable for a fracture or for short-term use for painful or unstable joints. Scotch cast is useful where a light, readily available splint is required. Plastazote is valuable where standard appliances cannot be used, e.g. for collars, back supports and footwear; it is especially useful for drop-foot resting splints. Hexcelite is useful

Table 12.5. Splinting materials for joints.

Material	Advantages	Disadvantages
Plaster of Paris	Cheap Malleable Easily applied Easily removed	Heavy Not waterproof Takes 12−24 hours to dry Not very durable
Scotch cast	Lightweight Easily applied Dries quickly Waterproof Malleable Durable	Sticky to apply Difficult to remove Not resilient
Plastazote	Lightweight Soft & comfortable Can be moulded	Oven required for splints Time-consuming to make Expensive
Hexcelite	Waterproof Dries quickly Lightweight Durable	Difficult to trim cylinder Not as malleable as POP
Thermoplastics	Lightweight Waterproof Durable	Time-consuming to make Very expensive

for making resting splints quickly. Thermoplastics are best for dynamic splints such as knee braces and lively splints.

Cervical spine   Collars can relieve pain caused by muscle spasm or nerve-root irritation. In patients with instability, plastic collars can be used in the shower or at the hairdresser while plastazote collars will permit even less movement and are suitable for patients with marked instability or neurological involvement. Patients with neck involvement should be advised to wear a collar in the car to reduce the risk of neurological damage from a whiplash injury.

Hands   During an acute flare, forearm resting splints are useful to reduce pain and support the hand in a functional position. They should hold the hand with the thumb in slight abduction and opposition. Ideally the wrist should be in 10−15° of extension with support under the carpal arch. The metacarpophalangeal (MCP) joints should be in comfortable flexion and the interphalangeal joints in some 5° of flexion. The splint should extend from the ends of the fingertips to some three fingers' width below the olecranon, with correction of ulnar or radial deviation. The splint can be fitted with two straps, one high on the forearm and the other over the wrist, but straps over the fingers can encourage subluxation of MCP and interphalangeal joints.

Working splints are used to relieve pain during activities and to increase function. When assessing hands one must consider the patient's feelings about splints: if he does not wish to wear one it is a waste of time and money to provide it. The splints can be made of inexpensive elastic material in standard fittings, such as Futuro, Spencer or Promedics. Alternatively, a cast can be made of the hand and a splint made of soft Persian or block leather or of thermoplastic. These are all relatively expensive and so are only appropriate for patients who find a splint of proven value and regularly use it. In addition, swan-neck splints, thumb stalls and ulnar drift splints can all be useful in certain patients. Dynamic splints are particularly useful after hand surgery: at rest the splint holds the joints in a corrected or over-corrected position to prevent shortening of soft tissues yet it still allows movement to take place.

Knees   Resting splints are provided for patients with active arthritis or flexion contractures. The splint should extend from just below the gluteal fold to some three fingers' width above the lateral malleolus. If the ankles are painful the feet can be included in the splint with the ankle in neutral position. When the knees have been damaged and are unstable, a knee brace may provide enough stability to permit weight-bearing and mobility. Several are available, including the Camp multicentric, Canadian (TVS)

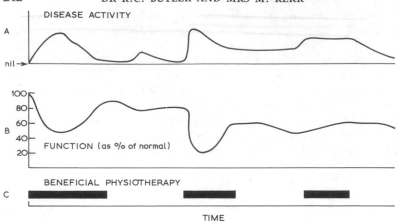

Figure 12.11. Schematic representation of the fulminating course of RA.

and thermoplastic types. Different braces will suit different patients: ability to put on the brace and cope with the fastenings is of prime importance.

Feet Patients should be advised about footwear. Shoes should be of adequate width and depth to avoid pressure lesions on the toes. Metatarsal insoles relieve pressure over metatarsal heads; valgus insoles will correct minor degrees of valgus instability and wedging or floating-out the heels can also provide stability. Off-the-shelf comfort-style shoes can help if ordinary footwear is unsuitable. Bespoke surgical shoes can be made from a cast of the patient's foot when there is advanced deformity, but are very expensive. During gait training the footwear should be reassessed regularly.

Serial splinting This can be applied to many joints but is most frequently used for the knee. When this is being undertaken the patient should avoid weight-bearing. A standard procedure is to treat the patient with hydrotherapy or hot packs followed by isometric quadriceps exercises to reduce muscle spasm. After analgesia and a muscle relaxant, such as diazepam, the leg is encased in a full-leg cylinder in as much extension as can be tolerated, and the patient then rests for 24–28 hours. Once the plaster is bivalved the back shells can be used as resting splints. After further hydrotherapy and exercises the procedure can be repeated and this can be continued until a satisfactory position is achieved.

Serial splinting is demanding for both patient and physiotherapist but can be very rewarding. A less demanding but longer-term method is to use full-leg flowtron splints. Intermittent

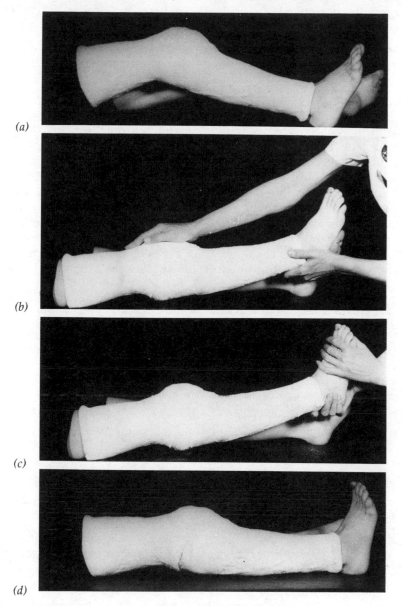

(a)

(b)

(c)

(d)

Figure 12.12. (a) Patient with a knee flexion deformity in a plaster-of-Paris cylinder; (b) the splint around the knee leaving a hinge anteriorly — correction has been effected, posterior aspects of the plaster separated; (c) correction maintained, awaiting a plaster bandage completion to hold the cylinder in a new position; (d) the completed cylinder with correction of the deformity.

pressure is applied for at least an hour 2–3 times a day in combination with hot packs, exercises and hydrotherapy.

Juvenile arthritis

Arthritis in childhood is uncommon, but not rare: there are probably some 12,000 affected children in the UK. Some forms of arthritis, collectively known as juvenile chronic arthritis (JCA), appear to be peculiar to childhood. In addition, some types of adult arthritis can affect children, e.g. rheumatoid arthritis, psoriatic arthritis and Reiter's syndrome. A classification of rheumatic disorders in childhood is shown in *Table 12.6*. Children with rheumatoid arthritis have progressive deforming arthritis with a positive test for rheumatoid factor ('seropositive') and radiographic evidence of erosions. The disease tends to be severe and progressive throughout life. The other adult types of arthritis run a similar course to that seen in the adult and will not be discussed here.

Table 12.6. Rheumatic disorders in childhood.

A. Juvenile chronic arthritis (JCA)

- Systemic type (Still's disease)
- Polyarticular type (five or more affected joints)
- Pauci-articular type (up to four affected joints)
  (a) Early onset in girls with positive ANF and uveitis
  (b) Late onset in boys with HLA–B27

B. Adult-type disorders which occur in childhood

- Rheumatoid arthritis (seropositive and erosive)
- Psoriatic arthritis
- Reiter's syndrome
- Ankylosing spondylitis
- Systemic lupus erythematosus
- Polymyositis and dermatomyositis
- Scleroderma

JCA: systemic type
This was the syndrome described by Still in 1897. Affected children are unwell with swinging fever, malaise, anorexia, lymphadenopathy, hepatosplenomegaly and rash. The rash tends to consist of a series of small erythematous patches which come and go in different sites over a matter of hours; it is often worse in the evening and brought on by a rise in temperature or a hot bath. The main differential diagnosis is from acute leukaemia, since

joint symptoms are often not prominent at the outset. Later, however, some 50% develop recurrent or chronic arthritis. The systemic features can respond well to NSAIDs, such as naproxen, but systemic steroids may be required. The condition typically has exacerbations and remissions over the years and tends to burn itself out when adult life is reached.

JCA: polyarticular type

Children with this form of JCA often have peristently active arthritis throughout childhood, although it tends to become inactive in the late teenage years. It can lead to considerable deformity and disability. The cervical spine is often involved, with limitation of neck movement and involvement of the temperomandibular joints commonly leading to micrognathia. Growth is often retarded and short stature is almost inevitable if steroids are used on a daily basis, although somewhat less likely if an alternate day regimen is used (Byron et al., 1983). Unfortunately, the arthritis is sometimes so troublesome that the use of steroids cannot be avoided. Drugs, such as gold, penicillamine and hydroxychloroquine, are often used with variable results, but physiotherapy is much more important and everything possible should be done to try to prevent deformities.

JCA: pauciarticular type

This group comprises a number of subsets. One subset is of young girls (onset 1–5 years) with positive tests for antinuclear factor (ANF) in their serum. These children are at high risk of developing uveitis, which can be asymptomatic yet lead to serious visual impairment. It is therefore vital that they are screened regularly by an ophthalmologist so that appropriate treatment can be started at the first sign of trouble. The arthritis can be troublesome in affected joints and, again, physiotherapy is very important since the arthritis generally abates as adult life approaches.

Another subset is of boys aged 10–16 years who have limited joint involvement, typically of the hip, knee or ankle. These boys possess the tissue type HLA-B27 and some, but not all of them, will develop ankylosing spondylitis in later life.

Physiotherapy

Long-term management of children with arthritis is complex and requires understanding and close collaboration between parents, doctors, nurses, physiotherapists, occupational therapists, social workers, teachers, educational psychologists, career advisors and social services. Co-ordination of activities in hospital, at home and at school is important to ensure that the child receives maximum benefit from treatment, with least possible disruption to home life and education.

The principles of treatment are similar to those used in the treatment of adults, but the key to success is a successful rapport built up between therapist, child and parents. Parents need to know about the disease and its implications so that they can take part in the management programme and help the child to mature in physical, mental and social terms in as normal a manner as possible.

Assessment and treatment   An approach to the assessment of inflammatory arthritis has been described for rheumatoid arthritis. Children with painful joints often respond by becoming quiet, irritable and withdrawn. They adopt antalgic postures and restrict movement in painful joints. Deforming contractures will develop in inflamed joints which are kept immobile (*Figure 12.13*). Lack of movement also leads to stunting of growth and poor muscle bulk.

Splints are used to rest actively-inflamed joints and can be used subsequently as resting splints to maintain joint alignment and prevent deformity. Where resting splints are used joints should be placed in functional positions. Splints must be comfortable for adequate compliance and ideally light yet effective. A working splint to stabilise a painful or unstable joint, e.g. a wrist splint, may permit daily activities such as writing which would

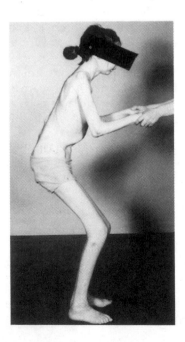

Figure 12.13. Severe deformities and muscle wasting in juvenile chronic polyarthritis.

otherwise be impossible. Serial splints may help to correct established deformity. Children with active JCA will often benefit from a period of rest in their splints during the day.

A programme of exercises should be instituted to build up muscle strength and put joints through a full range of movement. It is particularly important to exercise extensor muscles of the knees, hips and spine to prevent flexion deformities. Hydrotherapy is particularly valuable in JCA, since the hot water relieves muscle spasm and buoyancy permits activities such as walking and shoulder elevation to be relearned. In addition, it is usually good fun, which means that the child is particularly keen to co-operate with an exercise programme. Parents can be shown exercises which they can often then supervise in their local swimming pool. The child should be encouraged to use as normal a gait as possible and to avoid, for instance, walking with a limp, in a stiff-legged manner or with the knees and ankles flexed so that the heel does not touch the ground. Emphasis should be given to a normal heel strike and heel−toe sequence. Sport is a good form of exercise, and cycling and swimming should be encouraged, but it is generally advisable for the child to avoid contact sports.

Finally, it is important to re-emphasise that the parents must be involved in the whole process. Their co-operation is vital to ensure that splints are used and used correctly, that the child exercises regularly, and that medication is taken as directed. Ultimately, the disease will settle down and when that day comes the child should be able to face life with as little physical and psychological disability as possible.

References

Arnett, F.C., Edworthy, S.M., Bloch, D.A., et al. (1988). The American Rheumatism Association 1987 revised criteria for the classification of rheumatoid arthritis. Arthritis and Rheumatism, **31**, 315−323.

Bellamy, N. (1988). Methods of clinical assessment of anti-rheumatic drugs. Baillière's Clinical Rheumatology, **2**, 339−362.

Byron, M.A., Jackson, J. and Ansell, B.M. (1983). Effect of different corticosteroid regimens on hypothalamic-pituitary-adrenal axis and growth in juvenile chronic arthritis. Journal of the Royal Society of Medicine, **76**, 452−457.

Harris, E.D. (1990). Rheumatoid arthritis − pathophysiology and implications for therapy. New England Journal of Medicine, **322**, 1277−1289.

Ritchie, D.M., Boyle, J.A., McInnes, J.M., et al. (1968). Clinical studies with an articular index for the assessment of joint tenderness in patients with rheumatoid arthritis. Quarterly Journal of Medicine, **147**, 393−406.

Scott, D.L., Spector, T.D., Pullar, T. and McConkey, B. (1989). What should we hope to achieve when treating rheumatoid arthritis? Annals of the Rheumatic Diseases, **48**, 256−261.

Bibliography

Ansell, B.M. (1980). *Rheumatic Disorders in Childhood*. Butterworths, London.

Davis, B.C. and Harrison, R.A. (1988). *Hydrotherapy in Practice*. Churchill Livingstone, Edinburgh.

Hyde, S.A. (1980). *Physiotherapy in Rheumatology*. Blackwell, Oxford.

Kelley, W.N., Harris, E.D., Ruddy, S. and Sledge, C.B. (1989). *Textbook of Rheumatology*. 3rd edition. W B Saunders, Philadelphia.

Scott, J.T. (1986). *Copeman's Textbook of the Rheumatic Diseases*. 6th edition. Churchill Livingstone, Edinburgh.

Utsinger, P.D., Zvaifler, N.J. and Ehrlich, G.E. (1985). *Rheumatoid arthritis. Etiology, Diagnosis, Management*. J B Lippincott, Philadelphia.

13 The Spondyloarthropathies

J.J. Dixey and M. Kerr

Introduction

The spondyloarthropathies are a group of diseases brought together by their tendency to inflammatory arthritis of the spine or spondyloarthritis. As a group, they are fascinating for clinicians and scientists alike as greater understanding of these diseases provides strong clues as to the cause of joint inflammation. Study of their pathogenesis demonstrates a clear link between the environment and the host combining to cause disease. For instance, in reactive arthritis, joint inflammation occurs following gut or genito-urinary infection in those men or women carrying the HLA-B27 gene. Furthermore, as a group of disorders, the clinical picture or natural progression of disease is much more predictable than rheumatoid arthritis, where the disease pattern is more heterogeneous. For the physiotherapist, the spondyloarthropathies are most important as local therapy provides the mainstay of treatment, ahead of drug therapy.

Terminology

There is confusion about the classification of these conditions. In turn, they have been called rheumatoid variants, HLA-B27 disorders, and seronegative arthritis. Seronegative arthritis is too easily confused with seronegative rheumatoid arthritis (rheumatoid arthritis in the absence of rheumatoid factor) and implies that the lack of rheumatoid factor is in some way important in the pathogenesis of disease, which is not the case. So the term 'spondyloarthropathy' is preferable and is included in the American classification of rheumatic diseases.

Ten diseases are included in the spondyloarthritis group and are shown in *Figure 13.1*. The more important members of the group are ankylosing spondylitis, psoriatic arthritis, Reiter's disease and reactive arthritis and are considered separately below. The other less-common members all share clinical features with their senior partners. *Anterior uveitis* is an inflammatory disorder

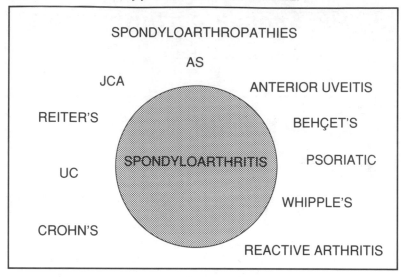

Figure 13.1. The ten diseases which comprise the spondyloarthropathy group (AS = ankylosing spondylitis, JCA = juvenile chronic arthritis, UC = ulcerative colitis).

of the eye characterised by acute and localised pain and loss of vision. It is included because a significant proportion of sufferers have or go on to develop ankylosing spondylitis. The chronic inflammatory bowel disorders, *ulcerative colitis* and *Crohn's disease*, are commonly complicated by spondylitis, but the activity of the bowel and spinal diseases are independent of one another. This is in contrast to a large mono- or oligo-arthritis, normally involving either knee or ankle, which can complicate either ulcerative colitis or Crohn's disease and mirrors the activity of the bowel disorder very closely. *Behçet's syndrome* is characterised by a triad of clinical features: recurrent oral and genital ulceration, chronic eye inflammation (posterior uveitis), and a large joint asymmetrical arthritis normally in knee or ankle. It is included in the spondyloarthritis group as sacro-ileitis is sometimes observed.

Behçet's syndrome is rare in Northern Europe and America, but is seen in the Mediterranean countries, especially Turkey. *Whipple's disease* is rare and should be considered when patients present with a large joint arthritis, chronic diarrhoea and considerable weight-loss. The cause is a microbial infestation of the small bowel, and it is an important disease to diagnose as the symptoms are eradicated with antibiotic therapy. The inclusion of *juvenile chronic arthritis* in this group is possibly more contentious, but ankylosing spondylitis and psoriatic and reactive arthritis do occur in childhood and are very similar to their adult counterparts.

Shared clinical features

The spine

As mentioned above, the tendency to inflammation of the spine is central to spondyloarthritis. The inflammatory process affects the sacro-iliac joints, the intervertebral discs and the apophyseal joints which articulate between the vertebral bodies (*Figure 13.2*). Typically, there is progression of disease with the sacro-iliac joints involved first, and then the thoraco-lumbar junction. The pathological process then spreads up the thoracic spine to the neck and down into the lumbar spine. Very often, the sacro-iliac joints are affected and the remainder of the spine is normal. In psoriatic spondyloarthritis, the sacro-iliac involvement can be asymmetrical and, rather than the orderly progression of disease up the spine described above, 'skip' lesions often occur.

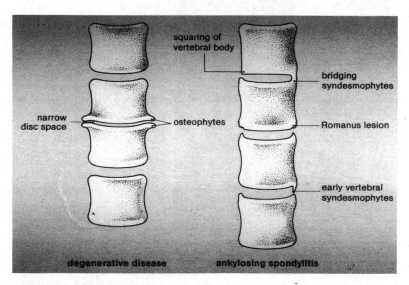

Figure 13.2. Anatomical drawing of the vertebrae in degenerative arthritis and ankylosing spondylitis (reproduced with permission from Gower Medical Publishing Ltd).

Enthesopathy

This is the inflammatory process which occurs at the junction of bone with either synovium, joint capsule, tendon or ligament. It is the central pathological event in spondyloarthritis and contrasts with rheumatoid arthritis where synovitis is foremost. In the spine, the enthesopathic process occurs at the point of attachment of the annulus fibrosus to the vertebral body, and the attachments of joint capsule to the margins of sacro-iliac and apophyseal joints. At first, an inflammatory infiltrate occurs, leading to bony erosion, followed by the laying down of fibrous tissue and finally bone. The result of this pathological event is the bony fusion of the intervertebral spaces and spinal rigidity so typical of ankylosing spondylitis (*Figure 13.3*). Enthesopathy also occurs outside the spine – a painful heel or plantar fasciitis is often the presenting symptom of a spondyloarthropathy and results from inflammation at the point of attachment of the plantar fascia to the calcaneum

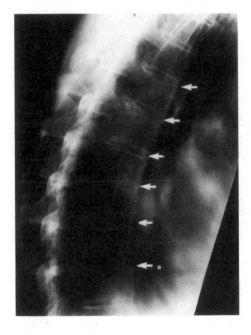

Figure 13.3. Radiograph showing bony fusion in ankylosing spondylitis.

Synovitis

The importance of enthesopathy has been stressed above, but synovitis in peripheral joints is also seen. In rheumatoid arthritis, a symmetrical involvement of peripheral joints is typically observed, but, in contrast, there is an asymmetric involvement of large and small joints in spondyloarthritis with fewer joints involved than in rheumatoid arthritis (*Figure 13.4*). The possible exceptions are the symmetrical involvement of hips seen in ankylosing spondylitis and the pattern of disease found in the rheumatoid-variant of psoriatic arthritis (see below). The synovitis is destructive, however, and the result, both clinically and pathologically, is indistinguishable from rheumatoid arthritis.

Skin

Clearly, the diagnosis of psoriatic arthritis is based on the characteristic rash and pattern of joint disease (sometimes the joint symptoms occur before the onset of rash). Skin involvement is, however, typical of the group of spondyloarthritis as a whole. Keratoderma blenorrhagica is a rash found on the hands and feet in reactive arthritis and is indistinguishable from pustular psoriasis. Genital ulceration occurs both in reactive arthritis and Behçet's syndrome.

Eyes

Aseptic inflammation of the eyes is a strong feature of these diseases. Acute conjunctivitis is a diagnostic finding in reactive arthritis; recurrent anterior uveitis frequently complicates ankylosing spondylitis and is relatively benign, and posterior uveitis occurs in Behçet's syndrome and is far from benign. Chronic iridocyclitis (a combination of both anterior and posterior uveitis) is a feared complication of juvenile chronic arthritis (Chapter 12).

Bowel

As mentioned above, the chronic inflammatory bowel disorders, ulcerative colitis and Crohn's disease, are complicated by spondyloarthritis. Mouth ulceration is an important feature of Behçet's syndrome, and reactive arthritis occurs after acute bowel infection with certain specific micro-organisms. Therefore, it has been suggested that a breakdown in the normal defence mechanisms at the bowel mucosa might be the central event in the pathogenesis of spondyloarthritis. A postulate supported by the recent demonstration of a high incidence of sub-clinical inflammation in the terminal ilium in patients with ankylosing spondylitis.

Familial tendency

Much emphasis is placed by rheumatologists on obtaining an accurate family history in an individual who presents with arthritis, because this knowledge can contribute to diagnosis. There is often clustering of rheumatic diseases in families, especially with spondyloarthritis. Not only do relatives suffer with the same disease, but they might have a different disease from within the

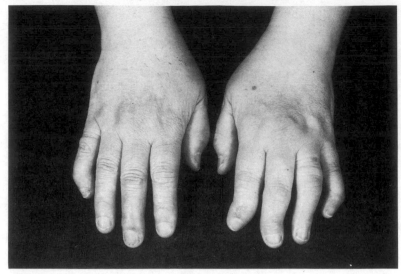

(a)

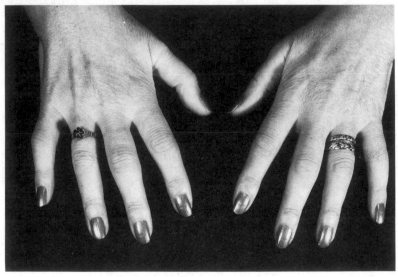

(b)

Figure 13.4. (a) Psoriatic hand demonstrating asymmetrical disease of PIP + DIP joints. (b) Rheumatoid hand with symmetrical involvement of PIP joints.

group of spondyloarthritis. This is illustrated in the family tree shown in *Figure 13.5*, where the index case or proband has ankylosing spondylitis and a number of his relatives suffer with spondylitis, psoriatic or reactive arthritis.

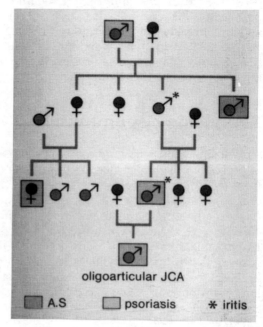

Figure 13.5. A family tree (reproduced with permission from Gower Medical Publishing Ltd).

oligoarticular JCA

A.S   psoriasis   * iritis

HLA-B27

The HLA (human leucocyte antigen) genes encode a group of globulins which are found on every cell in the body. These globulins or antigens act as a template or key for cell recognition by the immune system and, under normal circumstances, prevent self-destruction by the body's defences. HLA-B27 is one such gene and occurs in approximately 10% of the normal population, but is found in 90–95% of patients with ankylosing spondylitis. The incidence of HLA-B27 is also higher in other members of the spondyloarthritis group and is the strong genetic thread which links these diseases. Given the function of the HLA antigens described above, the higher incidence of B27 observed would suggest that there has been a breakdown of cell recognition by the immune system in spondyloarthritis resulting in disease. Furthermore, we now know that certain bacteria can trigger reactive arthritis and so, in spondyloarthritis, there is a clear link between host and environmental factors causing arthritis. How might the presence of HLA-B27 predispose to disease? Various theories have been proposed, the most accepted being the concept of molecular mimicry. There are, it is proposed, antigenic determinants on epitopes on the HLA-B27 globulin identical to those found on the surface of certain gut-associated bacteria. As a consequence of this 'mimicry', antibodies generated against the pathogenic bacteria are also toxic to cells expressing HLA-B27 and this breakdown in immunity produces arthritis. Many holes can be picked in this theory but perhaps further research into this and other theories will lead eventually to a better understanding of the role of the environment in the aetiology of arthritis.

Ankylosing spondylitis

Ankylosing spondylitis is a common disease whose true incidence is probably not known, as many of those with the disease suffer from a chronic 'bad back' or 'slipped disc' and are never formally diagnosed. It is an ancient disease, with study of human remains ('paleopathology') revealing evidence of the disease as far back as 4000BC. For reasons which are not understood, it is a predominately male disease (male : female, 9 : 1). Of all the rheumatic diseases, ankylosing spondylitis is an important disorder to diagnose because maintenance of good spinal posture is so vital for the long-term outlook.

Clinical features
The first symptoms normally appear in young men in their twenties. The onset can be gradual and insidious, with stiffening of the spine and pain, especially in the morning. Typically, the first complaint might be difficulty in putting socks on. Alternatively, the onset can be sudden, with an 'acute back' or the symptoms of sacro-ileitis. Sacro-ileitis causes pain that radiates from the buttock around to the front of the thigh (*Figure 13.6*) and is commonly mistaken for either sciatica or hip pain. It is not unusual for a patient with established spondylitis to give a history of recurrent bouts of sciatica before the diagnosis was made, pain which, in retrospect, was clearly sacro-iliac rather than neuralgic. Once established, spinal stiffness is predominant and symptoms become more chronic, but flares of spondylitis occur even after the disease has been active for many years. The course of disease is also unpredictable in that many patients will progress to full spinal fusion while others have mild symptoms and may never be diagnosed, as mentioned before. At its worst, pain is severe and poorly controlled with drugs but, once the spine has fused and movement is no longer possible, symptoms ease and the

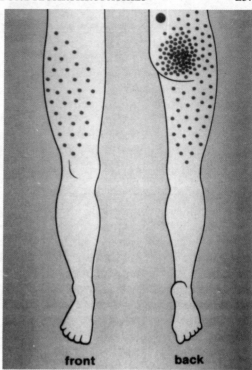

Figure 13.6. Diagram to illustrate sacro-iliac pain (reproduced with permission from Gower Medical Publishing Ltd).

degree of disability depends on the overall standard of spinal posture. Pains in the chest in spondylitic patients are frequently mistaken for angina, but are a feature of the disease: thoracic nerve-root entrapment gives radicular-type pain around the chest wall and the costochondral joints become inflamed, producing pain in the front of the chest and local tenderness. Enthesopathy (see above) contributes to diagnosis, as the finding of plantar fasciitis in a man with back pain would raise the likelihood of spondylitis. In severe disease, hips are commonly diseased and require replacement. The more peripheral joints can be involved and there may be complaints of pain in the base of the thumb or in the great toe. Occasionally, the first spondylitic symptom is unilateral swelling of the knee, particularly in juvenile disease.

Examination

A crucial part in establishing the diagnosis of ankylosing spondylitis is examination of the spine. At first, the only physical abnormality might be pain induced by stretching the sacro-iliac joints, or a subtle and small diminution in the range of spinal movement only apparent with careful examination. In more severe disease, there is vertebral tenderness localised to areas of active inflammation − or tenderness throughout the spine in acute flares. When posture has not been maintained, the classical deformities of spondylitis may be seen; loss of lumbar lordosis, pronounced thoracic kyphosis and hunchback with eyes pointing toward the floor (*Figure 13.7*). What are the physical features that might distinguish between mechanical and early inflammatory back pain? With mechanical pain, there might be localised vertebral and paravertebral tenderness, whereas in spondylitis, tenderness is localised to the sacro-iliac joints or over the thoraco-lumbar junction at first and then become more diffuse throughout the spine. Similarly, in mechanical pain, range of movement may be diminished in one section of the spine, whereas movement is reduced throughout the spine in spondylitis. Evidence of nerve-root entrapment would favour mechanical dysfunction, although sciatica can occur in spondylitis. However, physical examination

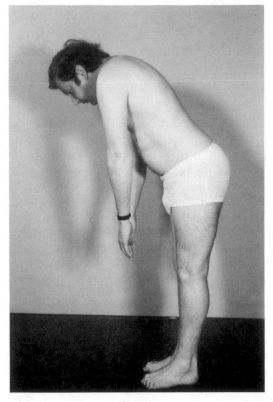

Figure 13.7. A middle-aged man with ankylosing spondylitis with a rigid lumbar spine and pronounced dorsal kyphosis.

alone is sometimes insufficient to establish the diagnosis, and investigations then become important.

Investigations

Blood tests are not particularly helpful. The erythrocyte sedimentation rate (ESR) is frequently elevated in spondylitis and should be normal in mechanical back pain, but is not specific. Frequently, the presence of HLA-B27 in the blood is considered diagnostic, but over-reliance on this genetic marker should be discouraged because up to 10% of spondylitics will be B27 negative. Radiology is particularly important in establishing the diagnosis. The earliest changes will be seen on isotopic bone scans, where increased uptake of the isotope over the spine and sacro-iliac joints is observed before abnormalities become apparent on plain radiographs. Changes on plain radiographs are diagnostic: the eroded appearance over the inflamed sacro-iliac joints; the small erosions or 'Romanus' lesion found on the vertebral end-plate at the T12/L1 level in early disease; and later, the typical new bone or 'syndesmophyte' formation from the vertebrae, with the syndesmophytes eventually fusing to form bony bridges between vertebrae (*Figure 13.8*). The newer imaging techniques are most exciting: computerized tomography (CT scanning) is a sensitive method for detecting early sacro-ileitis and magnetic resonance scanning (MR scans) will, it is hoped, provide more information in the future about the earliest changes in the spine.

Complications

The spondylitic spine is, not surprisingly, brittle and therefore the feared complication of the ankylosis is fracture. Spinal fracture can occur spontaneously or after relatively minor trauma. As a consequence, there is a significant incidence of tetraplegia or paraplegia in spondylitis. The fused neck is particularly vulnerable: spontaneous fracture occurs at the atlanto-axial level and normally results in sudden death; lower cervical fractures complicate whiplash injuries and spondylitic patients should be strongly advised to travel only in cars with correctly adjusted head restraints. There are various systemic complications of spondylitis which are fortunately rare: inflammatory dilatation of the aortic root leading to failure of the aortic valve; a higher incidence of heart block; and very occasionally secondary amyloidosis leading to renal failure. The eye and bowel complications of spondylitis are discussed above.

Treatment

Patient education and physiotherapy are the mainstay treatments for spondylitis: drug therapy and surgery are of secondary import-

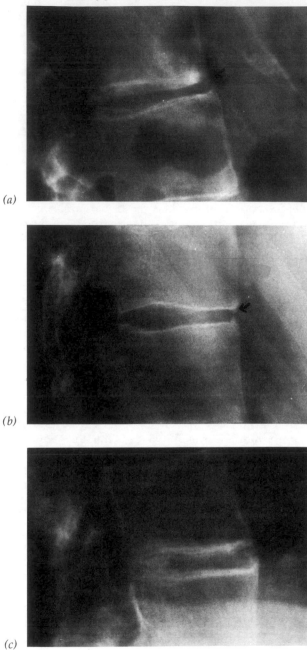

(a)

(b)

(c)

Figure 13.8. Serial X-rays of L1/L2: (a) Showing a Romanus lesion. (b) Syndesmophyte formation. (c) Bony fusion.

ance. There is little evidence that any treatment, physical or otherwise, prevents the progression to ankylosis. But there is firm evidence to suggest that local treatment, a rigorous exercise regime and education influence favourably the functional outcome and prevent spinal deformity. If, once the spondylitic process has completed its course, the spine is rigid, the outcome is surprisingly good as long as posture has been maintained. The maintenance of posture, therefore, is the crucial role played by the physiotherapist.

The spondylitic patient should be encouraged to attend classes, read the relevant literature and, most importantly, perform a daily exercise regime. The physiotherapist can also provide a helpful service by measuring spinal movement and the degree of deformity on a sequential basis. Non-steroidal anti-inflammatory drugs provide good symptomatic relief and are normally taken on a regular basis and well tolerated. If the modern NSAIDs are ineffective, phenylbutazone is indicated. Phenylbutazone was the first NSAID (apart from aspirin) to be introduced onto the market, but its product licence is now limited to use in spondylitis because the risk of the feared side-effect, drug-induced bone marrow suppression, is considered unacceptable for general rheumatological use. Specific anti-rheumatic drugs are of limited use in spondylitis.

Recent studies have indicated that sulphasalazine might be beneficial in early spondylitis, but its role in the treatment of a disease that is likely to be active for 20 or more years has yet to be identified. Hip replacement is the most commonly performed orthopaedic procedure in spondylitis. Spinal-corrective surgery is risky, but the outcome can be excellent when performed in specialised centres. There is potential risk to the cord, but this danger is often acceptable when posture is so poor as to impede function. Spinal irradiation was a highly effective treatment, but has now been largely abandoned because of the risk of iatrogenic leukaemia. Occasionally, in older patients with intractable disease, irradiation is still indicated.

Physiotherapy

Education is most important, especially when given to newly diagnosed spondylitics. Patients should be instructed about sitting and lying postures, and a daily exercise programme should begin at once. Self-discipline in exercise and posture should be stressed and encouraged in a positive manner. As a result of the education given by the physiotherapist, the patient should adapt his lifestyle while maintaining a normal existence. Annual measurements of height, posture and spinal movement are needed to document any progression of disease which might occur.

Assessment Spinal joints are principally affected. As spinal mobility decreases and the lumbar curve is lost, the thoracic spine becomes kyphosed. Hips and knees are flexed to maintain an even distribution of body weight. Straightening of the neck causes the hyperextension of the atlanto-axial joint and protrusion of the jaw. Spondylography is the best method of measuring spinal posture.

Spondylography The patient stands on the base of the spondylometer (*Figure 13.9*), as straight as possible, with heels touching

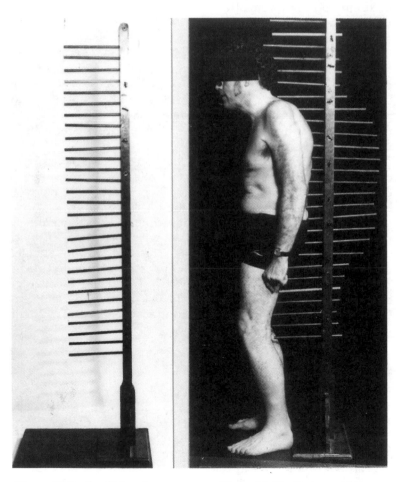

Figure 13.9. Spondylometer.

Figure 13.10. Patient with ankylosing spondylitis being measured with a spondylometer.

the base of the upright (*Figure 13.10*). Rods are spaced at 5cm intervals and are adjusted to make light skin contact over the spine. Measurements of the patient's overall height, level of the vertex, 7th cervical vertebra, posterior superior iliac spines and the head of the fibula are taken. The distance of protrusion of the rods from the upright is recorded and the measurements plotted on graph paper (*Figures 13.11* and *13.12*). For comparative purposes, spondylographs should be plotted annually. Serial photographs are also valuable for recording the progression of the disease.

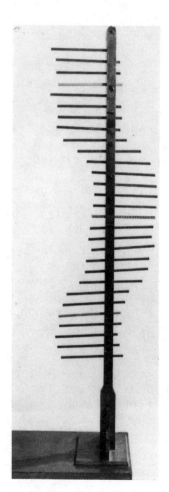

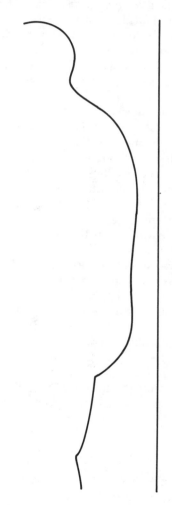

Figure 13.11. Outline of the posture on the spondylometer.

Figure 13.12. Spondylograph trace of the patient shown in Figure 13.10.

Measurement of spinal mobility   Cervical spine is measured separately with recordings made of active and passive ranges of flexion, extension, lateral flexion and rotation:

- *Thoraco-lumbar flexion and extension*: The sacrococcygeal junction and the spine of the 7th cervical vertebra are identified and the overlying skin marked. The distance between the two points is measured in the erect position, in full forward flexion, and in full extension. The difference between the measurements is an indirect indicator of spinal movement.
- *Lumbar spine flexion and extension*: The space between the 4th and 5th lumbar vertebrae and a point 10cm above are identified and the overlying skin marked. Again, the difference between the measurements taken at full flexion and extension is an indicator of spinal movement (Schober's index).
- *Lateral flexion*: The Schober's markings are extended laterally with a tape. The measurements on the right side measure left side flexion.
- *Rotation*: This is measured either in sitting to prevent pelvic movement — the patient turns his shoulders to either side and the angle created is noted — or in lying with hips and knees flexed — the pelvis is rotated on the spine and the angle created is noted.
- *Wall tragus*: This is a quick and worthwhile postural measurement. Heels must be against the wall and the body as erect as possible with the chin retracted.

Assessment of respiratory function   Involvement of the costovertebral joints in spondylitis results in limitation of chest expansion and a compromise of lung function. Chest expansion is measured at two levels — the xiphoid process (7th rib) and the nipple — and the difference noted between full inspiration and expiration. More formal measures of lung function can also be made using a spirometer.

Treatment   If untreated, ankylosing spondylitis can be a crippling disease with severe and predictable deformity and loss of mobility, but with appropriate management, patients are able to maintain a high level of independence. The aims of physical treatment are to retain spinal mobility, minimise deformity, and relieve päin. These aims are achieved mainly through active exercise.

    For the exercise programme to succeed, the patient must know the purpose of each exercise and be committed to a daily routine. The exercises should be simple, specific and require no apparatus. They will include mobilising exercises for the spine, hips and thoracic cage, posture correction and activities designed to improve muscle endurance.

Regular attendance in the department enables the physiotherapist to assess the patient and provide continuing advice about the importance of home exercising. Several patients may be treated together, as spondylitics respond well to group therapy.

Maintenance of mobility Movement of the spine may delay the rate of ankylosis, but not prevent it from occurring, so it is most important that the spine is moved daily through the full range of movement. Maitland mobilisation techniques can be used to free movement within the existing range. Although these techniques are suitable for any joint, they are particularly valuable for the facet and costovertebral joints and the type of mobilisation depends on the activity of the disease. Vigorous active exercises are performed wherever possible and it is advantageous to use a medium that supports body weight, allowing muscular effort to be devoted solely to producing movement. Support of the lower part of the body in axial suspension centred over the lumbar spine will allow flexion, extension or lateral flexion to be achieved by swinging to either side from a side-lying or lying position. Similarly, hip extension and abduction is encouraged.

Pool therapy is very beneficial: the warm water effectively reduces muscle guarding and improves joint mobility. Swimming, particularly breast stroke, is encouraged as this exercise not only improves endurance, but also promotes extension of the spine and mobilisation of the hip and shoulder girdle. Bad Ragaz patterns for arms, legs and trunk are effective in restoring mobility. Group treatments improve motivation and competition between patients which, in turn, encourage more sustained effort. Group therapy is also more economical in time for the physiotherapist.

Exercises to improve expansion of the thoracic cage and breathing are required to maintain lung function.

Minimising deformity If the spine ankyloses in a poor position, then function is impaired. Therefore, early and continued attention to good positioning is essential. Sleeping on a firm mattress is encouraged with one pillow to keep the spine extended. Adjustment of the height of chairs and work surfaces is advised to prevent stooping. A period of prone or supine lying will preserve hip extension. The wearing of spinal supports or prolonged bed rest is discouraged, because posture is threatened by weakening of the spinal muscles.

Relief of pain The symptoms of sacro-ileitis are often the initial reason for seeking medical advise in early spondylitis. Anti-inflammatory drugs are helpful, but pain associated with protective muscle spasm is relieved by hot packs or pool therapy. The pain from spinal joints is often alleviated by mobilisations, ultrasound

or TNS. Over-vigorous exercises and contact sports are best avoided by spondylitics, as the spine is brittle and prone to fracture and the resulting pain is difficult to treat with physiotherapy.
The outlook for the motivated patient who is well instructed is good. Out-patient physiotherapy is necessary when pain increases or further assistance is needed with the exercise programme. An admission to hospital is brought about by a flare of the disease with poor control of pain at home. Here physiotherapy involves an intensive period of the various treatments outlined, with education being a most important aspect of therapy.

Psoriatic arthritis

Arthritis occurs in 10–20% of patients with psoriasis. Why this particular complication of a common skin disorder happens is not known. Certainly, the characteristic plaques of psoriasis seen on the skin are not found in the joints. If the inflamed synovium is examined pathologically, the changes are very similar to those found in rheumatoid arthritis. As in the other spondyloarthritic conditions, a common genetic link is likely to be the relevant answer, as the skin and joint disease tend to run an independent course.

Clinical features
Five separate patterns of disease can be identified in psoriatic arthritis:

- Nail and interphalangeal joint disease.
- Persistent monoarthritis.
- Rheumatoid-variant.
- Ankylosing spondylitis-variant.
- Arthritis mutilans.

The most common, and fortunately the most benign, pattern of disease is localised swelling, which occurs at the distal inter-phalangeal joints in the fingers and toes, associated with florid and dystrophic nail changes. This is quite unsightly (*Figure 13.13*) but does not normally impede function or involve joints elsewhere. A monoarthritis usually involves either the wrist or knee and can be very destructive locally and unresponsive to treatment. The joint frequently presents before the skin disease, especially in children. Outlook is good as the lesion is amenable to surgical intervention. The rheumatoid-variant is often identical to rheumatoid arthritis, but without rheumatoid factor in the blood and,

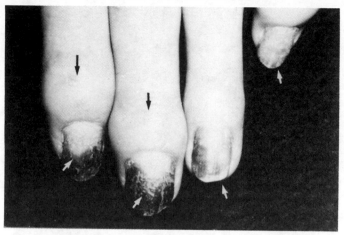

Figure 13.13. Nail and IP disease in psoriatic arthritis.

indeed, is probably rheumatoid arthritis with coincidental psoriasis. However, there is polyarticular psoriatic arthritis which is distinguishable from rheumatoid arthritis by the involvement of distal interphalangeal joints, a rather asymmetric pattern of disease, especially in the hands and feet, and cervical spine fusion.

This is an aggressive disease whose outlook is probably worse than rheumatoid arthritis. The spondylitic-variant again is similar to ankylosing spondylitis in most respects, with a high incidence of HLA-B27; in comparison, however, peripheral joint involvement is more frequent and the finding of unilateral sacro-ileitis and 'skip' lesions in the spine, should raise the possibility of psoriatic arthritis. Arthritis mutilans is a most aggressive disease affecting the small joints of the hands and feet. In the hands, the metacarpophalangeal and interphalangeal joints are destroyed and resorbed with instability and the fingers can be telescoped in and out like a concertina (*Figure 13.14*) and function is obviously poor. Fortunately, arthritis mutilans is rare.

Investigations

There are no serological markers for psoriatic arthritis, unlike rheumatoid arthritis. The sedimentation rate may be elevated but is a poor marker of disease activity. In polyarticular psoriatic arthritis, the configuration of joint damage seen on X-ray is similar to that in rheumatoid arthritis, but the finding of asymmetric changes and a periosteal reaction along bone shafts are distinguishing features.

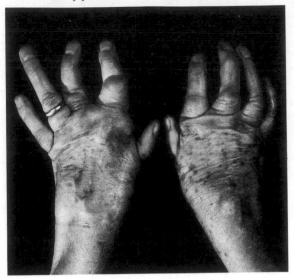

Figure 13.14. Arthritis mutilans.

Treatment

The principles of treatment are similar to the arthropathies that psoriatic arthritis mimics. Often, the skin disease is equally or more troublesome than the joint pains, and hospital treatment can be directed at both. Hence, the value of placing an ultraviolet source in physiotherapy departments. The principles of drug treatment are again similar to those of rheumatoid arthritis, but the role of specific anti-rheumatic drugs is less clearly defined. Treatment with gold and penicillamine is only occasionally effective, if at all. The verdict on sulphasalizine is 'open'. Methotrexate is the most effective treatment, both for skin and joints, and is the drug of choice. It is a cytotoxic drug and, therefore, can only be used in the more severe disease. Unfortunately, many patients with psoriatic arthritis have progressive and relentless disease, despite drug therapy, and here, physiotherapy and timed surgical intervention are important.

Physiotherapy

The physiotherapy depends on the type of arthritis the psoriatic arthropathy resembles. For instance, in the rheumatoid-variant, the treatment is the same as that for the parent disease. The management of skin and joints is usually separate.

Skin Topical therapy includes one or more of the following:

- Coal tar derivatives.
- Dithranol.
- Corticosteroids.
- Ultraviolet.
- Salicylic acid.

Coal tar, with or without salicylic acid, is beneficial in some cases and may be combined with ultraviolet. If not successful, dithranol (0.05% increasing to 2%) is indicated, but must be applied precisely on the lesions as it is a skin irritant. Dithranol is better for larger plaques, avoiding the face and flexor creases, and may be combined with tar baths and ultraviolet. This treatment is best given as an in-patient. Topical steroids are occasionally used for lesions on the head. Various shampoos are available for the scalp.

In severe cases, systemic therapy is required. Methotrexate, as mentioned above, has the added advantage in that it is effective for both joints and skin. The use of long-wave irradiation with a psoralen drug is very successful.

Reactive arthritis (Reiter's syndrome)

Many rheumatologists believe that reactive arthritis and Reiter's syndrome are the same disease. Others would diagnose Reiter's syndrome when the infection, which triggers reactive arthritis, cannot be identified. In this text, the two conditions will be considered as synonymous. Reactive arthritis is an aseptic arthritis triggered by an acute infection, either in the large bowel or genito-urinary tract at a site distant to the joint(s). The list of micro-organisms that can trigger reactive arthritis is growing ever longer (*Table 13.1*). There is a high incidence of HLA-B27 in those who suffer with reactive arthritis and so, in this disease, there is a clear link between the host (HLA-B27) and the environment (the infecting micro-organism) combining to produce arthritis. Therefore, not only is this disease important scientifically, but it is also the most common type of inflammatory arthritis in young people. How an infection outside the joint might cause disease within is not understood. Recently, fragments of the arthritogenic micro-organisms have been found in joint material obtained from patients with reactive arthritis. So it would appear that micro-organisms do travel between the site of the triggering infection and the joint, but neither how they do so nor whether they are viable on arrival is known.

Table 13.1. Micro-organisms implicated in reactive arthritis.

Enteric infections:
Salmonella typhimurium
Salmonella enteritidis
Shigella flexneri
Yersinia enterocolitica
Campylobacter jejuni

Genito-urinary infection:
Chlamydia trachomatis
Mycoplasma spp.

Clinical features

The triggering infection occurs 10–20 days before the onset of arthritis. In gut-associated reactive arthritis, there is normally a history of an acute diarrhoea from which the patient is just recovering at the onset of arthritis. Sexually associated reactive arthritis is normally manifest in men by a urethral discharge and history of new sexual contact. Very often, by the time the arthritis presents, the patients have already received antibiotics for non-specific urethritis diagnosed in a genito-urinary clinic. But in women, the triggering genital infection is frequently asymptomatic. Non-purulent conjunctivitis (*Figure 13.15*) at the onset of

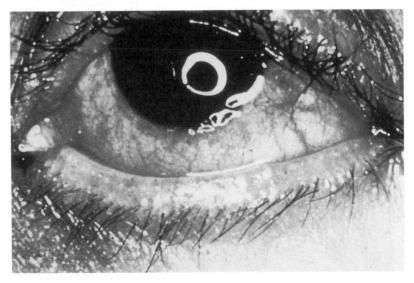

Figure 13.15. Conjunctivitis in a patient with Reiter's syndrome.

the arthritis is a further diagnostic feature (hence, the classical triad of Reiter's syndrome: urethritis, conjunctivitis and arthritis). Reactive arthritis is more common in men, so the presenting picture is of a young man with an acutely swollen knee, red eyes and history of penile discharge or food poisoning. The onset of arthritis is abrupt and the patients are often admitted into hospital to exclude a septic arthritis. Normally, knee and ankle are involved but an odd metatarsal- or metacarpal-phalangeal joint can become inflamed. The finding of plantar fasciitis in a man with unexplained arthritis would strongly implicate a reactive process. In men, a circinate balanitis on the penis and keratoderma blenorrhagica on the feet (a rash indistinguishable from pustular psoriasis, *Figure 13.16*) are the cutaneous manifestations. Rarely, the

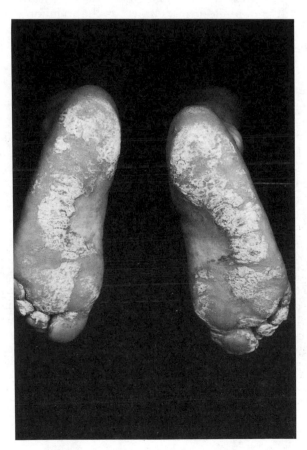

Figure 13.16. Keratoderma blenorrhagica.

arthritis is accompanied by systemic illness with high fevers, pericarditis and aortitis. In the majority, the arthritis resolves within 6 months and in 90% by a year. In 10%, the disease persists with a destructive arthropathy affecting small joints of hands and feet and, occasionally, spondylitis is seen. The presence of HLA-B27 is a risk factor for persisting disease.

Investigations

The presence of a leucocytosis in joint fluid (>50 000 cells/ml) and a prominent neutrophilic infiltration found on synovial biopsy, in the absence of joint infection, is typical of reactive arthritis, but these pathological features are by no means diagnostic because similar changes can be seen in early rheumatoid arthritis. The ESR is usually elevated and markedly so with the systemic complications described above. In the minority of case, antinuclear antibodies are present in the blood. It is worthwhile culturing both the gut and genito-urinary tract, as the triggering infections are often still active at the onset of arthritis. Further evidence of infection is available from measuring specific serological responses to micro-organisms in the blood.

Treatment

There is clearly a strong rationale for antibiotic therapy but, unfortunately, there appears to be no benefit. Similarly, the benefits of anti-rheumatic drugs are disappointing, but their use is limited by the knowledge that the majority of patients will improve without specific treatment. Recurrent aspirations of the knee with local steroid infiltration are frequently required and, if the disease persists, a surgical synovectomy may be indicated. Systemic steroids are given for the systemic complications.

Physiotherapy

In the acute stage, rest is essential with splintage of the severely affected joints. Supine and prone lying should be encouraged. Free active exercises should follow, with attention to back extension and postural advice, if the spine is stiff. Plantar fasciitis is treated with ultrasound and the provision of heel pads. Persisting disease resembles ankylosing spondylitis and should be treated in the same way.

14 Miscellaneous Inflammatory Arthropathies

R.C. Butler and M. Kerr

This chapter includes discussion of the crystal arthropathies; systemic disorders of connective tissue, such as systemic lupus erythematosus (SLE), vasculitis, infective arthritis and some less common diseases. These various disorders are less common than are osteoarthritis and rheumatoid arthritis, but are encountered fairly frequently in hospital practice and may require treatment by physiotherapists.

Crystal arthritis

This group of disorders comprises gout, pseudogout (chondrocalcinosis or calcium pyrophosphate deposition disease) and basic calcium phosphate (apatite) arthropathy.

Gout

Gout occurs more frequently in men than women in a ratio of about 6:1. It is rare before the age of 20 and in women is most uncommon before the menopause. It typically occurs in three categories of patient: young men with a strong family history of the disease; middle-aged men who drink too much alcohol; and elderly women on long-term diuretic therapy.

Gout results from an excess of uric acid, either due to excessive production or diminished excretion. Increased production occurs in obesity, polycythaemia and myeloproliferative disorders; in other patients there appears to be increased activity of the metabolic pathways by which uric acid is produced. Diminished excretion occurs with diuretic therapy and in chronic renal failure; many gouty patients without overt renal disease appear to have a reduced capacity to excrete uric acid. Urate is poorly soluble in tissue fluids and prolonged periods of hyperuricaemia (>0.45μmol/l) result in precipitation of urate crystals in synovium, cartilage, tendon sheaths and bursae. Aggregates of urate crystals over joints and tendons are known as tophi; they are typically yellow—orange in colour and non-tender, but can become acutely inflamed. They are often seen in the pulps and over the interphalangeal joints of the fingers, in the helix of the ear, in the olecranon bursa and around the great toe.

Clinical features

Acute gout This is an acutely painful condition in which symptoms of acute inflammation (pain, swelling, erythema, increased temperature and loss of function) develop suddenly and typically reach peak intensity within 24—48 hours. The great toe metatarsophalangel joint is affected in some 70% of cases, but knees, ankles, wrists and olecranon bursae of the elbow are also commonly affected. Acute episodes may be precipitated by trauma (explaining, perhaps, the frequency of great toe involvement), starvation, dehydration, surgery, an alcoholic binge or use of diuretics. Affected joints become exquisitely painful and tender, and the pressure of bedclothes may be unbearable. When lower limbs are affected walking may be impossible. Symptoms generally settle over a period of 1—3 weeks, sometimes with desquamation of overlying skin.

Acute gout is most commonly confused with septic arthritis and the two conditions can only be distinguished with confidence by aspiration and examination of joint fluid. Pseudogout, palindromic rheumatism, Reiter's syndrome and rheumatoid arthritis sometimes present similarly.

Chronic gout Since the advent of effective treatment for gout in the late 1960s, chronic gout has become relatively uncommon. It is still seen from time to time, typically in elderly ladies on long-term diuretic therapy, in whom tophi may be mistaken for Heberden's nodes, and in alcoholics. Tophi may also be confused with rheumatoid nodules or with xanthomata: lipid deposits found in patients with hyperlipidaemia (*Figure 14.1*).

Diagnosis A diagnosis of gout is usually made on the basis of the clinical features of an acute attack. Definitive diagnosis is achieved by identification of urate crystals in joint fluid by polarising microscopy. The vast majority of patients with gout have a raised serum urate, but so do significant numbers of asymptomatic persons so this test alone does not permit a diagnosis. X-rays show typical changes in advanced disease but are normal early in the course of the disease and are thus of limited use for diagnosis in most cases (*Figure 14.2*).

Associated diseases As noted above, gout may be a complication of diuretic therapy, myeloproliferative disease, renal failure or

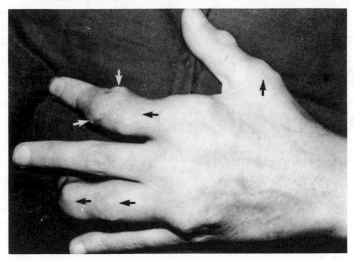

Figure 14.1. Tophaceous gout. Note *the sites of previous urate discharge.*

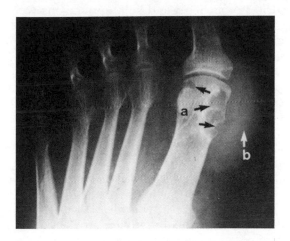

Figure 14.2. Radiograph of a foot affected by gout.
(a) Cystic and erosive change in the region of the
first metatarsophalangeal joint. (b) Soft tissue
swelling due to a tophus.

excessive alcohol intake. Hyperuricaemia leads to the excretion of increased quantities of urate in the urine and urinary calculi composed of urate occur frequently in untreated gouty patients. In addition, obesity, hypertension and hyperlipidaemia are more common in gouty patients than in the population at large.

Treatment

Acute attack One of the non-steroidal anti-inflammatory drugs (NSAIDs) will usually terminate an attack in 2—7 days. Indomethacin, naproxen and diclofenac are often used. Colchicine is an older drug with a different mode of action: it may cause troublesome diarrhoea, but some patients find it a satisfactory alternative to NSAID. Very rarely, an intra-articular steroid may be appropriate. The affected joint should be rested and the patient will usually insist on this in any case.

Long-term management Acute attacks can be treated as and when they occur or preventive therapy can be instituted. Preventive therapy requires long-term drug treatment and so should not be undertaken lightly. The usual indications are frequent attacks (more than two to three a year), chronic tophaceous gout, urinary calculi and renal disease. Allopurinol reduces the production of uric acid and is the drug of choice. It must not be started during an acute attack, since it may worsen it. Occasionally, acute attacks occur during the first weeks of allopurinol therapy so it is advisable for patients to take an NSAID or colchicine for 2—3 months after allopurinol is started. Before allopurinol became available, the uricosuric drugs probenecid and sulphinpyrazone were used and they can still be useful especially in those few patients who cannot tolerate allopurinol. They should not, however, be used in patients with renal failure or urinary calculi.

Physiotherapy In acute gout, immobilisation of the affected joint in a splint may be helpful, but little more can be done during the acute phase. In chronic gout, exercises to improve joint mobility and muscle function can be useful.

Calcium pyrophosphate deposition disease (pseudogout; chondrocalcinosis)

This condition may present as an acute arthritis similar to acute gout, hence the synonym pseudogout, or it may be an asymptomatic radiological finding, in which case it used to be known as chondrocalcinosis. Since the underlying problem in both instances is the deposition of crystals of calcium pyrophosphate in articular structures, the term calcium pyrophosphate deposition disease, or CPPD for short, is preferred.

Clinical features This condition tends to be seen in middle and later life and in a recent survey a third of patients in an acute geriatric unit had radiological evidence of the disease. An acute self-limiting arthritis similar to gout (pseudogout) is most commonly seen in the knee, but may affect the wrist, elbow, shoulder or ankle. It is sometimes associated with fever, and distinction from septic arthritis can be difficult on clinical grounds alone.

Alternatively, CPPD may be associated with chronic low-grade arthritis in many joints, with evidence of degenerative arthritis or a chronic inflammatory arthropathy similar to rheumatoid arthritis, but with negative tests for circulating rheumatoid factor. Most commonly, however, CPPD is an incidental radiological finding.

There is an association between CPPD and hyperparathyroidism, myxoedema and, less commonly, Wilson's disease and haemochromatosis, but in most cases the disease is idiopathic. Occasional pedigrees have been described with multiple affected family members, notably from Czechoslovakia, Chile and Quebec.

Diagnosis Radiology reveals calcification of fibrocartilage of the menisci of the knee, triangular ligament of the wrist and pubic symphysis. In addition, there may be calcification of the hyaline cartilage of the knee, shoulder, hip and sometimes other joints. Synovial fluid may contain crystals of calcium pyrophosphate and examination of joint fluid is the only certain means by which to distinguish this condition from gout and septic arthritis (*Figure 14.3*).

Treatment There is as yet no specific treatment for CPPD, although associated metabolic disorders will, of course, require treatment. Acute attacks of pseudogout respond to NSAIDs and

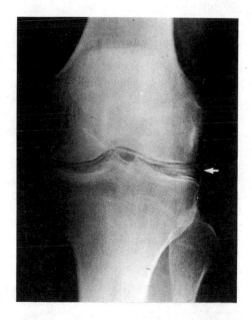

Figure 14.3. Radiograph of left knee joint showing chondrocalcinosis in a patient with pseudogout.

the more chronic forms of the condition may be helped by analgesic drugs or NSAIDs.

Basic calcium phosphate (calcium apatite) crystal deposition disease

Acute and subacute locomotor symptoms result from the deposition of basic calcium phosphate, or apatite, crystals in and around joints. Acute calcific peri-arthritis of the shoulder causes acute pain and limitation of movement, sometimes with overlying swelling, erythema and increased skin temperature. Similar acutely painful inflammatory episodes may affect the greater trochanter of the hip, the interphalangeal joints of the fingers and the tendon attachments of the collateral ligaments of the knee.

A destructive arthritis of the shoulder associated with large effusions and instability of the joint, known as Milwaukee shoulder, is also associated with large numbers of basic calcium phosphate crystals within the joint fluid. Some forms of destructive arthritis of the knee and hip also appear to be associated with such crystals (Dieppe et al., 1984). This condition may be diagnosed by the radiological features of the destructive arthritis and identification of crystals within joint fluid. There is no specific treatment, but NSAIDs are useful in acute attacks.

Systemic connective tissue disorders

These disorders have a number of clinical findings in common and individual patients may exhibit features which overlap several conditions.

Systemic lupus erythematosus

SLE is more common in women than in men in a ratio of about 10:1. There are perhaps 50 cases per 100 000 population, although milder cases may go unrecognised and the disease appears to be more common in some groups, such as Blacks and Chinese, than in Caucasians. It can present in childhood or in old age, but most cases present between the ages of 20 and 50. The clinical manifestations are variable and individual patients rarely show all the features listed below, but systemic symptoms, such as malaise, weight-loss and lymphadenopathy, are common. New clinical features may develop over a number of years.

Clinical features
- Rashes are common, the characteristic one being an erythematous area over the cheeks in a butterfly distribution, but rashes

may also affect the limbs and torso. Initiation or aggravation of the rash by sunlight (photosensitivity) is a typical feature and may lead to blistering of the skin. Discoid lupus is another type of skin lesion seen in SLE.

- Arthritis occurs in the vast majority of patients. It typically affects knees, fingers and wrists and is intermittent, migratory and symmetrical. It rarely gives rise to erosions although joint deformities may be seen.
- Mouth ulcers, usually painless, are common.
- Alopecia is often noticed by the patient and may sometimes be pronounced, either patchy or generalised.
- Raynaud's phenomenon is common, but it also occurs in other rheumatic disorders as well as in otherwise healthy people.
- Pleurisy is seen in about 45% and pericarditis in about 25% of cases.
- Renal disease affects up to 20% of patients, but varies in severity from mild proteinuria to severe glomerulonephritis with nephrotic syndrome and/or renal failure.
- Neurological involvement occurs in some 25% of patients. It varies from mild mood disturbance to psychosis, and convulsions or focal lesions including stroke.
- Recurrent miscarriage occurs in some patients with SLE.

Laboratory abnormalities Anaemia, leucopenia and thrombocytopenia are common. In addition, the disease is remarkable for the frequency of autoantibodies, i.e. antibodies directed against normal tissue components. Antinuclear antibody (ANF) is present in the serum of the vast majority of patients, but antibodies to double-stranded DNA are of greater diagnostic value. Other autoantibodies may be found and some of these tend to be associated with particular disease manifestations, see *Table 14.1.*

Table 14.1. Associations between autoantibodies and disease manifestations.

Autoantibodies	Disease manifestation
anti-RNP	Raynaud's phenomenon
anti-Ro	Sjögren's syndrome
anti-Jo-1	Myositis plus fibrosing alveolitis
anti-Phospholipid	Thrombocytopenia, miscarriage and thrombosis

Management Education of the patient is important since ignorance and misconceptions are common, even among health workers. In particular, patients must be told that sunlight may exacerbate their disease and advised to avoid strong sunlight and to use wide-brimmed hats and a high factor sunscreen lotion. In mild cases, treatment with NSAID may suffice, but where skin and joint problems are troublesome hydroxychloroquine can be useful. Corticosteroids may be needed in more severe cases, while cytotoxic drugs including azathioprine and cyclophosphamide are often used in patients with renal or neurological disease. Major organ involvement can be life-threatening and in previous years the disease was often fatal, but with recognition of milder cases and improved management, the 10-year survival in SLE in now some 90%.

Physiotherapy The arthritis of SLE tends to resemble that of rheumatoid arthritis, but is episodic and, as noted above, bone and cartilage destruction is rare and joint deformity relatively uncommon. The physiotherapist should teach the patient how to manage joint symptoms during acute episodes, concentrating on relief of pain, reduction of swelling and improvement of muscle strength. Generalised muscle tenderness and weakness may result from an associated myositis and may limit mobility during exacerbations. A carefully graded exercise programme may improve muscle strength and endurance.

Scleroderma

This is a connective tissue disorder characterised by thickening and fibrosis of the skin, which is often associated with involvement of internal organs. It is fairly rare, affecting some 10 new cases per million population a year. It is more common in women than men in a ratio of about 3:1, with the peak age of onset between 30–50 years.

Clinical features Severe Raynaud's phenomenon is a common presenting feature and a mild inflammatory polyarthropathy is not uncommon at onset. The skin becomes tethered to underlying structures so that it cannot be pinched up; on the dorsum of the finger this gives rise to sclerodactyly (*Figure 14.4*). Similar changes may occur on limbs and torso and, when the face is affected, restricted mouth opening is a common problem. Impaired mobility of the distal oesophagus often leads to dysphagia, reflux oesophagitis and stricture, and other manifestations of internal organ involvement include pulmonary fibrosis and pericarditis. Severe hypertension with rapidly progressive renal failure (scleroderma renal crisis) may develop suddenly and is commonly fatal.

Occasionally, calcific deposits (*Figure 14.5*) develop on the fingers, forearms and elsewhere, which may discharge. This is a characteristic feature of the CREST (Calcinosis; (o)Esophageal

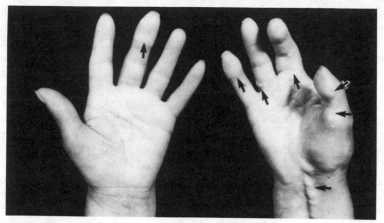

Figure 14.4. *Systemic sclerosis with multiple calcific deposits.*

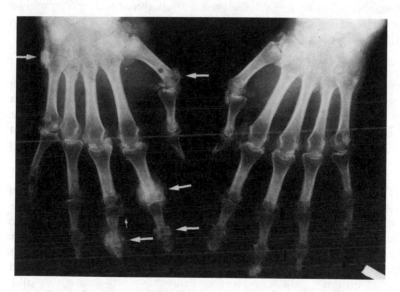

Figure 14.5. *Radiograph showing calcification in hands affected by systemic sclerosis.*

dysmotility; Sclerodactyly; Telangiectasia) variant of scleroderma, which generally has less internal organ involvement and a better prognosis than diffuse scleroderma.

The cause of the condition is unknown. Although the diagnosis is made on clinical grounds, many patients have a positive test for antinuclear antibody and two autoantibodies are often found in scleroderma: centromere antibodies, which are associated with CREST and a relatively good prognosis, and Scl-70 antibodies, which tend to be seen in patients with the more severe form of the disease. Drug therapy is disappointing, but penicillamine is often used and corticosteroids may be helpful for specific problems. Captopril has greatly improved the management of scleroderma renal crisis and cimetadine has reduced oesophageal problems.

Physiotherapy Progressive thickening and tethering of the skin of the fingers leads to restricted joint movement and muscle wasting with loss of hand function and disability. Physiotherapy plays a vital role in preserving mobility and in the prevention of contractures. Massage, passive stretching and active exercises all have their place, but must be instituted early before irreversible changes have developed.

Polymyositis and dermatomyositis

These conditions are characterised by a damaging inflammatory process in muscle, which leads to muscle weakness; in dermatomyositis there is in addition skin involvement. Myositis is fairly uncommon, with about five new cases per million population a year; women are affected about twice as commonly as men. It can occur at any age, including childhood, but the mean age at presentation in adults is about 50 years.

Clinical features The typical finding is muscle weakness, which is most obvious in proximal muscle groups; sometimes there is associated muscle pain and tenderness. The weakness leads to difficulty in climbing stairs and rising from a chair and patients may have difficulty in holding up their arms or in sitting up from a lying position. In severe cases, weakness can be profound and affect muscles of respiration. Polymyositis may occur as an isolated disease or in association with another connective tissue disease, such as SLE. The typical rash of dermatomyositis is an oedematous violet one ('heliotrope'), affecting the eyelids and extensor surfaces of the fingers, elbows and knees. In some adults dermatomyositis is the presenting feature of an underlying neoplasm, so all adults presenting with this condition need careful evaluation. Polymyositis in the child resembles the adult disease, but dermatomyositis in children is often associated with calcification of muscles and subcutaneous tissues and a vasculitis.

The diagnosis is made on the basis of clinical features and confirmed by elevation of serum creatinine kinase (CK) and muscle biopsy. Oral corticosteroids form the mainstay of treatment, but immunosuppressive drugs, such as azathioprine, are sometimes used in patients with severe disease.

Physiotherapy   Serial measurements of muscle strength and lung function are invaluable in the assessment of activity of the disease. During acute phases, rest is desirable and inflamed muscles should not be over-stretched; splinting may be valuable. Exercises should begin only as strength returns and they should be introduced gradually. Trunk muscles are often affected and mat work can give gratifying results.

Overlap connective tissue disorders

Some patients present with features of several connective tissue disorders, most commonly SLE, scleroderma and polymyositis. One such variant is known as mixed connective tissue disease, in which features of these three conditions overlap and are associated with marked Raynaud's phenomenon and a circulating auto-antibody known as anti-RNP. Initial studies suggested that the prognosis in this condition was better than in typical SLE, but more recent work has thrown doubt upon this.

Sjögren's syndrome

The term 'sicca syndrome' is applied to the co-existence of dry eyes (keratoconjunctivitis sicca) and dry mouth (xerostomia). This is known as primary Sjögren's syndrome when it occurs alone and secondary when it is associated with another inflammatory rheumatic disease, most often rheumatoid arthritis, SLE or scleroderma. Vaginal dryness is also a feature of the condition. Sicca syndrome is present in some 20% of patients with rheumatoid arthritis and leads to a sensation of dryness and/or grittiness of the eye, which may become red or even ulcerate. Impaired tear secretion can be confirmed by use of Schirmer's test paper and typical inflammatory changes can be seen on biopsy of minor salivary glands. Artificial tears, which may have to be used frequently, mouthwashes and vaginal lubricants are all useful. Patients with primary Sjögren's syndrome are at increased risk of developing lymphoma.

Polymyalgia rheumatica

This is a disease of older age and is relatively uncommon before the age of 60. Women are affected about twice as commonly as men. It is fairly common, with an annual incidence of about 35 cases per 100000 population aged more than 50.

Onset may be abrupt (overnight) or insidious, with a characteristic history of aching in muscles of the shoulder and hip girdles at night and disabling muscle stiffness in the morning, which makes it difficult for the patient to get out of bed. Muscles may be tender, but there is no wasting. Systemic features, such as malaise, anorexia, weight-loss and fever, may occur and occasionally patients develop arthralgia or arthritis, which may suggest a diagnosis of rheumatoid arthritis. The diagnosis is usually made on the basis of the history, but ESR and plasma viscosity are typically raised.

Oral corticosteroids are required to abolish symptoms and usually do so within 72 hours. The dose is then gradually reduced, but a significant minority of patients still require oral steroids 2 years after the onset of the disease. A few patients also have, or develop, symptoms of temporal arteritis (see below) with headaches and scalp tenderness; such patients need much higher doses of steroids to reduce the risk of visual failure.

Behçet's syndrome

This is a multi-system disorder of unknown aetiology characterised by the triad of oral and genital ulceration and relapsing uveitis. Arthritis occurs in some 50% of patients, but chronic deforming arthritis is rare. Other features, such as cutaneous vasculitis and focal neurological lesions, may occur. It is most often seen in Greece, Turkey and Japan, but also occurs in the UK, especially in ethnic groups.

Vasculitis

This term includes a heterogeneous group of disorders all characterised by vasculitis: inflammation within the walls of blood vessels. This inflammatory process often leads to thrombosis of the vessel with consequent ischaemia of the tissue it supplies, e.g. skin ulcer, and may weaken the vessel wall and cause haemorrhage. Classification of this group of disorders is notoriously difficult, but a practical guide is given in Table 14.2.

Polyarteritis nodosa is the best known of these conditions and is characterised by widespread vasculitic lesions, such as purpuric or necrotising ulcers on the legs, arthritis, neuropathy, renal involvement, gastrointestinal haemorrhage and scleritis. Lung involvement may occur in polyarteritis, but is even more common in Wegener's granulomatosis, in which cavitating lung lesions, sinusitis and renal failure are common. Churg−Strauss vasculitis resembles these diseases and is associated with pronounced eosinophilia. The vasculitis of rheumatoid arthritis is discussed in Chapter 12. High-dose corticosteroid therapy is generally required for these conditions and cyclophosphamide is often used, especially in Wegener's granulomatosis where it has greatly improved survival. Henoch−Schönlein purpura occurs in both childhood and adult life and is characterised by purpuric lesions on the lower limbs and buttocks, often with abdominal pain and sometimes gastrointestinal haemorrhage. This tends to be milder

Table 14.2. Classification of vasculitis.

1. *Systemic necrotising vasculitis*

   • Polyarteritis nodosa group
   • With granulomatosis: Wegener's; Churg—Strauss

2. *Small vessel vasculitis*

   • Henoch—Schönlein purpura
   • Cryoglobulinaemia
   • Drug-induced vasculitis
   • Vasculitis of RA, SLE

3. *Giant cell arteritis*

   • Temporal arteritis
   • Takayasu's arteritis

than the forms of vasculitis discussed so far, but can be life-threatening, especially when there is renal involvement.

Temporal arteritis may occur by itself or in association with polymyalgia rheumatica. The typical clinical presentation is with severe headaches and tenderness of the temporal arteries, which may be so pronounced that it is impossible for the patient to comb his hair. Jaw claudication also occurs. The main concern is that the ophthalmic artery may be similarly affected with the abrupt onset of irreversible blindness. High-dose steroid therapy must be started as soon as the diagnosis is made so as to reduce the risk of this complication.

Physiotherapy
There is no specific form of physiotherapy for patients with vasculitis. Arthritic symptoms can be treated along conventional lines, but ice should be used with some caution in view of the theoretical risk of further reducing blood flow through inflamed vessels. Treatments which raise core temperature may improve circulation to the limbs, but if heat is applied to a limb with vasculitic lesions the patient may experience an exacerbation of pain. Buerger's exercises may give some symptomatic relief.

Erythema nodosum

The lesions of erythema nodosum typically occur on the front of the shins and are extremely painful, raised, tender, red lesions each the size of a ten-pence piece. They may become confluent and resemble cellulitis and there is often an associated acute arthritis of the knees and ankles. The lesions are caused by a vasculitis affecting vessels in the subcutaneous fat and may be precipitated by drug hypersensitivity or infection with streptococci, Yersinia and numerous other micro-organisms. Sarcoidosis is another common cause when bilateral hilar adenopathy will usually be seen on chest X-ray, and inflammatory bowel disease is also associated with erythema nodosum. The lesions generally resolve within several weeks, but arthralgia may persist for several months and, although the use of NSAIDs will usually suffice, oral steroids may be required in severe cases.

Infective arthritis

Septic arthritis
This typically presents as an acutely painful arthritis of a large joint, such as the knee, hip or elbow. There is often overlying erythema and usually, but not always, a pyrexia. Septic arthritis is seen particularly in children, the elderly, those with pre-existing joint disease (especially rheumatoid arthritis) and in immunocompromised patients with malignancy or AIDS.

Symptoms are not always florid and if the possibility of sepsis is considered then it is vital to aspirate the joint at once and culture the synovial fluid. Septic arthritis is a medical emergency since the joint will rapidly suffer severe damage unless antibiotic treatment is started quickly. *Staph. aureus* is commonly responsible and *Strep. pyogenes* and *Strep. pneumoniae* are encountered fairly frequently. Gram-negative bacilli tend to be seen in immunocompromised patients, while *Haemophilus influenzae* is commonly responsible in childhood.

Gonococcal arthritis
This is now the commonest form of bacterial arthritis in the USA and some other Western countries (O'Brien *et al.*, 1983). Women are affected about four times as often as men and, as one might expect, it is most common in the 15–40 age group. It may present as polyarthralgia with fever or as an oligoarthritis, often of the knee and ankle with tenosynovitis of a finger. Characteristic pustular skin lesions may be seen on the distal limbs and the diagnosis can be confirmed by identification of the organism in synovial fluid, blood culture or from an appropriate orifice. Prompt therapy with high-dose penicillin is effective and sexual contacts should be traced, investigated and if appropriate treated for gonorrhoea.

Viral arthritis

Several different viruses are known to cause arthritis and undoubtedly further arthritogenic viruses will be identified in the future. Rubella commonly causes a transient arthritis and occasionally prolonged arthralgia; joint symptoms can follow immunisation as well as infection with the wild virus. Parvovirus causes an acute febrile illness with facial rash and rubella-like rash in children, and recently it has been recognised as a cause of acute arthritis in adults, which occasionally takes some months to disappear (Reid *et al.*, 1985). Arthritis is also common following infection with the hepatitis B virus. Patients infected by the HIV virus can suffer severe arthritis, but it is not at present clear whether this is due to the virus itself, to some other infective agent or to an abnormal immunological process.

Lyme disease

This was first noted in Lyme, Connecticut, in children who developed arthritis following a skin rash (erythema chronicum migrans) caused by a tick bite. It is now known to be an infection caused by the spirochaete *Borrelia burgdorferi*, which is carried by some wild animals, notably deer, and transmitted to humans via the tick (Steere, 1989). Cardiac and neurological problems may also occur. Chronic arthritis was seen in untreated patients, but most patients respond well to high-dose penicillin. It is fairly common in New England and sporadic cases are seen in the UK and Europe.

Arthritis associated with malignancy

In childhood, acute leukaemia may present as a polyarthritis and forms part of the differential diagnosis of juvenile polyarthritis. Occasional adult patients present with an inflammatory polyarthritis, usually seronegative for rheumatoid factor, which often remits with successful treatment of the underlying tumour. Hypertrophic osteoarthropathy with marked clubbing of fingers and tenderness of long bones around the wrists, knees and ankles may be associated with non-inflammatory effusions of the knees; it is usually due to carcinoma of the bronchus. Primary tumours can arise in bone, cartilage and synovium, but are fortunately uncommon. Metastatic deposits in bone may simulate arthritis but secondary depositis within the joint itself are very rare.

Haemophilic arthritis

Haemophilia A is caused by a deficiency of clotting factor VIII and haemophilia B (Christmas disease) of factor IX; they are inherited diseases which affect males and are transmitted by asymptomatic female carriers. Acute haemarthrosis is common and affects particularly the knees, elbows and ankles: pain, effusion and loss of movement occur suddenly and are sometimes associated with pyrexia (Arnold and Hilgartner, 1977). Haemarthrosis usually first occurs at 12–18 months of age, when the child begins to run, and attacks continue throughout childhood, but tend to abate in adult life. Recurrent episodes can lead to severe secondary degenerative arthritis. There may be premonitory symptoms of aching or pricking in the joints and these should not be ignored, since it is vital to institute treatment as soon as possible so as to reduce the risk of joint damage.

Essential treatment consists of infusion of the deficient clotting factor. Joint aspiration is usually part of the management of acute haemarthrosis, but in this condition it runs the risk of exacerbating the bleeding and must not be attempted before the clotting factor deficiency has been corrected. The affected joint should be immobilised, possibly with elevation, and ice packs may help. Once bleeding has been controlled, and generally after 24–48 hours, gentle range of motion and isometric exercises can be started. Affected joints must however be treated with respect since excessive exercise may lead to further bleeding.

References

Arnold, W.D. and Hilgartner, M.W. (1977). Hemophilic arthropathy. *Journal of Bone and Joint Surgery*, **59A**, 287–305.

Dieppe, P.A., Doherty, M., Macfarlane, D.G. *et al.*, (1984). Apatite associated destructive arthritis. *British Journal of Rheumatology*, **23**, 84–91.

O'Brien, J.P., Goldenberg, D.L. and Rice, P.A. (1983). Disseminated gonococcal infection. *Medicine*, **62**, 395–406.

Reid, D.M., Brown, T., Reid, T.M.S., *et al.* (1985). Human parvovirus-associated arthritis. *Lancet*, **1**, 422–425.

Steere, A.C. (1989). Lyme disease. *New England Journal of Medicine*, **321**, 586–596.

Bibliography

Kelley, W.N., Harris, E.D., Ruddy, S. and Sledge, C.B. (1989). *Textbook of Rheumatology*, 3rd edition. W.B. Saunders, Philadelphia.

Rheumatic Disease Clinics of North America (1988). *Systemic Lupus Erythematosus*, **14**(1), 1–252.

Rheumatic Disease Clinics of North America (1990). *Vasculitic Syndromes*. **16**(2), 251–497.

Scott, J.T. (1986). *Copeman's Textbook of the Rheumatic Diseases*, 6th edition. Churchill Livingstone, Edinburgh.

15 Osteoarthritis

D.J. Ward and M.E. Tidswell, updated by J.J. Dixey and M. Kerr

This is the commonest single form of arthritis and dates back to ancient times. Examples may be found in many different species apart from man. It is the end result of a series of changes which may be triggered by many different mechanisms, and several of these are now recognised. The arthritis is designated as *primary* or *secondary* depending upon whether a precipitating factor is known. As more causes are found, the incidence of the primary type diminishes.

Osteoarthritis is often regarded as a progressive process associated with getting older. There is, however, little evidence to support either an ageing or 'wear and tear' phenomenon. It should be regarded as the end result of abnormal mechanical, inflammatory, metabolic, physiological or pathological factors. There is no doubt that the incidence of the disease is higher in the elderly, but the clinical presentation may not be apparent for many years after the initial insult to the joint. During this time there is even the chance of reversibility if the initiating factors are corrected. It becomes obvious that recognition of these factors and their correction should reduce the incidence of osteoarthritis.

Terminology is confusing. Because the disease does not display such intense inflammatory changes as are seen in rheumatoid arthritis, there has been a tendency to call it 'osteoarthritis'. Although mild, and probably secondary, inflammation is present, however, and there seems little point in changing from osteoarthritis. Degenerative joint disease is unsuitable as also is hypertrophic arthritis (a reference to the new bone formation — osteophytes — seen in the disease) and none of these terms adequately describes the true nature of the process. *Osteoarthritis* is the term used in this chapter.

Epidemiology

Radiological evidence is much commoner than clinically recognisable disease. Symptoms may be present only in some 15% of those with radiological change, but after the age of 60 over 80% of the population will have some radiological evidence of osteoarthritis. Factors that trigger the disease may be present at birth or in early childhood, and even at the age of 20 there is a 10% incidence of radiographic abnormality.

It is equally as common in men as in women overall, but under the age of 50 there are more men, and over the age of 50 more women affected.

The disease occurs throughout the world. There is no climatic, geographic or racial factor involved. Differing prevalence for osteoarthritis of various joints is more likely to be related to cultural and industrial variations. For example, the squatting position more favoured by Asian communities may in some way protect the head of the femur and explain the lower incidence of osteoarthritis of the hip in Orientals.

Aetiology and pathogenesis

As already mentioned, classification of osteoarthritis is based on the concept of primary and secondary disease. This may not be a valid classification in that all cases could be regarded as secondary. Some authors would prefer to differentiate between multiple site involvement and the occurrence of osteoarthritis in only one or two joints. For now, however, we will retain the concept of primary and secondary though it must be appreciated that this situation will probably change.

Primary osteoarthritis
This includes:

- *Primary generalised osteoarthritis*. This occurs particularly in postmenopausal women and may be regarded as a hereditable form of the disease. Proximal and distal interphalangeal joints in the hands, the carpometacarpal joint at the base of the thumb, cervical and lumbar spine, knees and great toes are most commonly involved. Primary generalised osteoarthritis affects women more than men (ratio 10 : 1), presents at the time of the menopause, and is typified by more severe symptoms at the onset. During the acute onset the joints look inflamed and are red and tender. The acute phase may last for several months, but gradually osteophyte formation and deformity develop. Symptoms may be episodic and the patient sometimes has a mild generalised illness. In this disease, osteophyte formation is a pronounced feature. Heberden's nodes occur at the distal

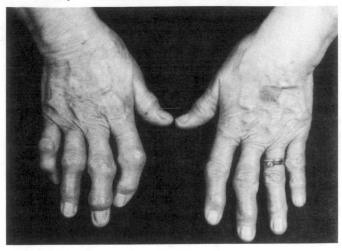

Figure 15.1. Heberden's and Bouchard's nodes in osteoarthritic hands.

interphalangeal joints in the hands and Bouchard's nodes at proximal interphalangeal joints (*Figure 15.1*).

- *Erosive interphalangeal osteoarthritis*. Again with involvement of proximal and distal interphalangeal joints, but with a different clinical and radiological pattern. The joints are subjected to attacks of inflammation with redness, tenderness and pain. Radiological changes include an erosive element and can mimic those seen in rheumatoid arthritis.
- *Idiopathic*. In many such cases, especially with hip involvement, there is probably an underlying cause which it may not be possible to identify as yet. Obesity is an important contributory factor, especially in women with knee involvement.

Secondary osteoarthritis

This may be initiated by a number of factors including:

- Developmental, e.g. hip dysplasia, slipped upper femoral epiphyses, osteochondritis dissecans, unequal leg lengths, etc.
- Inflammatory, e.g. rheumatoid arthritis and the spondylo-arthropathies.
- Infective, e.g. septic arthritis.
- Metabolic, e.g. gout, pseudogout, haemochromatosis, hydroxy-apatite crystal arthropathy (with chondrocalcinosis), Paget's disease.

- Traumatic, e.g. articular surface fracture, occupational (miners, sportsmen), hypermobility syndrome.
- Neuropathic.
- Endocrine, e.g. acromegaly.

In all these secondary cases either the stress on a joint becomes abnormal, or the ability of the joint to withstand normal stress is altered. Repetitive normal use of a normal joint does not cause osteoarthritis.

Attempts have been made to study osteoarthritis by inducing it in experimental animals. The results are interesting though difficult to explain. Immobilisation in plaster leads to cartilage degeneration. Overuse has not been shown to be associated with cartilage damage, unless there is considerable overloading as well. Altered forces across a joint will induce cartilage degeneration and this is reflected in the human following various injuries to joints. Instability leads to changes almost identical to osteoarthritis – for example, after cutting the anterior cruciate ligament of the knee, though this does not occur if the knee is immobilised in flexion postoperatively, again suggesting the importance of an alteration in the forces acting on the joint. Patellectomy can be shown to be followed by cartilage change and in the human the adverse effect of this procedure is well known. In these experimental models, the forces and stresses acting on a joint are altered. If the joint itself is rendered abnormal, then it loses its ability to absorb even normal stresses.

Congenital or developmental factors In the case of hip dysplasias, epiphyseal abnormalities, osteochondritis dissecans, etc., the joint is abnormal and there is an imbalance between the stresses on the joint and the ability to absorb those stresses. Scoliosis and inequality of leg length, however, alter the normality of forces acting on hip and knee. In both circumstances osteoarthritis ensues. In congenital hip dysplasia there is a shallow acetabulum that faces anteriorly and laterally and provides a poor cover for the femoral head.

Inflammatory factors After years of involvement by inflammatory disease, such as rheumatoid arthritis or one of the spondyloarthropathies, it is common to find that a joint develops more the changes of osteoarthritis with little or no excess of synovial fluid and no synovitis, but marked crepitus and sometimes osteophyte formation. Instability and lack of alignment are additional factors.

Septic arthritis can also cause sufficient damage to lead to osteoarthritis.

Metabolic factors   There are several so-called deposition diseases in which various substances may be deposited in cartilage. Haemochromatosis is often associated with chondrocalcinosis. Ochronosis is a rare disease in which homogentisic acid is deposited. In gout, urate crystals are deposited in the joint and in pseudogout, whether with or without general underlying disease, pyrophosphate crystals are identified. (There are several different conditions which may be associated with pyrophosphate crystal deposition, such as haemochromatosis, hyperparathyroidism, and many cases which are idiopathic.) In the 1970s it was realised that a number of patients diagnosed as having primary osteoarthritis had hydroxyapatite crystals in their joints and, although the role of these crystals has been the subject of much debate, it is possible that they are related to the development of osteoarthritis. Of course, in a number of the above situations, osteoarthritis may be due either to a post-inflammatory factor or a deposition factor − or even both.

Traumatic factors   Articular and peri-articular structures respond well to regular exercise and this has no part to play in the onset of osteoarthritis provided the joint mechanics are not altered. Obviously, correction of mechanical faults and proper rehabilitation after injury are very necessary; there is no doubt that minor injuries beset athletes and other sports people more frequently than those with more sedentary habits and as a result there is a higher incidence of osteoarthritis. Again, it is stressed that it is only in the case of trauma or biomechanical fault that this happens and not in the case of regular exercise.

Unusual activity (repeatedly) is known to lead to osteoarthritis (e.g., in the knees of coal miners). In the hypermobility syndrome, abnormal stresses are caused by the joint laxity allowing an excess of movement and this results in premature osteoarthritis.

Trauma, if it gives rise to micro-fractures in subchondral bone, if it causes a major fracture through the joint or if it results in dislocation, may in this direct fashion alter both the forces exerted on the joint and the ability of the joint to resist them.

Neuropathic   In the case of neuropathic joints there is a sensory loss from articular and peri-articular tissues with removal of the impulses necessary for the reflex activity required to maintain a joint's stability. The joint becomes relatively unstable and thus prone to osteoarthritis. Syphilis, syringomyelia and diabetes mellitus can result in such a neurological deficit.

Endocrine factors   Certainly acromegaly is associated with joint changes. In this condition there is an increase in growth hormone which results in changes in the cartilage and eventual osteoarthritis.

Diabetes mellitus and hypothyroidism have been said to carry an increased tendency to develop osteoarthritis but evidence is not very great.

Finally, one has to consider the role of obesity. It seemingly has little part to play unless a malalignment of hip or knee is caused by the sheer excess of tissue in the thighs. Other than this, however, it may well accelerate osteoarthritis of hip and knee arising from other causes, and especially if there is instability. The knee joint is the one most related to obesity.

Pathology

There are three obvious pathological processes. The first is the progressive destruction of articular cartilage, the second the formation of new bone at the margins of the joint (osteophytes) and the third, the formation of peri-articular bone cysts. The relationship between these processes is still not clear. It is a generally held view that the primary change occurs in articular cartilage and here the main biochemical change is a decrease in proteoglycans. The latter and collagen are the two most important substances necessary for the integrity and normal function of cartilage. The loss of proteoglycans and the consequences of a diminished amount in the cartilage are essential steps in the development of osteoarthritis. There is a loss of stiffness and elasticity that alters the effects of mechanical forces. The loss of proteoglycans also adversely affects cartilage lubrication. There is also a change in water content and the ability to absorb water. This latter fact may cause diffusion of degradative enzymes from synovial fluid. Histological studies show localised areas of softening in which the cartilage becomes irregular (fibrillation). Clefts develop and in time extend down to, and penetrate, subchondral bone with the formation of cysts. A continuing process of degradation results in fragments of cartilage being flaked off into the synovial cavity. These are phagocytosed and a mild inflammatory reaction is triggered. Eventually, bone may be completely denuded of cartilage and the bone-end become very smooth (eburnation). Until the final stage of the disease, reparative processes are taking place and in the early stages some, if not all, of the changes may be reversible.

New bone formation starts at the beginning of the disease, though the largest osteophytes are usually seen in those patients who have long-standing and slowly progressive disease. They may not be directly related to the cartilage destruction and could be dependent upon vascular changes. They may be responsible for some of the pain and restriction of movement experienced by the patient. The aetiology of bone cysts is unclear. Possibilities include extravasation of synovial fluid into bone or local bone infarcts.

The changes seen are common to all forms of osteoarthritis.

Clinical features

Patients complain of pain, stiffness, deformity and loss of function. The symptoms do not always correlate with radiological findings, e.g. there may be few symptoms even in the presence of marked radiological changes. The reverse is also true, and pain may be severe despite minimal clinical and radiological findings. Usually, there are increasing complaints over a number of years, but occasionally the history can be relatively short a matter of a few months only, despite extensive radiological disease.

Pain This is usually related to the joint involved, but in the case of the hip may be referred to the knee or to the thigh. With a combination of lumbar spine and hip disease, it can be difficult to isolate the site that gives rise to most pain.

The pain is described as dull and aching, but in erosive interphalangeal osteoarthritis it can be more acute. Acute pain and swelling occurring in a knee joint should always make one think of deposition of pyrophosphate crystals (pseudogout).

Pain is made worse by movement and, in the lower limbs, by weight-bearing and walking. Initially it is relieved by rest, but later in the disease rest pain can be severe and ultimately lead to disturbance of sleep.

Pain arises in structures that possess nerve endings and may result from micro-fractures in subchondral bone, increased venous pressure in subchondral bone and osteophytes, synovitis, capsular thickening and subluxation. After osteotomy it is said that pain relief may be due to lowering of the venous pressure and/or the severing of nerve endings.

Stiffness After resting, stiffness is a feature that lasts for about 15 minutes. It is never as marked a feature as in rheumatoid arthritis, but may occur in the morning after a night's sleep or after any prolonged use through the day. Patients learn to use their joints little, but often.

Deformity This is commonly observed in the hands and can be unsightly. In the lower limbs, flexion contracture of the hip and/ knee is due to protective muscle spasm and varus deformity is common at the knee (*Figure 15.2*). Due to the deformity and limitation of one joint, secondary change may occur in an un-

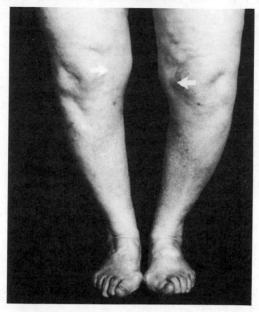

Figure 15.2. Obesity and osteoarthritis of the knees showing a varus deformity.

affected joint (e.g., flexion deformity and limitation of the hip secondary to long-standing knee disease with flexion).

In time, peri-articular structures thicken, varying degrees of subluxation may occur, and loss of congruity of the joint surfaces will limit movement, which may be further limited by the presence of large osteophytes.

Signs The signs found in osteoarthritis depend to a certain extent on the site of the disease. In easily accessible joints, bony thickening, sometimes with tenderness, may be evident, as may deformity, subluxation, instability, and limitation. Crepitus may be felt and heard when moving a joint (a fine or coarse creaking noise occasioned by irregular surfaces). Especially in the hip, a loud 'clunk' may be heard on movement, usually when there is a bone-on-bone situation. This sound can be heard from yards away, and a patient's approach may be heralded before he enters the room.

Investigations

Radiology In the initial stages the radiological appearance may be normal. Subsequently, the changes which are seen include:

- Joint space narrowing. This reflects the gradual disappearance of cartilage.
- Sclerosis (increased density) of bone beneath the cartilage as the process of eburnation takes place.
- Osteophyte formation at the joint margins.
- Cystic changes in the peri-articular bone. These are seen as translucent areas of varying size in close proximity to the joint. They can result in local collapse of bone.
- Deformity resulting from subluxation.
- The presence of loose bodies.
- Irregularity of bone surfaces. This may be made even more obvious by the collapse of bone cysts.

Osteophyte formation is a curious event. Although osteophytes are typical of osteoarthritis their presence *alone* does not imply that the other radiological changes will necessarily develop. Loss of joint space, subchondral sclerosis and the presence of cysts are perhaps more reliable indices of progressive cartilage destruction. Osteophytes related to the hip can occur in numerous different patterns and it is an interesting exercise to relate the differing sites of formation around the hip with clinical presentation.

Ankylosis is unusual and erosions are not seen except in erosive interphalangeal osteoarthritis. Radionucleide bone scans are a sensitive predictor of early osteoarthritis.

Laboratory tests There are no specific laboratory abnormalities in osteoarthritis, except in some cases of secondary disease in which there may be specific tests for the primary disease. The haemoglobin, white cell count, platelet count and erythrocyte sedimentation rate (ESR) are normal (except perhaps for a slight rise in the ESR during the acute phase of primary generalised osteoarthritis).

Tests for rheumatoid factor are usually negative, but the incidence of positive rheumatoid factors rises with age in the normal population.

Synovial fluid retains its viscosity and has a glairy mucous consistency. The protein content is rarely above 3g/100ml and the white count usually below 5.0×10^9/litre (often even less).

Medical management
From what has been said already it would seem that the most important approach should be a prophylactic one. Unfortunately, we are not yet able to achieve this goal, but continuing research into the mechanical stresses acting on a joint, the biochemistry of joint structures and the question of lubrication may radically alter

the approach to osteoarthritis in the future. Situations which place abnormal stress on the affected joint must be avoided and this may include obesity. Attention must be given to joint protection. Another approach to the question of prophylaxis is to identify the primary disease or condition that leads to osteoarthritis and apply effective treatment as early as possible.

Many patients will require no more than reassurance. The word 'arthritis' conjures up a picture of crippledom, and the fear of this must be dispelled. Fortunately, progression of the disease is usually slow and much of the patient's discomfort and disability can be relieved even though the pathological changes remain.

Rest relieves pain in the early stages, but induces stiffness. Too much rest is not a good thing, neither is too much exercise. A suitable balance between the two must be established and varies from patient to patient. How much rest and activity and what kind will vary according to the joint involved. Immobilisation is not as necessary as may occasionally be the case in rheumatoid arthritis. Often, a stick is the most effective treatment.

Drugs are frequently used, but constitute only one aspect of the treatment of osteoarthritis. The object is to use general measures and to avoid the need for drugs, but sometimes the latter are needed for symptomatic relief and to facilitate other approaches to treatment. Side-effects from drugs are frequently encountered and their use should be kept to a minimum. Pain and stiffness may be severe enough to justify the use of analgesics (paracetamol, salicylate, dihydrocodeine, etc.), and it is common practice to use non-steroidal anti-inflammatory drugs as well (see Chapter 12). Systemic corticosteroid therapy has no place in the treatment of osteoarthritis, but intra-articular or soft tissue injections may have a limited role. At least the latter may render the task of the physiotherapist easier. Other forms of medical therapy have been employed, but are of doubtful value and may be dangerous. This applies to irradiation therapy, various attempts at improving lubrication (e.g., intra-articular silicones) and intramuscular injections of extracts of cartilage. There is no single curative medication available. The use of drugs combined with physiotherapy and general measures related to the correction of abnormal stresses, and the treatment of primary disorders, should be satisfactory in the management of most patients. Reassurance is always required.

The disability created by osteoarthritis must be assessed, as well as its symptoms, such as pain or stiffness, and, as with rheumatoid arthritis, assessments must take into account the total environment of the patient. This should be easier than in rheumatoid arthritis, since a change in osteoarthritis is not as marked a feature and fewer joints are involved.

Surgical management

Over the last 20 years, joint replacement has resulted in a revolution in the treatment of osteoarthritis. Before hip and knee prosthetic surgery, osteoarthritis could result in significant functional impairment. But now, the outlook is much improved leaving cervical and lumbar disease the main source of handicap in osteoarthritis.

Physiotherapy

Patients present to physiotherapy departments with varying distribution and degrees of deterioration in the affected joints and are treated according to the stage of the degenerative process. For treatment to be effective, the basic principles of assessment, planning, implementation, evaluation and modification, followed by reassessment, are essential.

Assessment

A systematic approach is required in order to ensure that all relevant aspects of the patient's condition are considered. Careful recording of the findings of the assessment, treatment given and the patient's response is necessary. A great deal of information can be gained from the patient's notes, and the physiotherapy assessment should concentrate on those aspects of the patient's condition which concern the physiotherapist; these include pain, loss of function and joint stiffness.

Pain The level of pain experienced by the patient indicates the degree of joint irritability, but not necessarily the amount of joint deterioration. Information concerning the pain can be elicited by careful questioning of the following points:

- Site and distribution of the pain.
- Quality: burning, aching, throbbing, searing.
- Duration: permanent, persistent or intermittent.
- Triggering factors: weight-bearing, jarring, sustained stress; specific movement, rest, posture, weather, emotional state; no recognisable trigger.
- Relieving factors: rest, movement, postural adjustment, temporal adjustment; physiotherapeutic procedures, e.g. traction, application of external heat or cold, massage, manipulative procedures, resisted movements; analgesia.

Loss of function Damage to a single joint, such as a hip or knee, will have a significant effect on the patient's function. Although the patient may remain ambulant, he may have difficulty in negotiating stairs, bathing or certain aspects of self-care activities. Difficulties may be encountered in negotiating transport, as he may be unable to get on or off a bus or train and may have difficulty driving. If the patient is working, restricted mobility may cause problems. If the joints of the upper limb are affected, this may be disabling to the housewife or office worker and requires precision movements. The patient will be able to identify specific problems and treatment should be orientated towards their relief.

Joint stiffness   All affected joints display restriction of movement, and careful examination is required of the active and passive ranges so that the deficiencies may be noted. The quality of movement, point of pain limitation or muscle guarding should be noted and recorded. Movement must be localised to the joint under examination and care taken to prevent movement in adjacent joints augmenting that present in the affected joint.

Large joints are examined effectively using a goniometer to record ranges of motion, but small joints, e.g. of the fingers, can be measured by applying a malleable wire to the extensor aspect of the fingers, bending it to maintain contact with the skin through the range of motion and then transferring the trace of the wire to graph paper.

When examining joint movement, the physiotherapist must also check accessory movements at the joints involved. These movements are an essential part of normal movement and cannot be performed voluntarily in isolation. Restriction of accessory movements due to mechanical disruption of the joint surfaces will give rise to pain on movement and will preclude normal range or smooth quality of movement within the existing range.

Assessment is completed by noting the posture, identifying any deformity or asymmetry of limb lengths and testing the strength of muscles around the affected joints using the MRC scale.

Treatment

Once the patient's problems have been identified, treatment is directed towards improving function within the limits imposed both by the state of the affected joints and the requirements of the person's lifestyle. As always, successful management rests upon the co-operation and understanding of the person. Instruction in posture improvement, adequate rest in suitable positions, a programme of graded exercises, selection and use of appropriate walking aids, and dietary advice if obesity is present, will all continue to an easier way of life. The aims of treatment are:

- To control pain.
- To prevent further strain or damage to affected joints.
- To improve movements.
- To improve muscle power.
- To maintain or improve functional independence.

To control pain   Various physiotherapeutic techniques can be used to help relieve pain (in addition to any analgesics which may be prescribed):

- *Traction*: Distraction of joint surfaces, either manually or mechanically, either intermittently or prolonged, will reduce pain by relieving pressure on sensitive intra-articular structures. Protective muscle guarding is reduced and this will also ease the pain.
- *Heat*: Superficial or deep heat will relieve discomfort by reducing the protective muscle spasm. Hot packs, radiant heat, paraffin wax and short wave diathermy are all beneficial.
- *Cold*: Ice packs can be more effective than heat.
- *Ultrasound*: This is indicated when pain is centred on peri-articular soft tissues.
- *Interferential*: This is used for its analgesic and circulatory effects. It is able to be used in the presence of metal implants. Currents between 0–10Hz are used to provide muscle stimulation by a current, which is more comfortable than faradism. Care must be taken not to reduce pain and protective muscle guarding to the point where the patient will further damage affected joints by overactivity.
- *Hydrotherapy*: The warmth of the water and its buoyancy are helpful in relieving pain, particularly when weight-bearing joints are affected.

To improve movements   As there is no systemic involvement in osteoarthritis, vigorous techniques can be used to improve joint movement once the protective muscle spasm has been reduced (see above). Mobilisation may be active or passive:

- *Active*: Methods include the use of suspension therapy, pool therapy, and PNF techniques, such a hold–relax and slow-reversal hold–relax used in appropriate patterns.
- *Passive*: These techniques are used where mechanical dysfunction or alteration of the length of peri-articular soft tissues is limiting movement (*see* Chapter 7).

To improve muscle power   Muscle power can only be improved by active exercise. At each attendance the physiotherapist will select the appropriate starting positions, type and quality of resistance so that the patient works to the limit of his capabilities in order to hypertrophy muscle. Endurance will be increased by working muscles for a longer time against a submaximal resistance.

To maintain or improve functional independence By relieving pain and muscle guarding the patient's level of functional independence will improve; if problems remain the solution may lie in the use of an alternative method or, where this cannot be achieved, by supplying an aid.

When joint deterioration coupled with increasing pain become intolerable, surgery will be considered (*see* Chapters 16, 17 and 20).

Individual joints

For discussion of the spine, see Chapter 11.

Shoulder
Osteoarthritis of the gleno-humeral joint is uncommon as a primary event, but may occur secondarily after trauma or other joint diseases, such as rheumatoid arthritis. Extra-articular disease of soft tissues is by comparison very common (e.g., adhesive capsulitis, rotator-cuff syndrome and tendinitis with or without calcific deposits) and other causes of shoulder pain must be considered before a diagnosis of osteoarthritis is accepted (e.g., inflammatory arthritis, neurological and vascular lesions, referred pain, etc.). Osteoarthritis of the acromioclavicular joint is a rare cause of pain.

Elbow
This is an uncommon site for osteoarthritis, except after trauma.

Hand
The distal interphalangeal joints are the most frequently affected in the hand, with the clinically characteristic Heberden's nodes. These relate to osteophytes formed at the joint margin and are seen as prominences around the joint. Bouchard's nodes are similarly formed around the proximal interphalangeal joints, but occur less frequently (*Figure 15.1*). The osteophytic outgrowth may occur in one or two fingers, especially after injury, or simultaneously and spontaneously in all fingers. They are much more common in women and one must remember that activities requiring 'pinch' are more often undertaken by women. The loading set up by pinch is surprisingly severe. In the case of

women, one parent usually has had similar lesions, whereas in men, both parents will have been affected. Nodes appear at first in middle age. While they are growing, the fingers are painful and function is impaired. However, growth is complete after about 5 years. The pain goes, and function can be surprisingly good, even in the most gnarled hands.

Lateral deviation and flexion of the distal phalanx may be noted. Occasionally, cystic swellings will develop in association with the nodes (especially Heberden's nodes). They contain gelatinous material, can be painful and may burst. Treatment is not very satisfactory, but wax baths and intra-articular steroids may help.

Almost as common in the female is osteoarthritis of the carpo-metacarpal joint of the thumb (trapezio-metacarpal joint). The trapezium-scaphoid joint is also involved. This results in a squared appearance of the thumb with functional impairment. Patients find it very difficult to grasp objects and any function involving the thumb becomes painful and difficult. Excision of the trapezium or a silastic implant will give considerable relief, though it may take up to 6 months for power to return.

Erosive interphalangeal osteoarthritis gives rise to intermittent, apparently inflammatory, bouts of pain. Ankylosis is more com-mon than is the case with Heberden's and Bouchard's nodes and cartilage destruction is even more severe. Radiologically, erosions are present but this would seem to be a distinct entity and differs from both rheumatoid arthritis and classical osteoarthritis.

Let us consider the metacarpophalangeal joints. It has been taught that osteoarthritis involves the distal and proximal inter-phalangeal joints, but not the metacarpophalangeal joints. Ad-ditionally, rheumatoid arthritis involves the metacarpophalangeal and proximal interphalangeal joints, but not the distal inter-phalangeal joints. These are good guidelines. Occasionally, how-ever, radiographs will show evidence of osteoarthritis in the metacarpophalangeal joints. Is this primary, post-traumatic or post-inflammatory? The answer has not been resolved, but poses the question — are some typical osteoarthritic changes secondary to a mild unrecognised inflammatory arthritis? In other words, do we really know the true clinical spectrum of rheumatoid (or other) arthritis?

Finally, osteoarthritis in the hand may occur without other joint involvement or as part of a more generalised disorder. You must consider the hand as part of the whole. You must assess the disability, including the psychological as well as the painful distress. You must also realise that the discomfort and aesthetic displeasure are nothing in comparison with the disastrous con-sequences of rheumatoid arthritis involving the hand. The pain will diminish in time. The ugliness will not. The function will remain better than that in rheumatoid arthritis. Surgical treatment for the thumb can be very effective.

Physiotherapy assessment In addition to assessing the joint range and muscle power, it is important also to assess sensation and the functional use of the hand:

- *Range of movement*: Individual joint movement can be measured by moulding wire to the extensor aspect of the finger. Contact is maintained as the finger joints are flexed fully: a trace is taken of the position and transferred to graph paper. This is then repeated while the joints are extended.
- *Muscle power*: The intrinsic and extrinsic hand muscles should be tested individually, and graded using the MRC scale.
- *Sensation*: This tends to be diminished over the fingertips and is a contributory cause of hand clumsiness.

Treatment Paraffin-wax gloves will provide all-round warmth and are the most beneficial form of heat. The oiliness of the wax also lubricates the skin. Some patients may prefer immersion of their hands in a 50:50 mixture of crushed ice and water. Either form should be followed by mobilisation of the joints using traction, passive and active assisted movements.

Re-education of function requires particular attention to all grasping activities, gripping and precision movements. The needs of each patient must be known so that a rational treatment may be offered.

Hip

Osteoarthritis of the hip can be bilateral, but it is more usual for just one hip to be involved. Congenital dysplasia of the hip accounts for 25% or more of cases. Slipped capital femoral epiphysis is also a common cause and avascular necrosis (Legg—Calvé—Perthes' disease) may be responsible. Not to be forgotten is the possibility of a previous inflammatory arthritis, especially Reiter's syndrome or an atypical spondyloarthropathy. If severe enough, congenital abnormalities may present with symptoms in childhood, but a significant number may not and, in these cases, osteoarthritis of the hip will present as a disease of middle age.

Congenital hip dysplasia in a child results in a limp occurring as early as 2—3 years old. If the diagnosis is missed and there is only partial subluxation, the teenager will present with pain. In even less severe cases, osteoarthritis in middle age will be the presenting feature. The same sequence of events takes place in other congenital or developmental abnormalities. In some cases, symptoms related to the abnormality will start early, in mild form, and continue into adult life, emerging into the symptoms of osteoarthritis.

Congenital hip dysplasia is more common in females and a slipped upper femoral epiphysis is found more often in males.

Pain arising from the hip may be felt in the groin, lateral buttock or thigh and is not uncommonly referred to the knee. Internal rotation is the first movement to be impaired, but subsequently extension, abduction and flexion become restricted. Increasing adduction deformity leads to relative and then absolute shortening of the limb. The gait becomes antalgic (i.e., the body leans to the affected side during the stance phase of walking). The patient stands with the affected side elevated, but this can only be possible as a result of lumbar scoliosis developing and the heel will not meet the ground unless there is flexion of the knee on the unaffected side. A Trendelenburg gait is the result.

Trendelenburg's sign   This is an indication of the gluteal muscles' potential to abduct the hip when weight-bearing, and is positive if abduction is not possible.

To elicit the sign instruct the patient to stand on the affected leg and raise the other knee, as in marking time. Normally, the buttock of the raised leg rises higher than that of the standing leg. If the sign is positive, the buttock of the raised leg droops below the other.

Leg-length shortening may be apparent, as measured from the umbilicus (or xiphisternum) to the medial malleolus. True shortening is ascertained by measuring the distance from the anterior superior iliac spine to the medial malleolus on both sides.

It must be obvious that changes in the lumbo-sacral spine are a frequent consequence of hip disease. Scoliosis, changes in lumbar lordosis and osteoarthritis (e.g., of the facet joints) result from altered mechanical stress on the spine. It can be difficult to differentiate between pain that arises from the hip and that from lumbo-sacral spine disease, whether the latter be primary or secondary to the hip disease. This is an important aspect to take into account when considering hip surgery. Often pain is due to both conditions.

The contralateral knee is sometimes placed under undue stress and this will encourage the development of osteoarthritis here, again as a secondary phenomenon.

Paget's disease of the bone is quite common in the pelvis, and may be unilateral. In such a situation it is often associated with osteoarthritis of the hip and the questions are posed: Which condition is giving rise to the pain or is it due to both? Which condition should be dealt with first? Generally speaking, the osteoarthritis is more likely to be the source of most pain in this combination, but as surgery carries a danger because of the increased vascularity of bone in Paget's disease, the latter should be treated first (either by calcitonin, disodium etidronate or a combination of these).

Having regard for the above problems, osteoarthritis of the hip is usually a good condition to treat. Total hip replacement gives excellent results (*see* Chapter 17). Before surgery is considered, simple measures should be tried. These include weight loss (if obesity is evident), the use of a stick in the contralateral hand, local steroid infiltration of the trochanteric bursa, analgesia, traction and physiotherapy.

Physiotherapy treatment
Relief of pain During an acute inflammatory episode, complete bed rest for a few days with traction may be indicated, but usually less radical approaches will provide considerable ease. Application of ice or hot packs to the joint will reduce muscle spasm, and so reduce pain. Short wave diathermy is the deepest form of penetrating heat available in a physiotherapy department; while a significant number of patients will gain relief from its application, some find the pain exaggerated by it and will gain more benefit from radiant heat irradiation. Ultrasound, immersion in a treatment pool or repetitive exercise in a weight-relieved position may all help reduce protective muscle guarding and thus reduce pain.

Mobilisation of joints and prevention of deformity Once pain and protective muscle spasm have been reduced, mobilisation commences by passive or active means. It is advisable for the patient to spend some time during the day in a corrected position; prone is ideal, but this will be precluded in advanced cases by hip flexion deformity, and then the patient should lie supine with the hip extended as far as possible.

Maitland mobilising techniques of low grades when the hip is irritable, progressing to higher grades as irritability subsides, produce good results. Traction is also an effective passive measure.

Active extension and abduction of the hip can be encouraged using suspension apparatus to support the weight of the leg. Deep water exercises in the treatment pool and proprioceptive neuromuscular facilitation techniques are beneficial, particularly hold−relax and slow-reversal hold−relax in the extension, abduction and medial rotation pattern.

Strengthening of muscles Muscle contractions against a graded resistance using gravity, manually or by mechanical means are effective in strengthening muscle groups weakened by disuse or pain. Exercises may be performed in lying, side lying, prone lying, sitting or standing.

Gait re-education and posture correction A temporary raise may be required on the shoe of the adducted leg to equalise leg lengths and eliminate toe walking on that side or walking with a flexed knee on the contralateral side. Re-education may be started in the pool and progress to dry land with support from elbow crutches or walking sticks. A single walking stick in the contralateral hand will provide some weight relief.

A minimum of 45° of active hip flexion is required to climb stairs and as many patients cannot achieve this they should be taught to trail the affected leg in ascent and lead with it in descent. The non-affected leg will then take the strain of raising or lowering the body weight.

The patient should be reminded continually about his posture and any deviation corrected.

Functional independence Patients with an osteoarthritic hip may require training in functional transfers. In later stages of the disease, home adaptations may be needed to facilitate self-care, and the occupational therapist may be asked to advise about aids which will compensate for the lack of movement in the hip. These include a pincer-grip extension hand for picking up small objects from the floor; elasticated shoe laces; a half-step to aid climbing; and a high toilet seat raise.

Knee

Osteoarthritis may occur in the patello-femoral joint or in the medial or lateral compartments of the knee. Patello-femoral arthritis can occur on its own or following disease in the knee joint, and typically gives rise to pain anteriorly.

Initiating factors in osteoarthritis of the knee include fractures that involve the tibial plateaux and/or femoral condyles, instability (e.g. after ligamentous damage) and severe lateral deformities, and post-inflammatory states. Special instances include the development of arthritis after patellectomy, following a torn meniscus and in association with chondromalacia patellae. The incidence of change after meniscectomy is high and although a damaged meniscus that interferes with joint function has to be removed, care must be taken to ensure that the procedure really is essential. *Chondromalacia patellae* occurs in a younger age group (15—30) than patello-femoral osteoarthritis. There is pain with activity. Descending a flight of stairs or getting up quickly from a crouching position typically induce symptoms, which can be elicited also by passively depressing the patella in the femoral groove as a patient contracts the quadriceps. Symptoms tend to come and go, but can be severe. Eventually, osteoarthritis may supervene and the symptoms generally become more severe at this stage.

In the case of osteoarthritis of the knee, pain is more marked with weight-bearing and, initially at least, is relieved by rest. Transfers, kneeling and climbing stairs are especially likely to bring symptoms. Muscle wasting, especially of the quadriceps, is apparent. There is little or no evidence of soft-tissue swelling, but small effusions are common. The fluid is less inflammatory than that in rheumatoid arthritis, being more viscous and having a lower protein content and white cell count. There may be instability in both lateral and antero-posterior planes. Flexion becomes limited and it is common to develop lack of full extension. A varus deformity is more common than valgus and may be passively reversible only to reappear with weight-bearing. If the degree of varus deformity is less than 15°, then appropriate splintage (especially using a telescopic valgus-varus support (TVS)) might prevent progression in the degree of varus and in reversible cases perhaps improve mechanical forces with the hope of slowing down the arthritic process (*Figure 15.3(a)* and *15.3(b)*).

Crepitus is very commonly elicited. Locking or an acute exacerbation of pain may be caused by a loose body or a damaged meniscus.

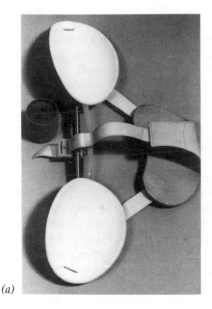
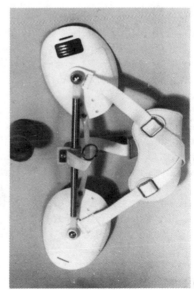

(a) (b)

Figure 15.3. TVS brace: (a) inner surface; (b) outer aspect.

Physiotherapy treatment

Relief of pain   Radiant heat, short wave diathermy, interferential, hot or ice packs encircling the joint may be used beneficially. Where there is nipping of the synovial membrane, traction will be of benefit.

Maintenance of movement and improvement of range   Patellar movements (distal, proximal and oblique) should be maintained by moving the patella passively in all directions. In severe lesions, manipulation under anaesthesia may be necessary, after which active exercise will be required to maintain the range gained.

Active exercises concentrating on establishing full extension of the joint are important. Pulley circuits, suspension therapy, hydrotherapy, particularly Bad Ragaz flexion and extension patterns, PNF techniques, etc., will all have a relevant part in the programme.

Strengthening of muscles   Although all the leg muscles may be weakened, it is the quadriceps muscles, and particularly vastus medialis, on which strengthening will be concentrated. This can be achieved by using progressive resistance on land or in water. The single most useful technique to employ is PNF, for it can improve quality of contraction, range of movement, power and endurance through being used in functional patterns.

Gait re-education   The gait should be analysed and corrected as required (*see* Chapter 2). Walking aids may be needed and the patient should be trained in their correct use. If both knees are affected, two sticks will be needed and the patient taught to use them as a normal four-point gait pattern; if only one knee is affected then a single stick used in the opposite hand is sufficient.

In severe cases it may be necessary to provide some form of orthosis (*see* Chapter 1). If external splintage is used particular attention must be paid to the maintenance of the quadriceps muscle strength.

Feet

Involvement of the hind foot is rare and is usually the result of injury. Conversely, the incidence of osteoarthritis of the first metatarsophalangeal joint (with or without hallux valgus deformity) is high. The joint becomes restricted and take-off during gait can be very painful. This state, progressing to hallux rigidus, can be alleviated by wearing thick, stiff-soled shoes or inserting a steel bar into the medial sole of the shoe. Osteophytes form and bursitis adds to the pain. Especially with hallux valgus, footwear becomes a problem and patients are happier in old shoes or slippers which have adapted to the deformed foot.

Bibliography

Davies, B.C. (1967). A technique of re-education in the treatment pool. *Physiotherapy*, **53**, 2.

Hollis, M. (1981). *Practical Exercise Therapy*, 2nd edition. Blackwell Scientific Publications Limited, Oxford.

Hollis, M. and Roper, M.H.S. (1965). *Suspension Therapy*. Baillière Tindall and Casell, London. (Now out of print but will be found in libraries.)

Hyde, S.A., *et al*. (1980). *Physiotherapy in Rheumatology*. Blackwell Scientific Publications Limited, Oxford.

Knott, M. and Voss, D. (1968). *Proprioceptive Neuromuscular Facilitation-Patterns and Techniques*, 2nd edition. Harper and Row, London.

Powell, M. (1981). *Orthopaedic Nursing and Rehabilitation*, 8th edition. Churchill Livingstone, Edinburgh.

Savage, B. (1984). *Interferential Therapy*. Faber and Faber, London.

Skinner, A.T. and Thomson, A.M. (eds) (1983). *Duffield's Exercise in Water*, 3rd edition. Baillière Tindall, London.

Wynn Parry, C.B. (1982). *Rehabilitation of the Hand*, 4th edition. Butterworths, London.

16 Osteotomy, Arthrodesis and Arthroplasty

M.D. Northmore-Ball

Introduction

The characteristics of the three types of surgical procedure are described prior to consideration of their application to joints of the lower limb.

Osteotomy means division of a bone. The use of the word as the title of a complete operation means that the whole purpose of the operation is to divide a bone (or bones) almost always in order to change its (or their) shape, alignment or length.

An osteotomy is also often an ancillary surgical step that occurs during other orthopaedic operations. In these cases an important ligament or muscle will need to be detached to give access to the operation site. Using this technique, access is achieved by detaching the piece of adjacent bone which carries the origin or insertion of the ligament or muscle. At the end of the procedure the piece of bone has to be reattached. The most well known example is probably an osteotomy of the greater trochanter to allow mobilisation of the glutei, as one method of gaining access to the hip in total hip replacement; similarly, osteotomies may be made through the acromion to gain access to the shoulder.

An osteotomy as an operation in itself is usually *indicated* to correct a bone deformity, where this produces significant pain, loss of function, or, rarely, for appearances alone. In the child (see Chapter 5) indications take into account the major changes that may be produced by later growth. An osteotomy is also very frequently performed deliberately to produce an abnormal shape in a previously normal bone, in order to alter the mechanics to treat a nearby condition, such as an un-united fracture or arthritis in a neighbouring joint.

The general principles of osteotomy technique are:

- To expose the bone surgically; the bone may be superficial (e.g., the ulna) or very deep (e.g., the anterior aspect of the spine).

- To divide the bone with an osteotome or saw.
- To remodel the osteotomy surfaces if required.
- To displace the bone ends to produce the desired change in shape, usually simultaneously approximating the newly shaped bone ends.
- Finally, to hold the skeleton in this new position by internal or external means.

Arthrodesis means surgical fusion of a joint and is *indicated* where significant pain, deformity or instability arises in an abnormal joint, and where it is felt that the resulting complete loss of joint movement is acceptable. With the advent of replacement arthroplasty (see below) these indications are seen much less frequently than in former times.

The general principles of arthrodesis technique are:

- To expose the joint surgically.
- Usually to dislocate the joint so as to expose the damaged joint surfaces.
- To bring these surfaces together in a position for best overall function, bearing in mind that the joint will no longer move.
- To hold the joint in this position by internal or external means.

A fundamental requirement for arthrodesis is that most if not all other joints should normally be mobile.

Arthroplasty is a non-specific term covering any surgical refashioning of a joint, with or without the use of artificial materials. It is *indicated* for pain, deformity or instability in a joint where loss of motion is considered unacceptable, and sometimes for the deliberate mobilisation of a previously fixed joint where this fixity, by itself, is the cause of significant symptoms (as, for example, in the mobilisation of a previously fused hip for intractable back pain).

There are three main types of arthroplasty, excision arthroplasty, interposition arthroplasty and replacement arthroplasty.

Excision arthroplasty

Here, one or both of the bone ends that form a joint are excised. The most common example is Keller's arthroplasty, excising the proximal end of the proximal phalanx of the big toe as treatment of a painful bunion. The resulting weakness and instability of the toe are not felt to be significant. The most well-known example in a large joint is the Girdlestone arthroplasty of the hip, now most commonly seen as an end stage following failed hip replacement (but see Chapter 17). After excision of the bone ends, the hope is that some form of flexible scar will form between them and therefore an attempt may be made to preserve the gap during the early stages of healing (with traction at the hip or a Kirschner wire in the big toe).

Interposition arthroplasty

Here the joint is opened, and something is placed between the bone ends. This may be a natural or prosthetic material or a prosthesis, and the bone ends may or may not be reshaped. Fascia lata was commonly employed for this; nowadays, silastic is quite often used. Examples are the Varian arthroplasty of the shoulder using a shaped silastic cup, and the now outmoded, but formerly widely used and quite successful, Mould Arthroplasty of the hip in which a Vitallium shell was interposed between the reshaped head of the femur and the reamed acetabulum. Arthroplasties of this type tend to require a prolonged period of vigorous post-operative rehabilitation, and suffer also from some unpredictability in the results.

Replacement arthroplasty

This has, to a large degree, superceded the other types of arthroplasty, as well as very greatly reducing the indications for osteotomy and arthrodesis in the treatment of symptomatic arthritis. Replacement arthroplasty of the upper limb is considered in Chapter 20 and of the lower limb in Chapter 17.

The hip

Osteotomy

Prior to the days of hip replacement, an intertrochanteric osteotomy was very commonly performed for osteoarthritis. The femur was divided with an osteotome, the bone ends allowed to fall into a natural position, and then the hip was immobilised in a plaster spica. This procedure (the McMurray osteotomy), though quite uncontrolled, gave a good result remarkably frequently and examples are still seen of patients, treated in this way many years ago, with continuing good function. Hip replacement has made osteotomy of the hip performed in this way virtually obsolete.

In younger people, however, joint replacement is now realised to have its own problems. Failed joint replacement in young people, followed by subsequent failed revision surgery, can produce a very serious problem with gross loss of the skeleton. This has brought about a renewed recent interest in osteotomy. On mainland Europe, osteotomy has continued to be practised, notably by exponents of the principles of Pauwels, who analysed the mechanics of the hip and the mechanical effects of specific alterations of hip-joint alignment. Carried out in this fashion, and using modern techniques of internal fixation (e.g. ASIF plates and screws) osteotomy can produce surprisingly good and predictable results, so that it can be a valid alternative treatment to joint replacement in very carefully selected younger patients.

The principle of osteotomy in the treatment of the young adult hip showing early or established arthritis, is to reduce the load per unit area on the abnormal hip surfaces by increasing the weight-bearing area and/or by reducing the total load taken through the surfaces, by improving the mechanical advantage of the muscles around the hip (notably the abductors), usually supplemented by defunctioning of some of the motor muscles, such as the psoas.

A very careful *pre-operative assessment* has to be made of the patient and the hip X-rays and this may need to include examination of the hip under a general anaesthetic, with screening, using an X-ray image intensifier.

Osteotomies of the acetabular or femoral sides of the hip, and sometimes of both, may be indicated. A common indication for a *pelvic* osteotomy is acetabular dysplasia, with deficiency anteriorly and superiorly of the acetabular roof. The osteotomy may then either redirect or enlarge the acetabulum. Redirection may be by inserting a graft in a transverse osteotomy just above the acetabulum (Salter), by dividing the ilium pubis and ischium, moving the whole block of bone bearing the acetabulum, or by division with a special osteotome of the subchondral bone all the way around the acetabulum, leaving the pelvic ring intact (Wagner). Enlargement of the acetabulum may be achieved in several ways, notably by the Chiari osteotomy in which the ilium is again divided above the acetabulum, but with displacement of the upper part laterally. *Femoral* osteotomy is usually carried out in the intertrochanteric region, the work of Bombelli being pre-eminent.

A *varus* femoral osteotomy may be done for supero-lateral arthritis where the acetabulum is normal, but where the femoral neck-shaft angle is increased. The varus will then increase the force, tending to make the femoral head move medially. A varus osteotomy requires the femoral head still to be spherical. A *valgus* femoral osteotomy may be done in quite advanced osteoarthritis and requires that the femoral head should have become flattened with medial osteophytes. The change to a valgus alignment completely alters the load-bearing fulcrum within the hip joint, moving it medially. Correctly indicated, these procedures can be remarkably effective (*Figures 16.1a, 16.1b, 16.2a, and 16.2b*). Varus and valgus osteotomies are usually combined with *extension* (i.e.,

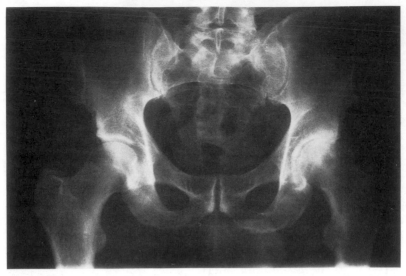

Figure 16.1(a). X-ray of the hips of a 55-year-old man showing severe osteoarthritis of the left hip.

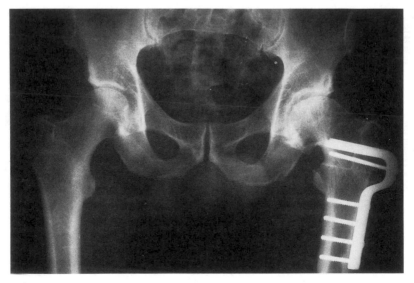

Figure 16.1(b). Appearance of the hips in Figure 16.2(a) 6 years following varus extension osteotomy. A thick layer of weight-bearing cartilage has appeared. The hip is almost completely free from symptoms.

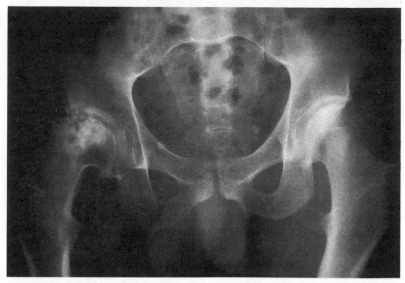

Figure 16.2(a). X-ray of a 26-year-old man with avascular necrosis of the right femoral head following steroid therapy for a bad head injury.

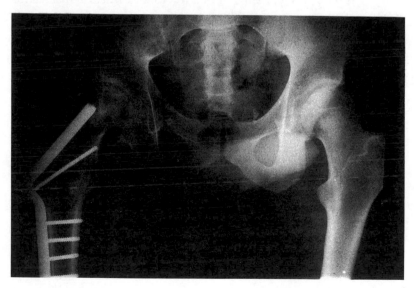

Figure 16.2(b). Appearances of the hip in **Figure 16.1(a)** *following valgus extension osteotomy. The femoral head has extensively remodelled and the patient has a major improvement in symptoms. The plate was later removed.*

allowing the hip itself to move into a slightly flexed position with the leg in normal position) and often need to be combined with *rotation* or with medial or lateral *displacement*. The overall alignment and length of the leg should be considered when planning osteotomies of this kind.

Post-operative management   This has to be individualised. For an intertrochanteric osteotomy the patient will usually carry out assisted active exercises of the hip from about 2 days post-operatively and will then get up, shadow-walking for some weeks. A sequence of special exercises is often desirable, with the early use of an exercise bicycle. A prolonged period of partial weight-bearing is then indicated, as (notably when used in the treatment of established osteoarthritis) this will give the best chance for regeneration of the damaged hip surfaces. This process, which has been confirmed histologically with the growth of islands of fibrocartilage in a previously denuded bony surface, is often confirmed by serial X-rays that show a gradual increase in thickness of the cartilaginous layer of the hip.

Arthrodesis
Arthrodesis has one main residual indication only. This is for the young person who is extremely young and active and who has an arthritic hip (typically the result of a fracture or fracture dislocation of the hip in an accident) which is very painful and has become very stiff. Such a patient will be able to cope with the limitations that a hip arthrodesis gives, and requires an absolutely durable surgical procedure. This indication is, however, rarely seen, most patients either having suitable localised conditions within the hip for an osteotomy, or having too great a residual motion in the joint for them to be prepared to sacrifice this by arthrodesis, preferring the relative uncertainties of a future with some other form of operation. An arthrodesis is now usually done using established ASIF techniques with a long cobra-headed plate running from the ilium above the hip down the lateral side of the femur. A concomitant pelvic osteotomy may be needed to give adequate bony contact for fusion to occur. This form of fixation allows very accurate positioning of the hip in about 20° of flexion and neutral or slight external rotation to be achieved, and at the same time does not require plaster immobilisation. A major advantage of the procedure is that, provided it is initially carried out appropriately, it is possible later to convert the arthrodesis into a total hip replacement.

Arthroplasty
Arthroplasty of the hip is nowadays confined, as a procedure for

treatment of arthritis, to replacement and this is considered in Chapter 17.

The *Girdlestone excision arthroplasty* is now confined to being an end-stage treatment for failed hip replacement. While many patients do have adequate function with this procedure, it does have severe limitations and is now done much less commonly than before (see Chapter 17).

The knee

Osteotomy

In contrast to the hip, *osteotomy* is frequently done as a treatment for arthritis in the knee, provided that it is of the degenerative rather than inflammatory type. Unlike the hip, the knee has three distinct compartments: medial and lateral tibio-femoral compartments and the patello-femoral compartment. The arthritic changes very commonly do not affect all three compartments equally, and the inference is that the compartments with the greatest arthritic change are being overloaded at the expense of the others. In the case of the two tibio-femoral compartments, it is often obvious which compartment is being overloaded, and a planned realignment of the leg to transfer some of the weight to the less-affected compartment can be expected to produce a good result. The underlying biomechanical principles and surgical technique are mainly associated with the work of Maquet. In the *typical case* the patient has a varus deformity, probably of long standing, is aged 65 or less, and has osteoarthritis confined to the medial side of the knee, often associated with arthritis of the patello-femoral joint, but with a normal lateral compartment. The patient's symptoms are such that major surgery is necessary, though this will have been preceded by a full course of conservative treatment and possibly also by an arthroscopy, with perhaps arthroscopic debridement.

Specific pre-operative investigations include a long leg weight-bearing X-ray. In a normal leg, the hip, knee and ankle lie on a straight line, giving an angle of about 7° between the axis of the tibial shaft and the axis of the femur, due to the medial offset of the femoral head in relation to the femoral shaft. With varus osteoarthritis, this is no longer the case. The actual angle of varus deviation can be accurately measured. A planned correction of this angle (plus 2° or 3° for a slight over-correction) can be worked out. With a valgus knee similar calculations can be made, though usually over-correction is not done.

The osteotomy may then be performed either in the upper tibia or lower femus, or occasionally in both, the choices mainly depending on whether the knee is varus, requiring a tibial osteotomy, or valgus, classically requiring a femoral osteotomy. A developmental sloping articular surface might require osteotomies of both, but this is rare. The double osteotomy, divided both the femur and tibia, but without accurate control of leg alignment; the operation is now done much less than formerly.

In an upper tibial osteotomy for a varus knee, the osteotomy is usually made at or just above the level of the tibial tubercle and can be done in several ways, commonly by a wedge removed from the outer side (perhaps with excision of the head of the fibula to gain good surgical access, as in the Coventry osteotomy) and taken to the medial side, or frequently using the so-called dome or barrel vault osteotomy, described by Maquet (*Figure 16.3*).

The advantage of this latter form of osteotomy is that the same shape of osteotomy can be done for any planned degree of correction, the bone ends remaining, in theory, congruent as the osteotomy is displaced. The fibula always has to be divided

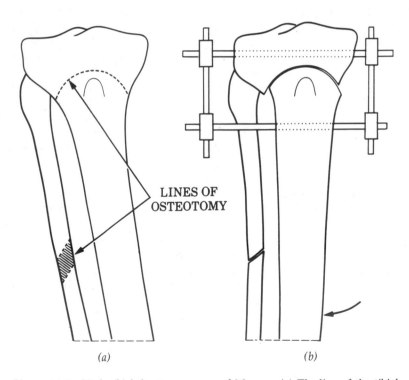

LINES OF
OSTEOTOMY

(a)   (b)

Figure 16.3. High tibial dome osteotomy of Maquet. (a) The line of the tibial and fibular osteotomies. (b) The correction achieved by rotating the distal fragment. Correction held under compression by an external fixation device.

as otherwise it splints the osteotomy and prevents proper displacement. The osteotomy then has to be held in the appropriate position. Plaster alone can be successful, but frequently this allows a subsequent shift with loss of correction, and impairment of the result, and nowadays some form of fixation is virtually universal. A closing wedge osteotomy may be fixed by staples; barrel-vault osteotomies are commonly fixed with an external fixator, either of Maquet type (*Figure 16.3*) or one of the new varieties of external fixator. When external fixation is used, immobilisation of the knee itself is not necessary, in principle a considerable advantage. Fixation may be needed for about 8 weeks.

While upper tibial osteotomy is usually a relatively simple procedure, the occasional complication of non-union may produce serious problems, and the change in shape of the upper tibia may complicate a later total knee replacement should this become necessary.

Patello-femoral arthritis The relation between symptoms and radiographic changes in patello-femoral arthritis is poor. Marked symptoms can be produced from the patello-femoral joint with plain radiographs showing no abnormality (though in some of these cases more advanced techniques, such as arthrography with computerised axial tomography or magnetic resonance scans, may show abnormalities in the articular cartilage, probably a precursor of radiographic changes), while patients are frequently seen with very severe radiographic changes, who state that symptoms are minor or have only recently arisen. The very common clinical problem of anterior knee pain, perhaps associated with patella malalignment, in the absence of frank osteoarthritic change, cannot be considered here. Symptomatic arthritis of the patello-femoral joint with fairly normal tibio-femoral compartments is not all that common. Simple conservative measures, washing out of the microscopic debris in the knee by arthroscopy, other arthroscopic surgical techniques, such as chondroplasty and drilling of subchondral bone in cartilaginous defects, and perhaps realignment procedures, have a very important place and will produce adequate relief in the great majority of cases.

Where these fail, relief may be achieved by a planned alteration of the mechanics by elevating the tibial tubercle. This may increase the lever arm in the extensor apparatus, thus reducing the compression force between the patella and femur during extension of the knee. This, as noted above, is a fundamental principle in the treatment of arthritis by osteotomy. More than about a 1.5cm elevation of the tibial tubercle (usually held by a small bone graft) can produce a serious difficulty with skin healing and the operation is not without its complications. Its place is therefore limited.

Arthrodesis

Arthrodesis of the knee is a much more satisfactory operation than arthrodesis of the hip, the loss of movement being much less of a handicap, and is still quite frequently carried out. The appropriate circumstances are where a young patient (often someone with secondary osteoarthritis following injury) develops such severe symptoms of pain and frequent instability that a radical cure for the condition is required. While many would have the view that such a patient should be treated by replacement, reserving arthrodesis for failure of the replacement, this group of patients remains one with a very good indication for arthrodesis. Formerly, patients with inflammatory arthritis affecting both knees might have one treated by replacement and the other by arthrodesis, but with recent improvements in replacement this would now seldom be done.

Probably the commonest present indication for arthrodesis of the knee is in the presence of a failed previous joint replacement, especially where this has been complicated by infection.

Surgical technique   Where a replacement has not previously been carried out, the ends of the femur and tibia are fashioned into two flat surfaces such that, when apposed, the overall alignment of the leg is correct with the centres of the hip, knee and ankle on a straight line. A few degrees of flexion is probably desirable. The bone ends are then held together with an external fixator. Union in such a case will usually be quite rapid, there being two large cancellous surfaces in contact.

Where there has been a previous replacement, the nature of the procedure will be governed by the type of replacement that has been removed. If this has been of the resurfacing type, then the same procedure as for a primary case is still appropriate. Where, however, as is commonly the case, a replacement of an earlier type has been used, these cancellous surfaces may have been lost. Many of these earlier implants invaded the upper tibia and lower femur such that, on removal, the bone ends resembled 'ice-cream cones'. Minimal surface areas are then left to bring into contact, and so the production of a sound arthrodesis may be very difficult or impossible. While the primary technique may still be appropriate, it will often be necessary to resort to other measures, such as, for example, the use of long Küntscher nails, preferably curved, running down the length of the whole leg. While a failed knee arthrodesis may produce an adequate false joint, so that the patient can still get about in a removable brace, this is by no means always the case, and very unsatisfactory uncontrollable instability may result.

Arthroplasty

Arthroplasty of the knee has had its indications radically reduced by the advent of replacement. It was formerly a common operation for tibio-femoral arthritis; the knee was opened and denuded areas of bone were drilled, and osteophytes removed. Through the drill holes in the subchondral bone, tufts of cartilage (as in the hip referred to above) had the potential for growing. This procedure must at best be unpredictable, however, and the technique is confined now to very early arthritic cases where the procedure is done arthroscopically. The arthroscopic technique enables immediate knee motion which is highly desirable.

The patello-femoral joint is perhaps the only major place where *excision arthroplasty* (i.e., *patellectomy*) is still used as a primary procedure. It was formerly felt to be an entirely benign procedure and was carried out with great readiness, but with the development of more conservative techniques, the indication for it in arthritis is now rather restricted. Also, as noted above, symptomatic patello-femoral arthritis is frequently associated with arthritis in the tibio-femoral compartments; if sufficiently advanced this will now usually be treated by knee replacement and in this procedure the patella may well be resurfaced (*see* Chapter 17). A common remaining indication for patellectomy is in the treatment of grossly comminuted patella fractures where reconstruction, even by modern fracture techniques, is not feasible.

The ankle and foot

Symptomatic arthritis in the *ankle* is usually due either to secondary osteoarthritis following a fracture, or to inflammatory arthritis. Except in rare cases, where there is a major angular deformity of the ankle following a fracture at or just above it, in which a supra-malleolar realignment osteotomy may be appropriate, the treatment, where conservative measures have failed, is in both cases by arthrodesis. The present state of replacement arthroplasty of the ankle is referred to in Chapter 17. Loss of motion of the ankle is obviously undesirable, but not such a great problem as with arthrodesis of the knee. The lower ends of the tibia and the talus are fashioned into flat surfaces, brought together and held, usually with an external fixator. It is critically necessary to align accurately the foot on to the tibia both in a varus/valgus sense and in a flexion/extension sense. A plantargrade position or, in women, a few degrees of flexion are required. Errors in positioning are a very common source of a poor symptomatic result.

Osteotomy and arthrodesis in the *hind foot* are sometimes needed in childhood for deformities due to developmental or neuromuscular abnormalities. In the adult, stabilisation of the hind foot by 'triple arthrodesis' of the sub-talar and mid-tarsal joints may be needed in inflammatory arthritis, and arthrodesis of the sub-talar joint may be required for badly symptomatic secondary osteoarthritis arising from displaced fractures of the calcaneum. Osteotomy, arthrodesis and arthroplasty all have a major part to play in the treatment of *forefoot* problems, particularly painful toe deformities in the adult. In the first ray, numerous varieties of osteotomy have been described at the proximal and distal ends for hallux valgus, sometimes in association with a varus first metatarsal. The Keller's excision arthroplasty of the base of the proximal phalanx for a painful bunion is the most common variety of excision arthroplasty. It frequently gives good results provided that the patient is not too young; interposition arthroplasty of the first metatarsophalangeal joint, using silastic, is often done. The fact that this material can wear when used as an articulating surface, with resulting undesirable effects due to wear debris, is now lessening its use.

Excision arthroplasty following removal of a silastic spacer, however, is usually satisfactory. Osteotomy of the proximal phalanx is sometimes used as a procedure for hallux rigidus in younger people and, in the treatment of hammer toes, interphalangeal arthrodesis and/or Kellerisation of the metatarsophalangeal joints is often needed. Good results from these procedures are as much dependent on an accurate assessment of the foot as a whole, particularly in relation to where the patient's symptoms lie, as on the details of the surgical techniques used.

Other sites

The spine
This subject is covered in Chapter 9.

The upper limbs
As in the leg, arthroplasty is nowadays almost entirely confined to replacement arthroplasty and this subject is fully covered in Chapter 20. There are occasional indications for osteotomy and arthrodesis; the following brief list is by no means exhaustive.

The shoulder   Osteotomy of the glenoid neck (Stamm) has been described as a treatment for supraspinatus tendonitis, resistant to all other measures. Rotational osteotomy of the upper humerus is sometimes required to improve arm function following Erb's palsy. Arthrodesis in the shoulder is by no means easy to achieve. The usual indication, though again a rare one, is a flail shoulder from a traumatic brachial plexus palsy.

The elbow   At the elbow, a badly displaced supra-condylar fracture in a child may later cause such a significant deformity, perhaps with ulnar nerve paresis, that a correctional osteotomy is required. Osteotomy of the olecranon is used as part of the surgical approach to severely displaced intra-articular fractures of the lower end of the humerus.

The wrist   At the wrist, congenital deformities and poor function due to a mal-united Colles-type fracture occasionally need a correctional osteotomy of the lower radius. Arthrodesis of the wrist may be required for post-traumatic arthritis or in rheumatoid arthritis.

The hand   In the hand there are several special indications for osteotomy and arthrodesis in primary, post-traumatic or inflammatory arthritis and in some congenital or acquired deformities, such as mal-union of fractures.

Bibliography

Bombelli, R. (1976). *Osteoarthritis of the Hip: Pathogenesis and Consequent Therapy*. Springer Verlag, London.

Liechti, R. (1978). *Hip Arthrodesis and Associated Problems*. Springer Verlag, London.

Maquet, P.G.J. (1984). *Biomechanics of the Knee*, 2nd edition. Springer Verlag, London.

Pauwels, F. (1976). *Biomechanics of the Normal and Diseased Hip*. Springer Verlag, London.

17 Lower Limb Joint Replacement

M.D. Northmore-Ball

In the lower limb, major joint replacement offers tremendous opportunities for radically decreasing patients' disabilities and improving function. In the hip and knee, several techniques exist which, if carefully followed, can be expected to give good results. Limitations of the procedures do, however, still exist and certain quite fundamental questions remain unanswered.

Implant design

This section deals with the design of total hip replacement implants. Many basic principles are, however, shared by hip and knee replacements; the reader will therefore need to refer back to this section when the knee is considered later.

Implant design may be subdivided into:

- Choice of base implant material.
- Geometry.
- Method of fixation.
- The materials used in the actual bearing.

Base material

It is usual nowadays for the base material of the hip replacement stem to be made of a metal, usually stainless steel, cobalt-chrome or titanium alloy. The manufacturer bases his choice on the material's strength, resistance to fatigue fracture, flexibility and biocompatibility. The first three of these choices depends heavily also on the geometry of the stem, as clearly, for example, a weak material might be adequate if the stem were thick enough; similarly, the flexibility of an implant, possibly desirable in allowing more uniform loading of the underlying bone, will be as dependent on the thickness of material as on its intrinsic flexibility. Some materials will be very good in some respects and very poor in others: titanium, for instance, is readily accepted by the body, but rather soft so that it readily abrades if motion occurs such that it makes contact with the skeleton. Metallic stems are not universal, one implant having the stem made of a flexible polymer strengthened with a metal core.

The *acetabular component* is usually made of the plastic, high density polyethylene. Plastic cups are commonly composite, the base material being used as one part of the bearing surface, but another material being used on the outside (*see* below). Polyethylene has the advantage of ready availability, a tradition of long use, and ease of manufacture. It is, however, not without its disadvantages (*see* Bearing material, below). Many cups are made of ceramic (notably aluminium oxide). These cups are usually in one piece so that the same material is used as the base material, for the bearing surface and on the outside. Ceramic, cups may have a very low wear rate. Ceramic, however, unlike plastic, is subject to fracture, as anyone knows from common domestic experience.

Geometry

The geometry of the *femoral stem* varies quite widely between implants. The femoral head may vary from 22mm (22.25mm was the original size chosen for the Charnley total hip replacement (THR)) to 38mm (*Figure 17.1*). The size of the head influences the

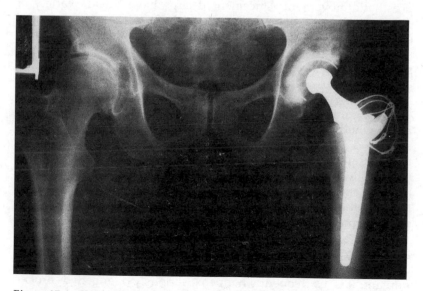

Figure 17.1. X-ray appearances of a classical Charnley cemented total hip replacement. The trochanter has been reattached with a cruciate wiring system and a Charnley staple clamp.

wear rate of the bearing and, in conjunction with the size of the prosthetic neck, influences the range of movement allowed by the components before the head lifts out of the socket. For given bearing materials, a small head tends to burrow further into the socket as wear proceeds. Wide variations also exist in the shape of the section of the stem within the remnant of the femoral neck. The femoral neck is commonly removed to a greater or lesser extent at surgery and the stem may have a collar which sits on the stump of the neck. The value of a collar remains contentious, some surgeons (e.g., Harris) considering it essential, while in the designs of others (e.g., Ling) it is completely absent. The underlying differences relate to where the load transfer is believed to be occurring in the system. In the Freeman (*Figures 17.2(a)* and *17.2(b)*) implant the femoral neck is retained, as it has been shown to have a very important influence on torsional stability of the stem in the femur (e.g., when the patient gets up quickly out of a chair). The shape of the stem itself is to some extent determined by the internal shape of the femoral canal, though the latter may be machined in certain cementless designs (e.g., into a cylinder rather than the natural more or less conical shape).

The *acetabular component*, if fixed by cement, is almost always hemispherical. The Charnley cup has a flange which is cut to fit the prepared skeleton to assist in cement pressurisation, and several implants have various parts trimmed away to facilitate prosthetic movement. Uncemented cups have a wide variety of different shapes, but are usually either hemispherical, partly conical, cylindrical and/or threaded. Wide variations in opinion again exist as to the correct shape; these opinions are only very slowly being backed up by experimental and/or clinical data.

Method of fixation

Component fixation is a subject dominated at present by a dispute about whether cement should or should not be used. The striking success of the early Charnley THR was produced by fixation of the implants with acrylic cement. Sir John Charnley persuaded patients with successful hip replacements to bequeath their hips back to him for histological analysis and this analysis showed that, in the majority of cases, the femoral cement is extremely well accepted by the body in the long term (e.g., for periods of up to 20 years), though less satisfactory acceptance was seen in the acetabulum for reasons which are still rather obscure. Cement can break up, however, especially when, with a less well-inserted implant, it is, as frequently happens, seriously overloaded. Broken cement is a cause (though only one, *see* below) of an osteolytic process leaching away the skeleton, a potentially serious problem. Thus, attention has been focused on this problem so that many

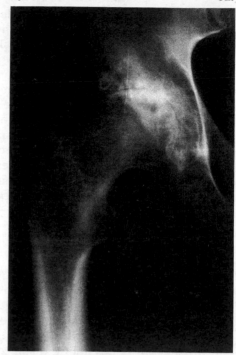

Figure 17.2. (a) X-ray of the right hip of a 49-year-old man, showing severe osteoarthritis. (b) Appearances following Freeman cementless total hip replacement. The special feature of the stemmed design of this implant is the preservation of the femoral neck.

(a)

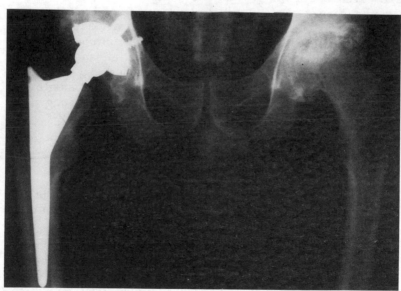

(b)

have the view that cement is an undesirable material to use for implant fixation and this has heralded a recent multiplication of cementless implant fixation systems. These rely on a 'press-fit', such that when the component is driven into a suitably prepared bed, it fits solidly. The press-fit can then be supplemented by various forms of rough or 'porous' surface, such as with beads (PCA) or mesh (AML). Fibrous tissue or, one hopes, bone may then grow into these surfaces. The reliability of this process is, however, uncertain. A recent promising development has been the use of bone crystal coatings (hydroxyapatite). Bone has been shown experimentally to grow preferentially up to such surfaces and it could be that the supplementation of a press-fit by hydroxypatite has an important future place. Certain commercially available hip replacements have it at present either on the stem or the cup.

Bearing material

The chief requirements of the *bearing surfaces* are that friction and wear should both be as low as possible. It has recently been realised that *wear products* arising from the surfaces may be harmful, perhaps seriously so; thus, some of the wear products of polyethylene have been found in the form of small particles of polyethylene in tissues a long distance from the hip itself. These products have the potential to produce osteolysis, as with cement particles. The combination of metal against plastic is time hallowed and effective, but will probably be improved upon in the future. Ceramic against plastic produces lower wear, and newer combinations (such as using polyurethane rubber) may almost remove wear altogether. Wear products and *corrosion products* may also be produced from around other parts of the implant. These will often be metallic, especially with porous-surfaced cementless implants, and there is the disturbing possibility that after a long time-lapse some of these particles might even be carcinogenic.

Hip replacement

Clinical indications

In the *standard* case, the patient has osteoarthritis, is middle aged or elderly, and is otherwise well: or is of any age, with inflammatory arthritis.

The main *symptoms and/or indications* for operation are pain, loss of hip movement, and loss of function, principally the ability to walk adequate distances, or a combination of these. The magnitude of symptoms that give a valid indication for THR depends on the individual case. In general, more minor symptoms may be accepted as an indication in the older patient. The pre-operative symptoms should always be tabulated and several systems for doing this exist. The author uses the Charnley modification of the D'Aubigne and Postel Hip Chart. In this system, six points each are given for pain, walking ability, and range of motion, normality being indicated by the figure 6. Patients are also classified into three different grades, A being a person with one arthritic hip, B with two arthritic hips, and C someone who has some other limitation, such that even with perfect hips there would always be a significant functional deficit, e.g. rheumatoid arthritis. The system allows for easy comparison with postoperative function. Secondary symptoms, such as analgesic requirements, the ability to put on socks or stockings, the use of walking aids, and the patient's gait (if walking is possible) without walking aids can also be recorded.

Once it is established that the patient has an indication for operation, a thorough *pre-operative screening* is needed. This includes a complete medical assessment, a specific search for potential anaesthetic difficulties, and then elimination as far as possible of potential sources of sepsis. These will include attention to teeth, skin lesions and other sources of remote sepsis. The condition of the peripheral pulses, and in a man a history of prostatism, also have to be evaluated, further specialist advice and/or treatment, e.g. from a urological surgeon, being not infrequently required. It is also good practice to have a series of routine screening blood tests done when the patient is seen in the out-patient clinic, as well as to have them grouped with an antibody screen and a urine clinitest.

As with pre-operative screening, certain aspects of the operation are designed to minimise the possibility of *complications*. These complications include infection, dislocation and loosening.

Infection A large multicentre international Medical Research Council sponsored study showed that joint replacement carried out in a laminar flow, ultra clean air operating theatre has half the chance of developing a deep infection than if carried out in an ordinary operating theatre, and that this figure is reduced to a quarter if all the surgical team are wearing total body exhaust suits or similar special clothing. Where facilities exist, this system should therefore be used. The reduction in infection is independent of, but summates with, a similar reduction produced by prophylactic antibiotics. Antibiotics are usually given systemically peri-operatively; some surgeons also add antibiotics to the bone cement.

Orientation to avoid dislocation   The components are carefully *orientated* using special jigs so that the range of motion allowed by their geometry comes within the motion likely to be allowed by the patient. If the orientation is such that the components come to the end of their range of movement while the patient still feels able to move the hip further (e.g. further flexion) then impingement of the prosthetic neck against one edge of the cup will occur, followed by the head's levering out from the cup, with the threat of *dislocation*.

Loosening   The subsequent complication of *loosening* is also, to a major degree, in the hands of the surgeon, and will depend greatly on how strongly the components can be fixed.

Venous thrombosis   It is good practice to use some form of prophylaxis against venous thrombosis, with its potentially lethal complication of pulmonary embolism. Available measures include systemic agents, such as anticoagulants and anti-sludging agents, and mechanical devices producing, directly or indirectly, regular emptying of the deep veins in the lower leg. Some of these devices can be used intra-operatively. Elastic stockings postoperatively are also commonly used, though their effect is uncertain.

Postoperative management
The patient is usually allowed to stand and walk within the first few postoperative days, sometimes from the day after surgery. This mobilisation is carried out with careful supervision by a physiotherapist. A frame is usually needed. Walking aids are then progressively reduced. It is very common for patients to be prescribed elbow crutches until 6 weeks from operation (especially for partial weight-bearing in the younger patient, *see* below), but two sticks may be all that is needed. At any time between 6 weeks and 3 months, it should be possible for all restrictions on function (again, considering a standard case) to be eliminated; improvement usually continues in a subtle way for many months. The end result should then be the 'forgotten hip'.

Further details on postoperative remobilisation are given in Chapter 16.

Hip replacement in special circumstances

In younger patients, it becomes increasingly likely that a hip replacement will wear out or come loose, or both, while the patient is still otherwise active. One view is that the standard operation should be carried out in such cases, with the full knowledge that reoperation (revision) will later be needed (see below). An alternative view, however, is that some other type of operation should be done. These include pelvic or upper femoral osteotomy, other rare forms of non-prosthetic operation, such as arthrodesis, hip resurfacing, replacement of the femoral side only with a bipolar component, and cementless THR.

For pelvic and upper femoral osteotomy and arthrodesis, *see* Chapter 16.

Some form of *prosthesis* becomes necessary if the hip clearly has unsuitable morphology, or where the bone is too soft (as in inflammatory arthritis) or contains large cysts, or where the joint is too stiff. The first priority for *prostheses* in younger people is that as little bone as possible should be removed, thus preserving it for further surgery later. This is the rationale for hip *resurfacing*, (*Figures 17.3(a)* and *17.3(b)*) in which a hemispherical cup is put on to the surface of the reamed femoral head, rather than having a stem down the femoral shaft. This procedure became very popular in the late 1970s, but a serious early failure rate became

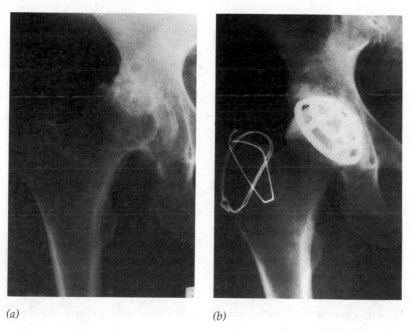

(a)   (b)

Figure 17.3. (a) X-ray of the right hip of a 44-year-old woman, showing severe osteoarthritis with collapse of the superior segment of the femoral head. (b) Appearances following Wagner hip resurfacing using high-density polythene acetabular component stiffened with a perforated metal backing and a ceramic femoral cup, both components being cemented.

apparent and, while to some extent these failures were due to incorrect design features not understood at that time, some of them were probably due to intrinsic difficulties in trying to resurface the head of the femur. Thus, the procedure was abandoned by most surgeons, but it has nevertheless been continued in a few centres with gradual improvements in the design. The author has the view that the procedure probably does have a place in the treatment of the young adult and that the indications might conceivably broaden with improvement in design and materials. Successfully carried out with a good design, the implant can produce a result similar to that of a total hip replacement, with preservation of bone such that the result of subsequent conversion into a total hip replacement is not greatly dissimilar from a standard case.

The clearest indication in degenerative hip disease for a *bipolar replacement* (i.e., one with a stemmed replacement of the femoral head only, in which a separate bearing within the femoral head reduces motion between the outside of the artificial head and the natural acetabulum) is for avascular necrosis of the femoral head,

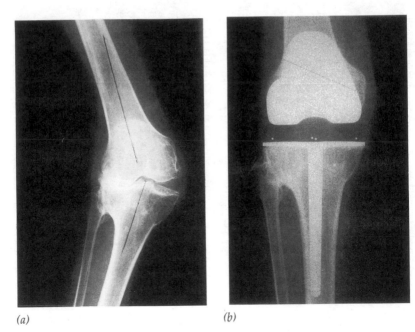

(a)   (b)

Figure 17.4. (a) X-ray of a knee showing severe osteoarthritis with a bad valgus deformity. (b) AP X-ray appearances following Freeman—Samuelson knee replacement of resurfacing type. The metal balls are markers within the plastic tibial component.

in which the acetabulum is normal. The commonest indication, however, is undoubtedly for fractures of the femoral neck in the elderly. This implant is then used instead of a Thompson or Austin Moore, and the additional bearing within the femoral head has been shown to reduce acetabular wear and penetration. Quite commonly, however, no procedure short of a *total hip replacement* will be adequate, the absolute indication for this being absence of the femoral head, such as when the patient has had a septic arthritis in childhood. This, then, is the chief currently accepted indication for cementless THR, as described above. It is, however, very important that the cementless THR used should be truly conservative of the skeleton; with some designs this is not the case.

A small group of patients, such as those with juvenile rheumatoid arthritis or with an old congenital dislocation, may require special components and/or bone grafting of the acetabulum.

The *postoperative management* of the above patients has to be individualised. It has been found that offloading the implant-bone interface for some time postoperatively increases the chances of thorough integration of the implant (as with the process of fracture healing) and therefore younger patients should be mobilised somewhat later and certainly kept partial or non-weight-bearing for the early postoperative weeks whenever possible.

Knee replacement

Implant design

The principles of materials, selection, fixation, bearing surfaces and wear are as for the hip. Fixation without cement has, in general, been found satisfactory with the femoral component of knee replacements, but less satisfactory with the tibia.

Geometry Modern knee replacements are virtually all of a resurfacing kind (*Figures 17.4(a)* and *17.4(b)*), hinges being outmoded. The generic term 'condylar' is often used, indicating resurfacing of both femoral condyles with one component and resurfacing of the upper tibia. The patella is also commonly resurfaced. The femoral component is usually of metal and the tibia of high-density polythene with a metal backing. The shapes of the surfaces adjacent to the bone vary widely between designs, pegs, stems, flanges, keels, and screws all being used. All seek to prevent prosthesis/bone movement.

The shape of the bearing surfaces also varies importantly, one essential determinant being whether the cruciate ligaments are retained or sacrificed. The anterior cruciate ligament is almost always removed (if still present); in many designs the posterior cruciate is retained. Tension of the posterior cruciate ligament influences the relative movement of the tibia and femur in flexion, which in turn influences the shape of the bearing surfaces. The shape of the bearing surfaces in turn influences the contact areas, the loading pressure, and plastic wear. The whole subject remains under active development at present. A group of knee replacements have a third element between the femora and tibia (the 'meniscal bearing') and this principle may represent an important advance, allowing fore-and-aft motion of the tibia, while retaining large bearing surfaces. This type of replacement, however, can only be used if the knee is not grossly deformed.

Where one side only of the knee is affected (most commonly in varus osteoarthritis) it is practicable to carry out a *unicompartmental replacement*, which allows total replacement later if required.

Clinical indications

In the *usual case*, the patient has osteoarthritis and is over the age of 60, or is a patient of any age with rheumatoid arthritis.

The *symptoms* are pain, instability (usually due to skeletal collapse) and loss of walking ability. Loss of knee movement is not in itself a good indication for replacement; the more distally one goes in the leg, the more acceptable loss of motion becomes. Simple conservative measures, such as quadriceps exercises and local symptomatic treatment, and simple surgical procedures, such as arthroscopy, dilatation, and arthroscopic debridement, may well be appropriate before a decision to replace the knee is made.

The symptoms should be *documented* with some form of chart, allowing comparison with the postoperative result. The author uses a modified version of the British Orthopaedic Association knee assessment chart. *Pre-operative screening* is as for the hip. Pre-operative investigations for knee replacement include a long leg weight-bearing X-ray, and for some designs a special X-ray of the pelvis with a radio-opaque bar to indicate the position of the hip.

At *operation*, carried out with a tourniquet and preferably in an ultra-clean air enclosure, the knee is opened through an anterior or antero-medial incision and the patella dislocated laterally. The bone ends are prepared using special jigs unique to any given design, to accept the chosen implants. The upper tibial surface is normally arranged perpendicular to a line drawn from the knee to the ankle, and the femoral component perpendicular to a line drawn from the centre of the knee to the centre of the hip. The latter line is usually at about 7° to the axis of the femoral shaft. As a second completely separate principle, the soft tissues have to be managed so that when the knee is fully extended the leg is stable to a varus or valgus force and in correct alignment (i.e., with the hip, knee and ankle in a straight line). This often requires lengthening of contracted ligaments medially or laterally. The knee also has to be stable when an antero-posterior force is put on the tibia with the knee flexed to 90° and the patella has to track correctly, for which purpose a lateral retinacular release may be required.

Flexion deformities have to be removed at surgery, usually by a combination of posterior capsular release and distal femoral resection.

The development of the soft-tissue balancing side of knee replacement has enabled knees with very severe pre-operative deformities to be replaced using a resurfacing type of implant, rather than a hinge.

Postoperative management

The knee may be kept still for the first few days, perhaps in a splint or plaster, or placed on a continuous passive motion machine. The latter devices, however, have not completely fulfilled their early promise. While some reports have shown a reduction in analgesic requirements and a more rapid return of knee motion with their use, the difference appears rather marginal, and there may be a tendency for recurrence of any pre-existing flexion deformity. The patient is allowed up, partial weight-bearing with crutches, some time within the first postoperative week. In-patient physiotherapy is needed, but physiotherapy is not usually required after the patient has gone home (see also Chapter 16).

Manipulation under anaesthesia   This is now needed rather infrequently, return of knee motion not usually being a problem if careful attention is paid intra-operatively to soft-tissue tensions in extension and flexion, and to patella tracking.

The ankle and foot

Ankle replacement

Usually carried out for rheumatoid arthritis, ankle replacement is technically possible, but in general the results have been poor. Nevertheless, it is possible that improvements in design will give this procedure a wider application sometime in the future. Arthrodesis (see Chapter 16) is normally considered preferable.

In the *foot* the metatarsophalangeal joint of the big toe is very commonly replaced, usually by some form of silastic interposition arthroplasty and not truly by a total joint replacement. The procedure is quite widely practised and can be effective, but silastic in contact with a rough surface is likely to abrade to an unacceptable extent. The results of failure in such a case, however, are a fairly good excision arthroplasty similar to a Keller's.

Revision surgery

This is a very large, and expanding, subject. Originally, failure of THR was almost always treated by excision ('Girdlestone' arthroplasty), but this is now extremely seldom needed and almost all failures (the patient being otherwise fit) can be treated by insertion of a further joint. The same now applies to the knee.

The chief indications for revision in the hip are mechanical loosening, deep infection, and recurrent dislocation; and in the knee, mechanical loosening, deep infection and instability. Combinations of loosening and infection and instability frequently occur. Each case has to be extremely carefully evaluated and special tests, such as isotope bone scans, computerised axial tomography and preliminary biopsy for bacteriological purposes, are frequently needed. Medical assessment also has to be rigorous as the operations take much longer to perform than a primary procedure. A very good case can be made for segregation of revision surgery into specialised centres, as the operations are often difficult, requiring special experience both from the surgeon and the theatre team, special equipment, and often special implants. Unless every care is taken, the complication rate is liable to be substantially higher than in primary surgery, and units carrying out this work frequently have referred to them patients who have already had one or more previous revisions. Each revision is, of course, more difficult to do than the one before.

Revisions are usually carried out in one operation, the previous components and cement, if present, first of all being removed, a thorough debridement then being done and new components, with or without cement, then being inserted. Sometimes, in revisions for infection, an interval of some weeks is allowed between these two steps. Bone grafting either with autograft or allograft bone (for which purpose a bone bank is needed) is frequently required and sometimes striking improvement in the skeleton can be achieved. The postoperative course is always slower than in primary surgery, patients usually being kept in bed for 1 week in a straightforward revision, for 3 weeks in a revision for deep sepsis and sometimes for longer periods than this where extensive bone grafting has been done. Subsequently, they may need to be partial weight-bearing for quite a long period.

With suitable attention to detail, revision surgery, even though taxing for the patient and the surgical team, can produce improvements in patients' well-being and function even more striking than in primary surgery.

Bibliography

Black, J. (1988). *Orthopaedic Materials in Research & Practice*. Churchill Livingstone, Edinburgh.

Charnley, J. (1979). *Low Friction Arthroplasty of the Hip*. Springer Verlag, London.

Freeman, M.A.R. (1980). *Arthritis of the Knee*. Springer Verlag, London.

Ling, R.S.M. (1984). *Complications of THR*. Churchill Livingstone, Edinburgh.

Morscher, E. (ed.) (1984). *Cementless Fixation of Hip Endoprostheses*. Springer Verlag, London.

Proceedings of Knee Society (1989). *Clinical Orthopaedics and Related Research*, **248**, 2–157.

18 Physiotherapy Following Surgery to the Lower Limb

A. Biggs

Patients admitted to hospital for surgery to the lower limb present with similar problems:

- *Pain* — this is a consistent feature and may have been severe and disabling for several years. The severity, type and distribution of pain will influence the surgeon's choice of procedure; also, the patient's perception of pain and response to it will influence postoperative management and ultimate recovery.
- *Dysfunction* — pain will lead to disordered movement and dysfunction results. The patient may develop hypermobility with associated instability in other joints as a result of protecting the painful one, or the joints may become stable but stiff.
- *Stress* — most patients are apprehensive about hospital admission, the surgery proposed, and the possibility of further pain, and also worry lest the results of surgery are not those expected or desired.

Surgery to the lower limb has three primary aims: to relieve pain, improve function and, in most cases, to increase range of movement.

The patient is admitted a few days prior to surgery for medical examination, pathological and radiological investigation and physiotherapy assessment. During this time the patient meets the doctors, nurses, physiotherapist and occupational therapist, who comprise the rehabilitation team. Successful rehabilitation requires the full co-operation of the patient and commences during this pre-operative time, as all members of the rehabilitation team discuss their roles and responsibilities with the patient.

This pre-operative assessment period also allows the physiotherapist to establish a rapport with, and gain the confidence of, the patient. The patient has the opportunity to discuss any worries, expectations and hopes. The physiotherapist uses the time to assess the patient's condition and to discuss the patient's role in the rehabilitation programme, in order that the maximum benefit is gained from the planned surgery.

Both subjective and objective assessments by the physiotherapist are required.

The subjective assessment includes identification of the patient's perception of pain, its type, distribution, severity, duration and relieving factors. A functional history is taken which gives insight into the patient's life style and identifies any difficulties encountered on a regular basis with regard to activities of daily living, such as dressing, bathing, cooking and eating. The patient's home circumstances are investigated to determine the type of home, e.g., flat, bungalow or multistoried house, which will determine the patient's need for competence on stairs postoperatively and indicate any possible adaptations to the house that may be required to support independence. The help of family and friends is ascertained, as is the patient's mobility outside the home. The physical abilities are different for driving a car, being a passenger or having to cope with public transport.

Information gained from the subjective assessment may indicate the need for involvement of other members of the team, e.g., the social worker or occupational therapist, who should be asked to see the patient where particular problems exist.

The objective assessment centres on the physical examination of the patient and, as some form of walking aid will be required after the operation, examination of the upper limbs, the trunk and the other lower limb are as important as the examination of the area on which surgery is to be performed. A holistic approach by the physiotherapist is required.

The importance of assessing the physical state of the rest of the body that supports the area of surgery cannot be overstated and all patients admitted for orthopaedic surgery to the lower limb are taught a scheme of exercises designed to assist venous return, to reduce the likelihood of development of deep vein thrombosis and chest complications and to keep the patient's level of activity stable. This routine of maintenance exercise, which must be practised by all patients frequently and regularly following surgery, includes:

- Deep breathing exercise.
- Foot and ankle movements in the full range of both legs.
- Isometric exercises of quadriceps and glutei of both legs.
- Active exercise to the joints of the non-operated leg.
- General arm and trunk movements.

Physiotherapy relevant to specific surgical procedures to the lower limb is determined by the type of procedure used, the surgeon's preference and the condition of the patient.

Each patient has individual abilities and limitations dictated by the response to surgery and ultimate potential for rehabilitation. The physiotherapy outlined in the remainder of this chapter provides guidance to the therapist for appropriate postoperative achievement. Modification of the programmes identified to meet the patient's individual needs will be necessary.

The hip

Surgery to this joint includes total hip replacement, excision (Girdlestone) arthroplasty and arthrodesis.

Total hip replacement

For clinical indications for total hip replacement, see Chapter 17. Physiotherapeutic management depends on the type of operation and the surgical approach used. Charnley total hip prostheses are most frequently used and, during surgery, the greater trochanter of the femur, with its muscle attachment, is detached and later wired back onto the femoral shaft. It is, therefore, important to maintain hip abduction and avoid adduction until healing occurs in the soft tissues around the joint and at the greater trochanter.

If a posterior approach is favoured, hip flexion should be limited postoperatively to approximately 45°, to avoid the possibility of dislocation, which will occur if undue stress is put on the structures of the posterior aspect of the joint. When sitting out of bed, the patient inclines backwards, thereby maintaining limited hip flexion.

Many surgeons now perform joint replacements without using cement as an interface between the bone and prosthesis. This retards the rate of postoperative rehabilitation slightly, as the patient initially takes less weight through the affected limb and uses crutches for a longer time. However, the tight fit of the femoral prosthesis in the shaft of the bone provides a more stable result for the majority of patients.

Pre-operative physiotherapy Prior to surgery the procedures involved and postoperative management are explained to the patient. Subjective and objective assessments are completed and the scheme of maintenance exercises taught. The subjective assessment is outlined above and the objective assessment should include the following:

• Observe the patient's gait to determine the pattern of gait, whether or not there is a limp and whether or not the patient uses walking aids.

- Observe the posture, and record any abnormalities.
- Check mobility of the lumbar spine and record any alteration of the lumbar curve.
- Check the active and passive range of motion in both hips and record any inhibiting factors, such as pain or stiffness.
- Test the muscle strength and note any wasting of muscles on the affected limb.
- Identify the presence of pain and whether it occurs at rest or on weight bearing.
- Note the presence and extent of deformity of the joint.
- Note any inequality of leg length, measured with the patient lying supine, the pelvis level and feet slightly apart. *True* leg lengths are determined by measurement from the anterior superior iliac spine to the tip of the medial malleolus of the same side. *Apparent* leg lengths are determined by measurement from the umbilicus or tip of the sternum to the tip of the medial malleolous on each side.

Postoperative physiotherapy The sequence of postoperative activity will be the same for all patients, although their individual rates of recovery will vary according to the surgeon's preference and the patient's condition. Patients return from theatre to be nursed supine for approximately 24 hours, during which time postoperative chest care and maintenance exercises are practised. Following initial postoperative recumbency, the patient is placed in a semi-recumbent position with his legs held in abduction by means of a Charnley wedge placed between them. Alternatively, the abducted position may be maintained by placing the legs in troughs.

Once the patient is in the semi-recumbent position, the physiotherapist assists production of small range hip flexion and abduction movements and flexion of the knee on the affected side.

Provided normal progress is maintained after 48 hours, a postoperative check X-ray is performed and the wound inspected. If the wound is satisfactory, drainage tubes are removed, and if the X-ray proves satisfactory, weight-bearing can commence.

Weight bearing commences before the patient is allowed to flex the hip freely, and so care must be taken to protect the hip on the operated side from falling into adduction and flexion, as this position is unstable and the joint may dislocate. A safe method of transfer from inclined lying to standing is as follows:

- The patient moves to the side of the bed nearest to the operated hip, with the physiotherapist supporting the leg in an abducted position.
- The legs are gently swung over the edge of the bed, the physio-

therapist maintaining the position of abduction and minimal flexion on the operated side. The patient is now sitting on the side of the bed.

- The physiotherapist then assists the patient to push up from the bed to a standing position and the patient supports this position with a walking frame.

Provided the patient's balance is satisfactory, weight transference and exercises for balance can now be performed prior to walking a short distance. The patient is then returned to bed, reversing the procedure for getting up outlined above.

Exercise regimes, balance and walking are progressed within the patient's tolerance, and by the fifth postoperative day hip flexion should have increased sufficiently to allow the patient to sit out of bed for a short time. Active and assisted active exercises are progressed in range and power, which assists the return to general mobility and independence.

When able, usually by the end of the first week, the patient should be allowed to dress and complete self-care with little or no assistance. Support during walking is reduced as the patient progresses from walking frame to elbow crutches. By the end of the first week the patient is expected to walk safely with crutches without supervision and should be increasing both the speed and the distance walked as confidence returns.

The physiotherapist maintains a supervisory role during this time, evaluating the patient's performance at each visit and progressing the rehabilitation programme appropriately.

Careful observation of the limb to give early warning of any circulatory problem is necessary. Pain in the calf, restriction of dorsiflexion of the ankle or persistent swelling of the limb could be indicative of circulatory complications, which would affect the rate of the patient's rehabilitation and should be reported to nursing or medical staff when first observed.

Any difference in leg length is corrected with the appropriate height of shoe-raise prior to finalisation of gait rehabilitation, to ensure the patient uses equal stride length and has even timing. Posture is noted and any correction required is given. It is essential that the patient is taught to rise from a chair of appropriate height, to get in and out of bed safely and to negotiate steps, slopes and stairs prior to discharge.

To ascend stairs safely, the patient holds the bannister with one hand and both crutches in the other, the second crutch being held in a horizontal position. The patient supports his body weight on the crutch and bannister and raises the non-operated leg to rest on the step above the one on which the crutch and operated leg stand. The patient extends his hip and knee on the non-operated side and the crutch and leg from the lower step rise to join the other leg. The process is repeated until the ascent of the stairs is completed. To descend stairs, the procedure is reversed. The bannister is held with one hand, the two crutches held in the other. The crutches and operated leg are lowered to the step below and, when stable, the non-operated leg is lowered to join the operated leg and crutch. This sequence is repeated until descent of the flight of stairs is completed.

In the absence of a bannister, the patient uses the second crutch for support and undertakes the sequence of movements as described above.

As 90° flexion at the hip and knee is required to place a foot on the step above, it is possible that it will be 3 months before the patient can negotiate stairs using alternate feet.

When competent in all these activities, the patient is discharged from hospital having been given the following advice:

• Rest is essential, particularly during the first few weeks following discharge.
• The new hip should be treated with care to allow the healing processes to be completed.
• Flexion of the hip beyond 90° and adduction beyond neutral must be avoided, as must any twisting of the body on the hip.

This produces some restrictions of activity which are to be adhered to during the total healing time. To allow healing to progress satisfactorily, the patient should therefore:

• Avoid bending the hip too far. He should sit on a chair that allows the knee to rest lower than the hip. He should not bend to tie up shoe laces, or use alternate stepping to ascend or descend a flight of stairs.
• The patient must not cross his legs when sitting or lying and, when lying on his side in the bed, he must lie on the operated side.
• When turning round, the patient must not swivel feet, but must use a series of small steps to turn the body.

It is probable that the occupational therapist will check the patient's performance for a full range of functional activities and will provide, and teach, the use of aids where they are required.

The wound should be healed after 12–14 days, when the sutures are removed and the patient is discharged from hospital. The patient is seen by the surgeon in his out-patient clinic approximately 6 weeks after surgery and, provided all is progressing normally, the patient will progress from elbow crutches to sticks, which are then retained for a minimum of 3 months. Provided patients have received adequate rehabilitation instruction post-operatively, out-patient treatment should not be necessary.

Excision arthroplasty — Girdlestone

This operation is rarely seen nowadays, as failure of total hip replacement and other surgery can now be treated by revision of the original procedure (see Chapter 17) which, although having a longer rehabilitation time, will give patients a better result than would be obtained by the use of excision arthroplasty. Excision arthroplasty is usually a salvage procedure involving removal of the femoral head and neck. It may be used in elderly people when all other surgical procedures have failed to alleviate the underlying hip problem (see Chapter 16). Pre-operative physio-therapy is as for a total hip replacement. Postoperatively, the patient will be on bed rest, usually in skeletal traction, for ap-proximately 6 weeks, so the scheme of maintenance exercises assumes an important role. As soon as the pain in the hip starts to subside, movement of the affected hip can commence in traction. Once traction is removed, the patient can be mobilised with crutches.

Non-weight-bearing crutch walking for several months is pre-ferred, to enable fibrous material to fill the joint space. This will provide stability of the joint and reduce shortening of the leg on the operated side. As these patients are usually elderly, non-weight-bearing walking may not be possible and patients will require a shoe raise to balance the leg lengths if early weight bearing on the operated side results in excessive shortening of the limb.

The patient is discharged as soon as independence on crutches is achieved. Eventually, the patient may progress from crutches to walking sticks, but it is rare for the patient to walk without any aid following this operation.

Arthrodesis

This is the surgical fusion of the joint and has now been superceded as improvements in joint replacement surgery and the develop-ment of revision surgery have removed the need for it in most cases. On the rare occasions that it is performed, it is used to relieve pain in the joint, provided that only one hip is affected and adjacent joints are in such good condition that they can compensate for the loss of movement that results from this pro-cedure (see Chapter 16).

The method of fixation to encourage fusion may be internal, external or a combination of both, according to the surgeon's preference.

Pre-operative physiotherapy is as for total hip replacement, with emphasis being placed on assessment of the mobility of the lumbar spine and the knee, ankle and foot of the affected leg. For optimum function postoperatively, the hip joint will be arthrodesed in 15–20° flexion, 10° abduction and 5° lateral rotation, and the patient returns from theatre with the joint immobilised in this position.

Following a short period of bed rest, during which time the patient practises the scheme of maintenance exercises, the patient is taught non-weight-bearing crutch walking. Once the patient is independent, mobile using crutches and the wound has healed, discharge from hospital is assured. Splintage is removed once the arthrodesis site has united and the patient continues guided rehabilitation until full weight-bearing is permitted and normal activities are resumed.

Upper femoral osteotomy

This procedure is performed to relieve pain, correct deformity and to maintain or improve the mobility and stability of the affected limb. For details of the clinical indications and procedures, see Chapter 16.

Patients who undergo this surgery are often younger than those who require total joint replacement for, although they complain of severe pain, there is found to be little or no joint destruction. The different types of osteotomy are reviewed in Chapter 16 and the surgical technique and method of postoperative fixation will vary according to the surgeon.

Pre-operative assessment follows the same pattern as that for total hip replacement.

Postoperatively, the sequence of rehabilitation is similar to that for rehabilitation following total hip replacement, with the surgeon identifying the time when patients may mobilise with crutches. The surgeon will also determine if weight is to be taken through the operated side, when this will be allowed and how much is permitted. Discharge from hospital is permitted when the wound has healed, usually about 2 weeks after surgery.

The patient will remain non-weight-bearing on crutches for 4–6 months and will benefit from hydrotherapy if a pool is available. Once union has occurred, walking sticks may replace elbow crutches and the patient will continue the programme of rehabilitation until full weight-bearing is allowed and normal activities undertaken.

The knee

Surgery for this joint includes total knee replacement, hemiarthroplasty, arthrodesis and ligament reconstruction. Although the postoperative rehabilitation for patients following surgery to the knee will vary, the pre-operative physiotherapy assessment is common to all surgical procedures that involve the knee and is here described fully for total knee replacement only.

Total knee replacement
This section should be read following study of the knee replacement section in Chapter 17. The operation is performed for the patient who presents with severe pain, deformity and joint instability and, such is the progress in this type of surgery, there are many options available. The majority of surgeons use a small amount of cement to fix the tibial component of prosthesis, but increasingly the femoral components are being held by their fit into the bone without cement.

Pre-operative physiotherapy Prior to surgery, the procedures involved and postoperative management are explained to the patient.

Subjective and objective assessments are completed and the scheme of maintenance exercises taught (see p. 341); particular emphasis is placed on the need for regular exercise of quadriceps. The subjective assessment is outlined on p. 341. The objective assessment should include the following:

- Observe the gait and note the pattern and whether or not aids are used.
- Observe the posture and record any anomalies.
- Identify any deformity or instability present in the knee, on weight-bearing or non-weight-bearing.
- Measure both the active and passive ranges of motion of both knees and note any inhibiting factors.
- Observe any muscle wasting.
- Measure the power of contraction of the quadriceps.
- Identify the state of mobility of the patella.
- Note any swelling of the limb.
- Record the presence of pain at rest or on weight bearing.

Postoperative physiotherapy Following surgery, the patient returns to the ward with the limb splinted in plaster of Paris, a pressure bandage or a pressure bandage and canvas splint. The foot of the bed is elevated to aid venous return and minimise swelling. The scheme of maintenance exercise is performed by the patient frequently during waking hours, with emphasis on the necessity for vigorous foot and ankle movements and quadriceps exercises. Following removal of the wound drainage tubes and subject to a satisfactory check X-ray at approximately 48 hours postoperatively, partial weight bearing walking may commence with, initially, a frame being used for support.

On average, knee flexion commences on the fifth day following reduction of the dressing and inspection of the wound. Some surgeons will encourage earlier mobilisation of the knee and others will limit the amount of flexion allowed for some days, until the wound is healing well. It is imperative that the patient should gain and then maintain full knee extension with strong contraction of the quadriceps prior to discard of splintage during walking.

Active flexion and extension exercises are performed regularly throughout the day, working initially with the heel supported on a sliding board. As control and strength improve, these exercises can be performed over the edge of the bed, the heel initially supported by the physiotherapist to minimise pain. The range of movement achieved should be measured and recorded daily.

The patient progresses through active-assisted, to active and active-resisted exercises, using facilitatory techniques if required to increase range of movement, muscle strength and joint stability. The aim is to have a fully active extension of the knee, good quadriceps control of position and easy flexion to 90°.

Throughout this rehabilitation period, the patient is instructed in the use of crutches and undergoes gait re-education.

Sutures are removed 12–14 days following surgery and, provided the patient has quadriceps control in extension and 80–90° knee flexion, discharge from hospital is arranged. Treatment as an out-patient is encouraged until no further improvement is noted.

Some patients progress more slowly and benefit from a longer period in hospital. If the wound is healing well, hydrotherapy will be of value, particularly in the encouragement of knee movement.

Patients who are slow to gain knee movement may require manipulation under anaesthetic. It is useful if the physiotherapist can observe the procedure, as treatment is commenced immediately in an attempt to maintain and later increase the acquired range. Ice packs are effective in the reduction of any swelling and for the relief of pain following manipulation. Active exercises are used to maintain the range achieved under anaesthetic.

Out-patient physiotherapy is arranged to continue the rehabilitation programme for these patients and is maintained until they have full functional recovery, have an active range of pain-free movement and full muscular stability of the knee.

Hemi-arthroplasty

This type of joint surgery includes the McIntosh knee prosthesis and bi-compartmental tibio-femoral replacement, as well as hemi-arthroplasty. It is indicated when the patient complains of pain in the medial or lateral aspect of the knee.

The pre- and post-operative management follows the same regime as for total knee replacement. However, the rate of improvement during rehabilitation is much increased.

Arthrodesis

Provided that the adjacent joints are freely mobile, this operation may be the surgery of choice in patients who have problems that affect one joint only, and it is performed more frequently than arthrodesis of the hip (see Chapter 16).

Pre-operative physiotherapy assessment is as described before, with particular consideration being given to mobility of the other joints of the limb.

Postoperative physiotherapy Following surgery, the patient returns to the ward with the arthrodesis site immobilised by internal fixation, external fixation or a combination of both. Commonly, a plaster-of-Paris cylinder is used for external fixation. The patient will practise the scheme of maintenance exercises prior to mobilisation, with non-weight-bearing crutch walking. The precise timing for mobilisation will depend on the patient's condition and the surgeon's wishes. Should the patient's age preclude non-weight-bearing crutch walking, a compromise situation of toe touching may be necessary.

Once the wound has healed and the patient is independent on crutches, discharge from hospital is arranged. Splintage is removed when the fusion is solid and the patient continues rehabilitation until he is pain-free in full weight bearing activities and has made a full functional recovery.

There is little shortening of the limb following this surgical procedure and it is unlikely that a shoe raise will be required.

Ligament reconstruction and/or augmentation

This is a new field of surgery, so treatment protocols are still developing as the surgical technique develops; results from this procedure are encouraging (see Friedman and Ferkel, 1988).

Surgery is performed when the joint instability is proven to result from ligamentous laxity, particularly affecting the anterior cruciate ligament. It is a condition the most often occurs in young athletic people.

The ligament may be reconstructed using either an autogenous graft or a prosthetic graft, of which there are several varieties, all with different treatment protocols.

Prior to treating these patients the physiotherapist must determine the surgeon's preferred protocol, so the following regime is presented for guidance only. Pre-operative assessment follows the procedure for all knee surgery, described on p. 348.

Postoperatively, the patient will practise the maintenance scheme of exercise with the exclusion of movements to the operated knee. The patient is mobilised on crutches, which will be retained for approximately 3 months, the patient progressing from non-weight-bearing to weight-bearing when the surgeon permits.

Supervised gentle non-weight-bearing knee flexion is started after approximately 3 weeks and the knee may be slow to mobilise during the first 6—8 weeks. Patients are discharged when fully mobile and independent with crutches, and continue treatment as out-patients. After a further 3 months, vigorous rehabilitation is started with emphasis on building up the power of quadriceps and hamstrings to support the operated knee. Rehabilitation continues until the patient is fully independent and has returned to all previous activities. Sporting activities may be introduced approximately 6 months after surgery.

In practice, physiotherapists must follow the surgeon's individual protocol for management of this situation.

Lower femoral/tibial osteotomy

An osteotomy is performed to relieve pain and correct deformity at the joint, this being done in the region of the distal end of the femur or the proximal end of the tibia (see Chapter 16).

The site of osteotomy and fixation of the bone ends depends on the deformity present and the surgeon's preference. Fixation of the operation site may be achieved with staples, compression clamp, cast brace or plaster-of-Paris cylinder. The site of operation and method of fixation will dictate the speed of the patient's rehabilitation.

Pre-operative physiotherapy is as for total knee replacement.

Postoperative physiotherapy

This involves routine maintenance exercises, with emphasis on foot and ankle movements and exercises for the quadriceps.

Once good muscular control by the quadriceps has been achieved, the patient may get up and mobilise with crutches, the degree of weight bearing being determined by the surgeon.

All external splintage is retained for 6–8 weeks or until bony union has taken place, when mobilisation of the knee is started. If a plaster-of-Paris cylinder has been used for postoperative fixation, a back splint may be required for walking when knee flexion commences, as the ability to extend the knee may be lost for a short time.

The use of the cast brace, staples or compression clamp as fixation for the operation site enable knee mobilisation to be commenced soon after surgery is performed, if the surgeon agrees.

Patients are discharged from hospital when independent on crutches, returning as out-patients for removal of the splintage and further rehabilitation to restore full knee function and independence.

The ankle

Because of the complexity at this joint, satisfactory joint replacements have not yet been developed. The surgery of choice therefore is arthrodesis. Similar rehabilitation programmes are followed for each type of procedure.

Pre-operative physiotherapy

Assessment must include the following components:

- Examination of gait, its pattern and use or not of aids.
- Assessment of the range of movement of the ankle and subtalar joints.
- Measurement of muscle power and joint stability.
- Identification of any muscle wasting.
- Documentation of the presence of pain on weight bearing or at rest.

Postoperative physiotherapy

Following arthrodesis of the ankle, surgical fusion is held by internal, external or a combination of both types of fixation. This is retained for 6–8 weeks until bony union has occurred, at about which time the patient is re-admitted to hospital for a short stay to have any external fixation removed, after which the patient is discharged when seen to be independent.

The foot is supported in the surgeon's choice of splintage and held in high elevation to minimise swelling. Routine maintenance exercises are started as soon as possible. Once the drainage tubes have been removed, at about 48 hours, the patient may sit out of bed with instructions to keep the leg elevated whenever possible. The commencement of weight bearing is determined by the surgeon and, once this is permitted, forefoot mobility is encouraged and the patient mobilised with the aid of crutches.

As the pain decreases, the patient will increase the amount of weight bearing on the joint, gradually progressing to full independence, firstly on crutches, then with the aid of one stick. The patient gains confidence not only walking on the flat, but also in walking on slopes, up and down steps and on uneven ground.

The patient is usually discharged from hospital within 2−3 weeks postoperatively, with out-patient physiotherapy organised where necessary.

Reference

Friedman, M.J. and Ferkel, R.D. (1988). *Prosthetic Ligament Reconstruction of the Knee*, Saunders, Philadelphia.

19 Biomechanics of Shoulder Movement

J.H. Patrick

Shoulder movement can be considered in three main sections, depending on functional anatomy. The true synovial shoulder joint is that articulation between the glenoid and the head of the humerus. The sterno-clavicular joint and the acromio-clavicular joint are also synovial joints of the shoulder girdle, and allow clavicular movement which occurs every time the arm is elevated (as personal testing will easily prove). These arthrodial joint movements will be described in some detail below. The other 'joint' is not a synovial one, but is equally important for shoulder function. Movement of the scapula round the chest wall is necessary for elevation of the arm and shoulder; it is controlled by muscle action and, since movement occurs, it has been named the scapulo-thoracic 'joint' or articulation.

All four joints work together synchronously to permit very free three-dimensional movement. The shoulder is very mobile, unlike the deep, stable hip joint. The large surface for articulation produces a most versatile range of motion, especially for the hand. The shallow glenoid fossa has suspended from it the humerus, with stability provided by soft tissue, muscles, ligaments and a joint capsule – in normal circumstances, a highly effective joint. Versatility allows rapid conversion from a heavy weight-lifting function to bowling or painting a ceiling; and in every part of prehensile activity we act to stabilise our shoulder and arm to allow the hand its great range of essential tasks, be it working or in activities of daily living across a spectrum which includes maintaining personal hygiene right up to the violinist plying his bow.

No apology is made here for the mention of the hand as an essential part of shoulder movement. The hand has been graphically termed the 'organ of the upper limb'; its function very much depends upon the contribution of shoulder movement.

Figure 19.1 (the shoulder anatomy) clearly shows the anatomical structure, a large humeral articular surface, a shallow glenoid cavity (of the scapula) having one third of the surface area of the

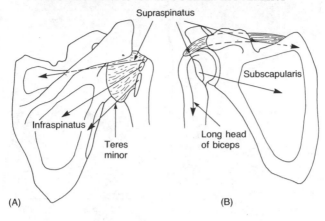

Supraspinatus

Subscapularis

Infraspinatus

Teres minor

Long head of biceps

(A) (B)

Figure 19.1. Posterior (a) and anterior (b) view of the bones of the shoulder with the rotator-cuff muscles that stabilise the shoulder joint.

opposing head. The glenoid depth is increased by the labrum of fibro-cartilage which ensures stability (shoulder dislocation is an uncommon event), but allows movement. The scapula is said to 'glide' around the rib-cage, rotating with the clavicle about a sternal point of origin. The muscles of the shoulder region become tendinous around the gleno-humeral joint and these tendons 'blend' in with the joint capsule (*see* 'rotator-cuff' in *Figure 19.1*).

Functional positions are legion; at rest the arm is dependent and the humerus can be considered to be vertical. The glenoid faces the head at a slight angle, ready for three patterns of motion – elevation, internal and/or external rotation and horizontal flexion and extension. As an example of shoulder joint movement, solely elevation will be considered here. The other movements have been evaluated and complete accounts can be found in other texts.

Elevation

Raising the arm from the trunk, from the resting position, is called abduction (which itself needs further explanation). Scapulo-thoracic motion and movement of the humeral head within the socket also occur in this movement. In *Figure 19.2* abduction is occurring in the trunkal coronal plane. We must know that the plane of the joint is 30° anterior to the body median or coronal plane. Thus elevation first means a movement of the arm towards the body coronal plane by horizontal extension, then movement

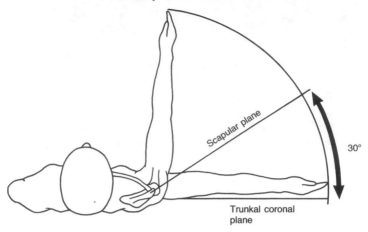

Figure 19.2. Planes of arm elevation: neutral, flexion, and abduction.

into *true* abduction (away from the trunk). Eventually (*Figure 19.3*) there will be impingement of the greater tuberosity of the humerus on the acromium. If external rotation of the humeral head is possible (under the influence of infra-spinatus contraction), then the greater tuberosity is rotated laterally and clears beneath the acromium. We can check this for ourselves by maximally medially rotating our own humerus, then attempting elevation − the arm only gets up to 90°. Consequently, a plea is made for using the scapular plane for basic testing of arm elevation, so that more accurate communication about motion ranges in patients can be made between us all.

The gleno-humeral joint accounts for 120° of arm elevation. The remainder comes from the coincident movement of the scapula where a turning moment exists (*Figure 19.4*). Initially the scapula rotates little beyond the first 60° of arm elevation; e.m.g. (electromyogram) studies have shown synchronous muscle activity in the upper portion of trapezius muscle, the serratus anterior, and levator scapulae. These 'pull' the scapula forwards and laterally; the glenoid face faces ever more upward and outward as a result. This facilitates the movement and, as importantly, dissipates the forces applied when falling on to the outstretched hand. Then shock-absorption becomes of paramount importance. This recoil mechanism, described by Carter Rowe (Rowe and Sakellarides, 1961), is not widely appreciated, but is a hugely successful mechanism in preventing damage from pushing or pulling, lifting, or after indirect blows to the shoulder. Clearly, during recoil, muscles

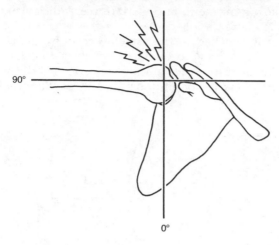

90°

0°

Figure 19.3. Abduction without external rotation allows impingement of the tuberosity against the acromion.

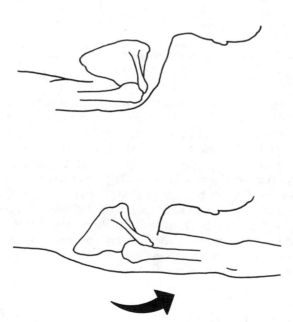

Figure 19.4. Turning moment in scapulo-thoracic movement and humeral rotation.

contract to allow movement, and work (force × distance) is done, dissipating the energy applied.

The scapula is attached to the skeletal 'core' by the clavicle at the sterno-clavicular joint to allow the clavicle to rotate (*Figure 19.5*). The fulcrum of the scapulo-thoracic glide is at this joint, the clavicle *rotating* along its longitudinal axis three-dimensionally.

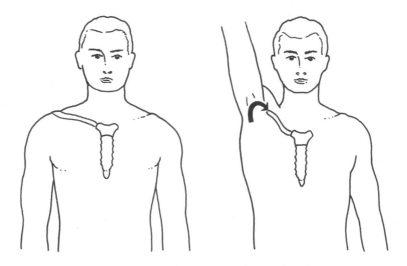

Figure 19.5. Clavicle rotation during elevation.

During abduction the resultant forces between the humeral head and the glenoid can be resolved mathematically and are found to be nearly 0.8 times the body weight (Popper and Walker, 1976). By other calculations, reinforced by e.m.g. studies, it can be shown that the rotator-cuff, especially the supraspinatus, is used to depress the head and 'stabilise' it in the centre of the ball and socket. This is of great importance, clinically, if rotator-cuff injuries occur, since the fulcral point of the gleno-humeral joint will change dramatically during abduction (the latter occurring by deltoid muscle action). If the humeral head moves excessively upward on the glenoid, then the deltoid action is severely compromised. Why is this?

Shoulder muscles

We are aware that the deltoid is in three parts and is the main abductor of the shoulder. It has central, anterior and posterior

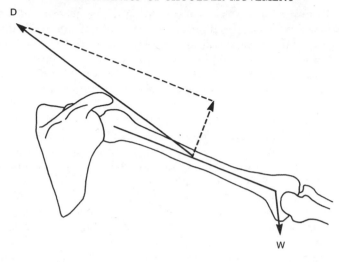

Figure 19.6. The resultant of the deltoid force acting on the shoulder joint.

portions. When considering equilibrium of the shoulder joint being held in abduction (*Figure 19.6*) the most significant muscle action is by deltoid and only small errors will be introduced by ignoring subscapularis, infra-spinatus and teres minor. Inman *et al.* (1944) have shown that when supporting the weight of the arm 'W' the line of action of the deltoid is shown as 'D'.

These are the forces being applied to the shoulder, except when the arm is hanging beside the trunk (then its weight is supported by the configuration of the joint surfaces and by the capsular and coraco-humeral ligaments). The muscle forces will vary in magnitude and direction as the arm is elevated. Calculations of the value of 'D' will thus change, but all depend upon the lever arm of the point of centre of mass of the whole upper limb. At 30° of elevation, the distance of the mass centre to the fulcrum point in the shoulder joint is *less* than when the arm is elevated to 80° or 90°.

Taking an approximate position for the centre of mass at just above the elbow, you can see in your own arm that that point moves progressively further away from the centre of the joint. (Imagine a perpendicular passing through the centre of your shoulder and think of the distance that the elbow moves away from that vertical line. That is the lever arm.) The principles of moments applied to levers can be further explored in Chapter 1.

As the distance increases, so the moment arm increases *requiring* extra muscle activity (or demand torque). In order to maintain equilibrium, the typical value of torque required to keep the arm elevated at 30° is about 8Nm; at 90° of elevation this has increased to about 16Nm. Mainly, this is provided by the deltoid, which, as a power-producing muscle, is *multipennate* to allow many more muscle fibres to be present within the same volume. Also, our consideration of lever length can be pursued to explain how the deltoid manages, as a relatively small muscle, to continue exerting its force in such a variety of shoulder positions. We realise that the greater the leverage a muscle has, the greater and more effective is its turning moment.

From our discussion earlier, we know that the lever length is the perpendicular distance between the muscle's line of pull and the fulcrum of motion (*Figure 19.7*). The shoulder fulcrum is kept at the centre of the shoulder joint by the combined action of the supraspinatus and rotator-cuff muscles, so that as the middle deltoid abducts the arm, the *perpendicular distance* of the muscle's

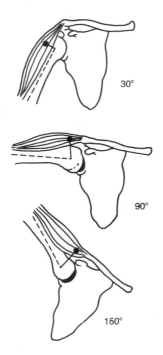

Figure 19.7. The mechanical leverage of the muscle equals the distance between the longitudinal muscle axis and the centre of gleno-humeral rotation. It is modified by the degree of arm elevation.

action to the centre of the gleno-humeral joint increases, the deltoid and upper humerus being beautifully designed to accomplish this task. As the arm is moved upward the deltoid muscle line of action progressively changes – always increasing its lever arm and thus efficiency. The different parts of the deltoid assist in elevation in similar ways at different times, the anterior being most useful at about 60° of scapular plane abduction, the posterior part being most effective above 120° of elevation.

Reference again to *Figure 19.6* will allow us to realise that the deltoid force 'D' acting to elevate the arm may be considered to have two components of force – one directed horizontally as a compressive force, driving the humeral head into the socket (in this it assists the supraspinatus muscle). The other is a vertical component lying along the line of the face of the glenoid – as a *shear* force – which is thus attempting to destabilise the joint by producing an upward movement of the humeral head. This is opposed somewhat by frictional forces, but also by the 'inferior' parts of the rotator-cuff muscles (the infraspinatus, subscapularis and teres minor). These contract synchronously with the deltoid (again shown by activity – e.m.g. studies) preventing this upward slide. In disease states, a high humeral head can often be found radiologically; in some pathological states, impingement of the rotator-cuff on the acromium can occur, producing symptoms.

The supraspinatus is virtually a horizontally positioned muscle (*Figure 19.1*). It passes from the supraspinous fossa of the scapula to the greater tuberosity of the humerus. Unsurprisingly, it produces mainly a compressive force between the two bones. Attrition rupture, or arc syndromes caused by loss of blood supply to the tendon just below the acromium, allows the compressive force to fall, and the humeral head can then 'ride-up' the glenoid face, worsening the impingement and leading to loss of elevation (or deltoid abductor) power. It is probable that the production of this compressive force is a more important function of the muscle than its elevation capability. However, some patients with complete deltoid denervation can fully elevate the arm, admittedly with great loss of power. The other cuff muscles actively contract to keep the head in the socket centre, pulling the humerus to allow it to pass under the acromium during elevation. This is not the complete picture though – e.m.g. studies have shown that the subscapularis and infra-spinatus have other less synchronous contractions and functions.

Mention was made earlier about the scapulo-thoracic articulation. That there is rotation of the scapula around the chest wall is indisputable; how, though, is this brought about? We know that by this motion the abduction–elevation movement is possible, since the glenoid face is rotated to face ever more upwards during elevation (*see Figure 19.7*). The scapula, though, also has to keep the shoulder and arm in position by possessing a posture of its own. This occurs through the deep fascia of the neck, which inserts on to the clavicle, acromium and spine of the scapula. Also, the levator scapulae and the upper trapezius muscle contract to resist any downward pull on the arm or hand (*Figure 19.8(a)*).

There are several large muscle groups which have been identified as being active in the production of scapular rotation. The trapezius is functionally divided into upper, middle and lower sections, to which are added the rhomboids and serratus anterior. These muscles (and others − for example, the pectoralis minor and levator scapulae) have individual actions used in some of the greatly versatile actions of the shoulder during sports activities, instrument playing, lifting, and even writing. These will not be discussed. Rather, we shall concentrate on the force couples which exist to assist scapular motion. In *Figure 19.8* we can clearly see that the upward rotators of the scapula are the upper fibres of the trapezius.

Less obvious is the action of the upper segments of serratus anterior (a muscle clothing the *deep* surface of the scapula and

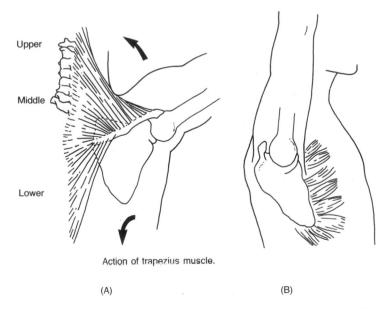

Action of trapezius muscle.

(A)   (B)

Figure 19.8. (a) *Trapezian muscle in three parts: upper, middle, and inferior·* (b) *serratus anterior muscle slips.*

attached to the chest wall). Careful thought will allow under-standing of how the upper part of serratus contracting with the upper part of trapezius will pull the acromium and scapula upward and rotate it forward around the chest wall. Clearly, the sudden action of these powerful muscles will need to be opposed, and the rhromboid muscles achieve this objective. The lower trapezius segment provides assistance in this stabilisation, and similarly contraction of these more posterior—inferior muscles (including the lower rhomboid) will control posterior scapular movement during descent of the arm.

Scapular rhythm

The two main articulations described above, acting with a rotating clavicle, allow subtle or fierce movements under load for the shoulder. A rhythm is recognised, and disease in any of the elements described can upset this rhythm, leading to various degrees of disability. The role of the physiotherapist is commonly to treat various shoulder pathologies, along quite traditional lines. From this account we may perceive that while the individual parts of shoulder activity have been investigated, and are now largely understood, such is the enormously complex interrelation-ship of the actions of the muscles employed, that we would not be surprised if our patients are not always happy after treatment. Often the rhythm is broken permanently because of muscle weakness or disease in the articulation. Control of so many muscle contractions, acting synergistically, can become faulty. In spite of the great possibility for error, it is some comfort that few patients have cause for complaint about their shoulders.

References

Inman, V.T., Saunders, J.B., De, C.M. and Abbott, L.C. (1944). Observations on the function of the shoulder joint. *J. Bone Joint Surg.*, **42**, 1.
Popper, N.K. and Walker, P.S. (1976). Normal and abnormal motion of the shoulder. *J. Bone Joint Surg.*, **58A**, 195.
Rowe, C.R. and Sakellarides, H.T. (1961). Factors related to recurrences of anterior dislocations of the shoulder. *Clin. Orthop.*, **20**, 41.

20 *Surgery and Associated Physiotherapeutic Management of Conditions that Affect the Upper Limb*

R. Jones and A.M. Jamieson

Introduction

Joint replacement in the upper limb was developed following the success of total hip replacement in the lower limb. Because of the anatomical variations of the joints involved, and the predominence of rheumatoid arthritis as an indication for surgery, there were problems with the early designs. For example, the Dee elbow hinge did not withstand the tortional stresses and early loosening at the bone — cement junction occurred, with ensuing failure of the prosthesis. Metal hinges that were used for metacarpophalangeal joint replacement were liable to cut out of osteoporotic bone in rheumatoid patients. The use of unconstrained joints and silastic has now given more predictable results.

Indications

Although still in the early stages of development, joint replacement in the upper extremity may be indicated in a small group of patients who have severe and persistent pain, limitation of movement and loss of function in one or more joints. The operation is primarily performed to relieve pain, but may lead to an increased range of movement and improved function. An additional benefit in the hand may be to improve the cosmetic appearance in rheumatoid disease. One must remember, however, that if there is little pain and good function, despite marked deformity, then joint replacement is contra-indicated. In some patients the disease process may have led to marked absorption of bone around the joints, leaving little bone stock into which to insert a prosthesis.

Other patients frequently have multiple joint disease and careful assessment is needed to see whether replacement will actually benefit the patient.

Physiotherapy

Successful postoperative rehabilitation requires the patient's full cooperation. This is achieved by the physiotherapist illustrating for the patient the functional improvement expected of surgery, explaining the physiotherapeutic procedure to be used at each stage of rehabilitation, and entering into a partnership of care with the patient to achieve the maximum therapeutic benefit from surgery.

The universally acceptable pre-operative assessment for these operations is identified below and in the following section; individual postoperative regimes are indicated where necessary.

Preoperative functional and physical assessment

This should be made and recorded prior to surgery. Both the affected side and the unaffected side should be assessed, as follows:

- The ability to take the hand to the mouth.
- The ability to dress and to attend to personal toilet, with or without aids.
- The ability to take the hand to the head to comb the hair.
- The ability to carry out normal activities or occupation.
- The active and passive ranges of movement.
- The presence of pain on movement and/or at rest.
- Muscle power throughout the limb.
- Atrophy of muscle due to nerve involvement.
- Posture of the joint in the contour of the shoulder.
- Impairment of other joints.
- Loss of sensation.

Shoulder arthroplasty

Indications

Some conditions requiring shoulder replacements are:

- Primary osteoarthritis, where the head becomes surrounded by marginal osteophytes. In advanced cases the glenoid cavity may result in posterior subluxation of the humeral head. Usually the rotator cuff is intact.

- Secondary osteoarthritis, e.g. following avascular necrosis due to sickle cell anaemia; also recurrent dislocation.
- Rheumatoid arthritis, which often affects the rotator-cuff in severe cases. Often the acromio-clavicular joint is affected and is excised at the same time.
- Old traumatic injuries, e.g. displaced fractures and fracture dislocations. These are difficult to rehabilitate due to contractures and scarring of the muscles, and to injuries to nerves.

Types of arthroplasty

There are various types of arthroplasty, but basically all of them work on the ball and socket principle.

Varion silastic cup   This is an interpositional arthroplasty in which a silastic cup is placed over the humeral head, separating it from the glenoid. It is a simple operation and improves motion by removing pain (Varion, 1980). Experience has shown the head must be placed concentrically, for if it is deformed, the silastic cup often fragments and leads to failure of the arthroplasty (Spencer and Skiring, 1986).

Neer total shoulder II   This is an arthroplasty which has a metal alloyed head at the stem, cemented inside the medullary cavity of the humerus. The glenoid component is high density polythene with a metal backing fixed to the neck of the glenoid (*Figure 20.1*). It has been used in rheumatoid disease, osteoarthritis and also following severe fractures of the humeral head. It can give a good range of movement when the rotator-cuff is intact; however, often in rheumatoid disease mobility is attenuated, but the increased range of rotation will still significantly improve function of the limb (Neer, 1982).

Physiotherapy

Physiotherapy will vary with the type of prosthesis, the surgical approach and the conditions of the structures surrounding the joint. When the rotator-cuff is intact, less protection of the joint will be required than when there is a tear in the rotator-cuff which requires repair or reconstruction (the shoulder will then be protected and treatment delayed until healing has occurred).

Guidelines for postoperative management were developed by Neer to support the operative process of his arthroplasty. These are used extensively in hospitals that follow his regime and are reproduced below.

After surgery, the arm is immobilised in a firm bandage or in a sling worn under the clothes, for a length of time that varies according to the individual surgeon's preference. During immobilisation, hand, wrist and finger movements are encouraged.

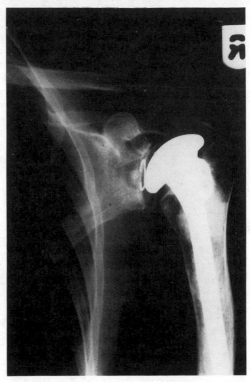

Figure 20.1. Neer II total shoulder.

Following approximately 5 days of immobilisation, a programme of exercises is commenced. All movements of the shoulder joint are exercised, except for lateral rotation. This movement is left until 6 weeks postoperatively, when all the soft tissues have healed and thus will prevent dislocation. The elbow will be stiff and need gentle movements. Shoulder shrugging and isometric exercises are commenced to maintain tone, the resistance given by the therapist at first; then the patient is taught to use the good arm or an immovable object such as a wall, or a door jamb (*Figures 20.2–20.7*).

Pendulum exercises in standing (*Figure 20.8*) and active-assisted exercises (*Figures 20.9–20.12*) are designed to maintain and increase motion. It is important to note that in each exercise, the operated arm is assisted by the good arm or by a pulley. The assistance is necessary to give maximum early return of motion and yet avoid excessive strain on the repaired muscles. The use of the arm is encouraged in daily activities.

Progression is made to active exercises, which strengthen the shoulder muscles and increase range through a programme of progressive strengthening techniques and facilitatory techniques.

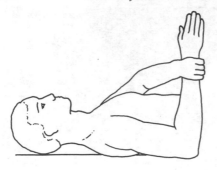

Figure 20.2. **External rotators:** *Lying on the back — with the elbows flexed to 90° and held close to the body, grasp the wrist of the operated arm with the good hand, attempt to move the operated hand outward, and resist motion with the good hand. Do not allow the operated arm to move.*

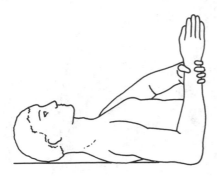

Figure 20.3. **Internal rotators:** *Lying on the back — with the elbow flexed to 90°, grasp the wrist of the operated arm with the good hand, attempt to move the operated hand inward, and resist any motion with the good hand.*

The patient may also attend hydrotherapy. Treatment with the progressive exercise programme may continue for 3 months. The patient is encouraged to resume normal activities with simple home exercises.

Elbow complex arthroplasty

Total elbow replacement
The increasing knowledge of the biomechanics and kinematics of the elbow and the development of biomaterials have produced a significant transition since the early days of elbow joint arthroplasty. New implants and techniques continue to be developed, but elbow joint arthroplasty still remains a salvage procedure.

Indications Total elbow replacement is indicated for patients with advanced rheumatoid arthritis where joint destruction precludes procedures such as synovectomy or excision of the head of the radius, or where there is trauma or tumour, or for those

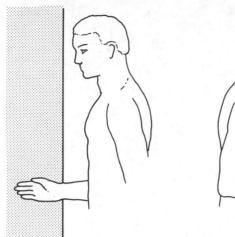

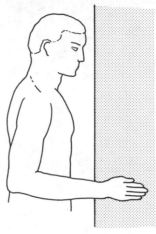

Figure 20.4. **External rotators:**
*Standing – with the elbow flexed to
90° and held close to the body,
attempt to push the hand outward
against a door jamb.*

Figure 20.5. **Internal rotators:**
*Standing – with the elbow flexed
to 90° and held close to the body,
attempt to push inward against a
door jamb.*

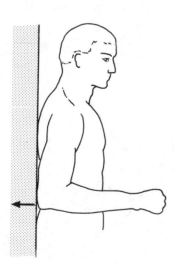

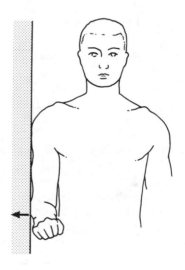

Figure 20.6. **Extensors:** *Standing –
with the elbow flexed to 90° and held
close to the body, attempt to press it
backward against the wall.*

Figure 20.7. **Middle deltoid:**
*Standing – with the elbow flexed to
90° and held close to the body,
attempt to move it out to the side
against the wall.*

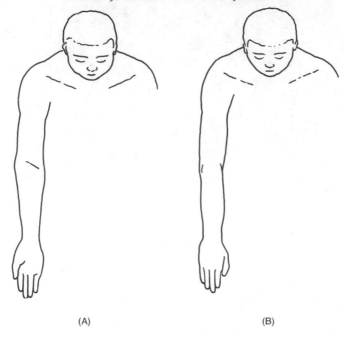

(A)   (B)

*Figure 20.8. **Pendulum exercises:** Standing — (a) bending over at the waist, circle the arm outward, with the palm facing forward; (b) bending over at the waist, circle the entire arm inward, with the palm facing backward.*

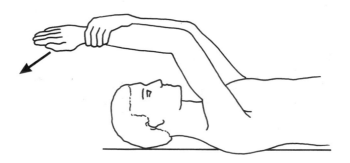

*Figure 20.9. **Assisted forward elevation:** Lying on the back — grasp the wrist of the operated arm with the good hand and reach for the forehead and up overhead.*

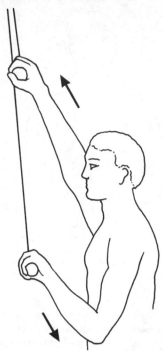

Figure 20.10. **Pulley
exercises:** *Standing — the
good arm supplies the power
to bring the operated arm as
near to the pulley as possible.*

patients who have bilateral elbow ankylosis. The operation is
performed primarily to relieve pain, restore and maintain mobility
and improve stability, thereby improving function. It is contraindicated if the shoulder on the same side is ankylosed, if there is
infection, or if the limb has to perform tasks that involve weight
being taken through the joint.

Souter total elbow
This is an unconstrained joint with a metal alloy humeral component which is cemented within the humeral condyles; a high-
density olecranon component is cemented into the proximal ulna
(*Figure 20.13*). This arthroplasty usually gives good function, but
some residual fixed flexion of the elbow is common. Some patients,
as with many other elbow arthroplasties, develop an ulnar nerve
neuritis (Souter *et al.*, 1985).

Physiotherapy A full pre-operative assessment must be carried
out and recorded.

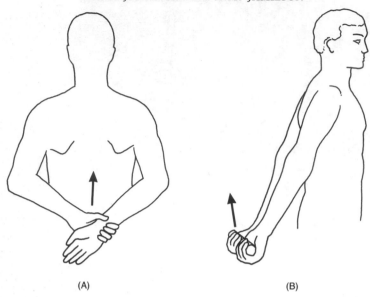

Figure 20.11. (a) **Assisted internal rotation:** Standing − clasp the wrist of the operated arm with the good hand behind the back, and slide the hands up and down. (b) **Assisted hyperextension:** Standing − grasp a stick with both hands behind the back and push backward, with the good arm supplying the power.

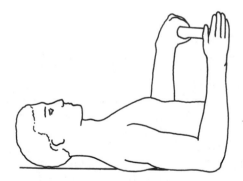

Figure 20.12. **Assisted external rotation:** Lying on the back − with the elbows flexed to 90° and held close to the body, push the operated hand outward, with the good arm supplying the power through the use of a stick.

After surgery, the arm is supported in a pressure bandage and a plaster posterior shell, and the limb is elevated. The degree of flexion is determined by the type of prosthesis and the surgical technique. Hand and wrist movements are encouraged. Mobilis-

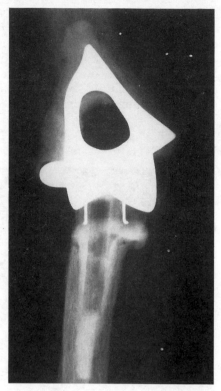

Figure 20.13. A Souter elbow.

ation begins according to the surgeon's wishes. This is often at 5 days postoperatively, if wound healing is satisfactory and post-operative oedema has subsided. Active assisted exercise begins for half-an-hour twice per day. The posterior back shell is retained between each exercise session for up to 2–4 weeks until the triceps is secure and the tissues around the joint are healed. At this stage, pronation and supernation should be avoided due to the possibility of dislocation. Flexion and extension may be as-sisted by the use of a slippery board. Ice is very effective for the control of postoperative swelling. Gradual immobilisation con-tinues until functional movement has been achieved.

A complication of the elbow replacement is ulnar nerve paresis and, therefore, any alteration in sensation and/or muscle weakness of the ulnar nerve must be noted. The patient must be advised against overloading the elbow joint by lifting or carrying awkward or heavy objects or by using the arm for weight bearing (as when using elbow crutches or a walking stick).

Swanson's silastic replacement of the radial head

The silastic radial head (*Figure 20.14*) prosthesis mimics the shape of the bone and has a stem which fits inside the proximal part of the radius; this acts as a spacer between the neck of the radius and the capitalum of the humerus. It is sometimes used as an alternative to simple excision of the fracture fragments when displaced comminuted fractures of the radial head have occurred.

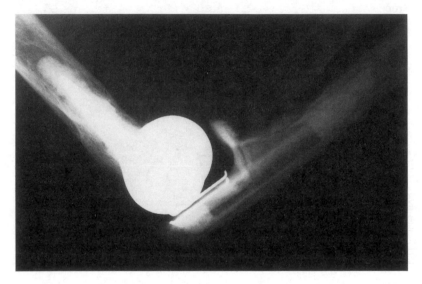

Figure 20.14. A Swanson radial head.

Wrist and carpus

Arthrodesis of the wrist

The rheumatoid wrist can be very painful and deformed with subluxation of the carpus from the articular surface of the distal radius. Arthrodesis gives good pain relief, stability is gained and hand function improves. However, the grip that remains is a simple power grip, or baggage grip. Sophisticated activity of the hand requires ulnar deviation and this movement is lost following arthrodesis.

Physiotherapy Following the operation, the arm is elevated to minimise swelling and shoulder and elbow active exercises are begun, along with gentle finger exercises. The wrist is fixed either by internal fixation, an external fixation device or an external splintage, e.g. plaster of Paris, or a combination of these methods, until fusion is sound. When fusion has taken place functional activities are encouraged.

Total wrist arthroplasty

A silastic wrist replacement acts as a flexible spacer between the radius and the carpus (Swanson, 1973). It aims to provide a pain-free, stable but mobile joint in patients who require some pain-free movement to the wrist because of occupational or recreational needs. For example, patients who suffer from rheumatoid arthritis often have stiffness, instability, pain and deformity that affect hand function. A few degrees of wrist movement can increase the reach of fingers by several centimetres and so improve hand function.

The absence of extensors of the wrist is a contra-indication to replacement surgery. The stability of the implant, either silastic or total joint replacement, is dependent on an adequate balance of the wrist prime movers, and an imbalance due to rupture or weakness creates forces which prejudice the long-term survival of the implant.

Patients who have a replacement rather than fusion find that they have a more sophisticated grasp, but do have limitation of the power grip.

Following the operation, the hand and wrist are supported in a voluminous dressing and plaster splint, and the arm is elevated to minimise swelling. After 3–5 days a plaster-of-Paris cast or a Hexolite splint is made, with the wrist in a neutral position; this is worn for approximately 2–4 weeks to allow soft-tissue healing. The patient is encouraged to exercise actively the shoulder, elbow, and fingers on the affected side in as full a range as possible. When the cast has been removed, active and active assisted movements are given to increase the range of flexion and extension and to improve muscle power. Normal activities within the ability of the patient are resumed as soon as possible.

Trapezium

Women often develop carpo-metacarpal arthritis at the base of the thumb; in such cases, excision of the trapezium may give good results, but there is usually some shortening of the thumb. The Swanson silastic implant fills the space of the excised trapezium and the stem fits inside the medullary cavity of the first metacarpal (*Figure 20.15*). The soft tissues are usually reinforced to prevent complications of subluxation of the prosthesis into the subcutaneous tissue.

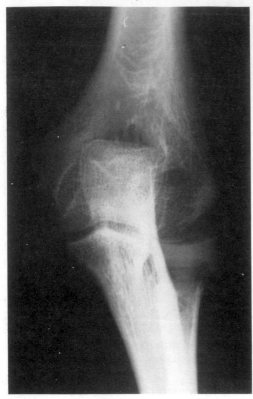

Figure 20.15. A Swanson trapezium.

Lunate
In Kienböck's disease, the lunate undergoes fragmentation and can lead to arthritis of the wrist joint. The silastic lunate is placed between the scaphoid and the triquetrum, and provides pain relief, as well as preventing the development of arthritis.

Scaphoid
The features of the scaphoid can sometimes lead to avascular necrosis of the proximal pole with some collapse. A Swanson silastic scaphoid can be used as an interpositional arthroplasty between the lunate and the trapezium to try to prevent the development of osteoarthritis, see Figure 20.16 (Swanson, 1970).

Silastic implant of the metacarpophalangeal joint
Joint replacement of the metacarpophalangeal joint is indicated for patients who have severe and persistent pain due to destruction of the joint surfaces, and present with the deformity of ulnar

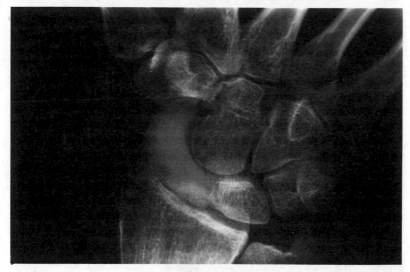

Figure 20.16. A Swanson scaphoid.

deviation due to subluxation or dislocation of the joints caused by rheumatoid arthritis. In some cases, quite gross dislocation may be associated with good function and little or no pain. Therefore, in itself dislocation is not necessarily an indication for surgery, which may improve the cosmetic appearance of the hand but do little or nothing to improve the function. The operation is performed to provide a stable joint and improve mobility, but primarily to relieve pain.

The joints are designed as flexible hinges with stems that fit inside the medullary cavities (*Figures 20.17* and *20.18*). Corrective surgery of the soft tissue is undertaken at the same time to give a good cosmetic appearance to the hand. The function of metacarpophalangeal joint replacement is usually good when there is no involvement of the proximal interphalangeal joints, replacement of which does not usually give as good a functional result as a prosthesis at the metacarpophalangeal joint (Swanson, 1972).

Complications Loosening of a cemented prosthesis can occur and may lead to revision arthroplasty or possibly to conversion into an arthrodesis. The flexible silastic hinges can fatigue and fracture, but in many cases, because they act as spacers, no loss of function occurs. The rheumatoid patients, especially those on steroid therapy, are more susceptible to infection and loosening of the prosthesis because of osteoporosis of the bone. If this

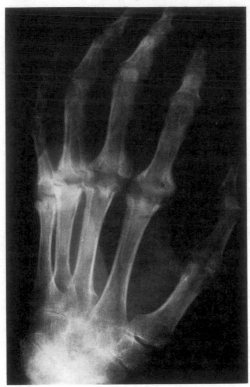

Figure 20.17. Swanson metacarpophalangeal joints.

happens, they usually require removal of the prosthesis and appropriate antibiotic treatment. It may be necessary to carry out salvage operations, such as arthrodesis.

Physiotherapy   The silastic implant provides an internal inert flexible splint which stabilises the excisional arthroplasty. This enables meticulous rebalancing of the soft tissues, which control early postoperative movements. The protection provided by the lively splintage allows the formation of the capsule around the implant, permitting stable movement with pain relief and improved function. The cooperation and involvement of the patient in the rehabilitation programme is essential after surgery. No joint can be treated in isolation and the range of movement in the shoulder, elbow and wrist must be maintained to prevent any tendency for a shoulder–hand syndrome to develop.

After surgery, the hand is supported in a pressure bandage to help minimise swelling in elevation. Postoperative treatment will

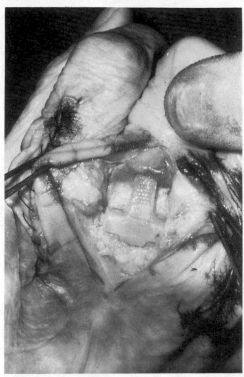

*Figure 20.18. Operative
view of a flexible hinge.*

vary according to the wishes of the individual surgeon. One
treatment regime is reproduced below.

After 24 hours postoperatively, the bandage is reduced and a
resting splint is made, still maintaining elevation. At 48 hours, a
lively splint (*Figure 20.19*) is made to restrict flexion to 30° and, at
the same time, to encourage flexion and extension within that
range, but also to permit movement at the interphalangeal joints.

Swelling may be reduced by the use of ice and Flotron in high
elevation. Between periods of exercise in the lively splint and
reducing the swelling, the resting splint must be worn; it must
also be worn during the night. Exercises, passive and active
assisted, are encouraged for all the joints, to minimise swelling
and encourage movements.

After approximately 1–2 weeks, the patient is allowed home,
but must attend frequent physiotherapy. The lively splint will
need readjusting of the rubber band slings placed over the proximal
phalanges that guide the alignment of the digits into the correct

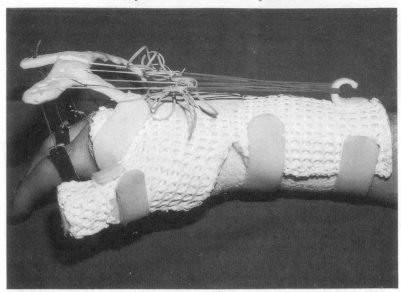

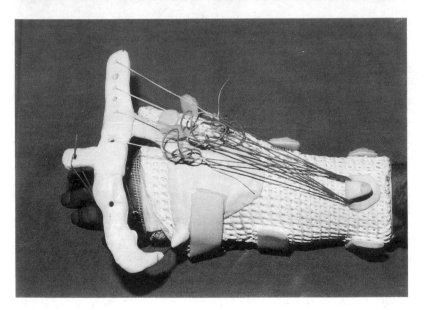

Figure 20.19. Swanson's outrigger — Note the bar with holes along its length through which elastic bands with finger loops are threaded. This splint may be altered easily by adding extensions to gain the desired effect. To correct any ulnar drift, the angle of the outrigger pulls through the elastic bands, beginning in neutral and progressing radially as hand function improves.

position to prevent recurrence of ulnar deviation. The tension of the rubber bands must be tight enough to support the finger and yet loose or flexible enough to allow 70° of flexion at the meta-carpophalangeal joints. Constant readjustment must be made to find the correct position.

Specific exercise periods to increase the range of movement and increase the strength of the flexors and intrinsic muscles of the hand are started. If at all possible, 70° of flexion should be achieved by the end of the third week, because the reconstructed joints start tightening up during the second postoperative week and will be quite tight by the end of the third week.

Active physiotherapy and occupational therapy to increase range and muscle strength, and to improve function, must occur at specific times during the day. The patient is encouraged to practise these exercises frequently. If, however, there is persistent exten-sion lag, a tendency to flexion contracture, or ulnar deviation of the fingers, the lively splint should be retained. Active treatment should be continued for about 3 months or until there is adequate flexion to permit the patient to grasp small objects and to use the hand for careful normal activities.

Conclusion

Joint replacement in the upper limb can lead to alleviation of pain and improved function. However, once surgery has been carried out and the wounds have healed, physiotherapy is the mainstay of treatment for producing good results. Rehabilitation programmes are aimed at obtaining optimum joint movement with increased muscle strength and at avoiding the development of stiffness.

References

Neer, C.S. (1982). Recent experience in total shoulder replacement. *Journal of Bone and Joint Surgery*, **64A**, 319–337.

Souter, W.A., Nicol, A.C. and Paul, J.P. (1985). Souter–Strathclyde arthroplasty of the rheumatoid elbow. *Journal of Bone and Joint Surgery*, **67B**, 154.

Spencer, R. and Skiring, A.P. (1986). Silastic interposition arthroplasty of the shoulder. *Journal of Bone and Joint Surgery*, **68B**, 375–377.

Swanson, A. (1970). Silicone rubber implants for the replacement of the carpal scaphoid and lunate bones. *Orthopedic Clinics of North America*, **1**(2), 229–309.

Swanson, A. (1972). Disabling arthritis at the base of the thumb. Treatment by resection of the trapezium and flexible (silicone) implant arthroplasty. *Journal of Bone and Joint Surgery*, **54A**, 456—471.

Swanson, A. (1973). Flexible implant arthroplasty for arthritis disabilities of the radiocarpal joint. A silicone rubber intra-medullary stemmed flexible hinge implant for the wrist joint. *Orthopedic Clinics of North America*, **4**(2), 383—394.

Varion, J. (1980). Interposition silastic cup arthroplasty of the shoulder. *Journal of Bone and Joint Surgery*, **62B**, 116—117.

21 Fractures – Clinical

P.B.M. Thomas

Introduction

The word fracture is used to describe any kind of damage produced in a bone by an applied force. The damage may range from an undisplaced crack to complete disruption and shattering of a whole bone. While some fractures are so minimal that they cannot even be detected on normal X-rays, others are so gross that their presence is obvious from the deformed appearance of the limb. The force required to produce a fracture varies greatly from one person to another – the femur of a fit athlete may momentarily withstand loads in excess of one hundred times his own body weight, while the femur of a chairbound old lady may fracture as she attempts to walk. There are many interrelated factors which determine the strength of bone and, as people age and become inactive, their bones become progressively weaker.

Mechanism of injury

The way in which a bone fractures is often related to the way in which violence is applied. The footballer who receives a kick on the shin may well sustain a transverse fracture of the tibia, but the torsional force applied when a skier falls with faulty bindings will result in a long spiral fracture of the tibia and fibula. The cat burglar, unexpectedly disturbed, will probably fracture both calanei when he jumps from a first floor window, while the house owner who punches him sustains a fracture of the right fifth metacarpal. Some fractures may even be produced by the violent contraction of a muscle. These avulsion fractures were once seen in patients who received electroconvulsive therapy, and they still occur occasionally in epileptics and athletes. Just as the type of fracture may indicate the mechanism of injury, so the description of a certain type of accident will suggest the possibility of a particular fracture.

Diagnosis

Röentgen's discovery in 1895 revolutionised the treatment of fractures to the extent that almost all fractures are now recognised and treated by reference to X-rays. Before the discovery of X-rays, fractures were diagnosed by examination and categorised by the dissection of amputated limbs and cadavers (*Figure 21.1*). We sometimes forget the importance of a careful history and examination, but the history will often reveal a mechanism which is known to cause a certain type of fracture. Gentle examination will reveal swelling and tenderness around a fracture and may also reveal deformity or a wound. Most fractures are associated with some degree of damage to other structures and a careful examination will confirm or exclude abnormalities of the vascular or nerve supply. An examination will also help in deciding which X-ray view to request. X-rays 'see' the bone from one direction only and a fracture may, therefore, be missed on a poorly planned X-ray. It is only the fracture lines which run perpendicular to the X-ray plate that show clearly, so most bones are X-rayed in two planes at right angles to each other.

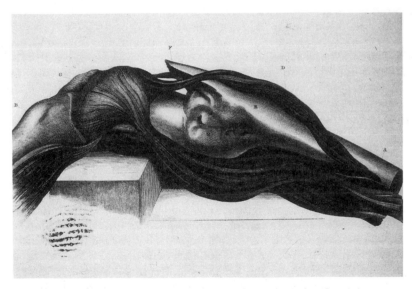

Figure 21.1. Dissection of a femoral fracture from Sir Astley Cooper's treatise, Fractures and Dislocations *(1824). The healed fracture proves that the patient survived the injury, but the malunion would have shortened the leg and interfered with the quadriceps muscle.*

Occasionally, a radio-isotope bone scan will reveal a fracture which cannot be seen on X-ray. Scaphoid fractures are sometimes detected in this way. If a fracture has occurred through a carcinomatous deposit, then an isotope scan may reveal other deposits in the skeleton. Tomograms are X-rays, taken with a moving tube and plate, which blur everything except the structures at the centre of their rotation. This technique produces 'cuts' in different planes through the bone and will sometimes demonstrate a fracture which does not show clearly on a conventional X-ray.

A computerised axial tomogram, or CAT scan, uses X-rays from which are produced computer-reconstructed sections through the body; this is often helpful in delineating fractures of the spine, pelvis and acetabulum. It is even possible, in certain centres which have the software, to produce three-dimensional pictures from a CAT scan. These are very useful in planning the reconstruction of complex pelvic and acetabular fractures. When an injured joint is aspirated, liquid marrow-fat is sometimes found floating on the surface of the blood and synovial fluid. This indicates that there is a fracture line running into an articular surface.

A fresh fracture is usually exceedingly painful, so examination and X-rays must be performed with great care.

The pathology of fresh fractures

Although most fractures are recognised by the pattern of bony damage seen on X-ray, bone is only one of the many structures which may be disrupted. The amount of damage sustained by soft tissues is roughly proportional to the degree of violence. If a force was slowly applied to a bone until it cracked, the surrounding tissue would sustain minimal damage. This is mostly because the bone would not have continued deforming after the fracture had occurred. Unfortunately, most violence which results in a fracture will continue after the bone breaks. The X-ray is thus only the last frame in a film in which the bone ends were displaced during the accident and have returned to a position of equilibrium. If a motorcyclist hit a car at 80m.p.h. and sustained a fractured femur, the film might have shown that his leg flailed and twisted wildly during the accident, although at the end it looked approximately leg-shaped again. This violent distortion of tissues causes stretching and tearing of all the structures around the bone.

The periostium covering the bone will tear first, and may be stripped back for some distance. Muscle will be stretched, bruised or sliced by sharp bone ends, and nerves and blood vessels may be contused or torn. An artery which appears to be in continuity may still not conduct blood because of damage to the intimal lining, and nerves not actually divided may cease to function for several months while an axonotmesis recovers. Finally, the bone ends may become covered in road dirt or grass. All this occurs in the short space of time before elastic recoil brings the tissues to rest.

The initial zone of damage may be quite extensive. During the first few days after injury, however, the zone of damage appears to increase. Severely traumatised muscle will die immediately, but less severely damaged tissue will begin to swell as the inflammatory phase of healing begins. Skin which was stretched during the injury may develop 'fracture blisters' after a day or two and skin that looked reasonable to begin with may subsequently become black and dead.

Fractures with a wound in the skin are called 'compound', and those without are called 'closed', but a high-velocity closed fracture may still be surrounded by more tissue damage than a low-velocity compound fracture. As a rough guide to treatment, compound fractures are graded as follows:

- Grade I, wound less than 2cm.
- Grade II, wound greater than 2cm.
- Grade III, severe soft-tissue damage.

Grade III compound fractures are sometimes further subdivided according to the degree of tissue loss or contamination.

The physiology of bone

Bone is a remarkable tissue. Although it appears inert, its various components are removed and replaced continuously, so that the whole skeleton is effectively renewed every few years. Bone is designed to withstand stress and, in fact, thrives on it: normal or physiological stresses stimulate bone to remain strong. New bone is laid down along lines of stress and this phenomenon, known as Wolfe's Law, accounts in part for the ingenious structures of bones. If the pattern of stress changes, then the bone will slowly remodel to accommodate it. The body is very economical. If the stress on a bone is reduced, then it will become weaker as mineral and bone matrix are taken away. This disuse osteopenia is seen in astronauts who have spent time in weightless conditions and, more commonly, in people confined to bed. The bone mineral is sometimes removed so quickly that a patient may develop kidney stones of calcium after a few weeks in bed. Overstressing bone may also cause trouble. Athletes and soldiers on long marches may repeatedly stress bones beyond their physiological limit, which may cause weakening and an eventual stress fracture. This is unusual, however, and bone, like most tissue, is maintained by use.

Fracture healing

Fracture healing occurs by two distinct processes which happen sequentially. The first is the callus response and the second is remodelling. In normal physiological bone healing, the callus response occurs in the first few weeks and continues for a few months, while remodelling begins over a few months and continues for several years.

The callus response

Bones are structural and the callus response is nicely designed to re-establish structural strength as quickly as possible. The fresh fracture is initially surrounded by a haematoma and by the remains of damaged tissues, such as periosteum and muscle. Over the first few days this begins to become organised by the influx of specialised cells and within a week or two callus begins to appear. On X-ray, the callus is first seen as a faint fluffy opacity surrounding the fracture but lying outside the original boundaries of the bone. As the strength of a tube is proportional to its diameter, by forming outside the bone this shell of callus is well placed to hold the ends of the fracture steady.

Callus is made of immature woven bone and does not have the sophisticated structure of mature bone. As the purpose of callus is to prevent relative movements of the bone ends, it continues to form only until it is strong enough to prevent that movement. The production of callus is therefore initiated and maintained by movement. If there is no movement at all, then no callus will form, but if movement continues, then the blob of callus will carry on growing in an attempt to stop it. If the agitated patient, insensate from a head injury, shakes his fractured femur around on traction, a huge ball of callus will form.

But if a fracture is held rigidly with a plate or fixator, then callus will not appear at all. This paradox of fracture treatment will be enlarged upon later.

Callus is a 'one-off' response. If it does not occur within a few weeks of injury it will not occur at all, and movement later on will not induce it to appear (*Figure 21.2*).

Remodelling

Once the movement at the fracture ends has been brought to rest by callus, the slower process of remodelling begins. The process is the same as that which reshapes bone to respond to changing patterns of load. Mature bone is made up of lamellae and interlaced by the microscopic tubules of the Haversian system. Osteons are organised groups of cells which move through the bone, constantly removing and replacing it. By the same process, the woven bone formed in the callus phase is also slowly replaced by mature bone. The callus response is directed by quite gross movement, which it ultimately controls. The remodelling process is directed by the pattern of stress distribution and ultimately redistributes

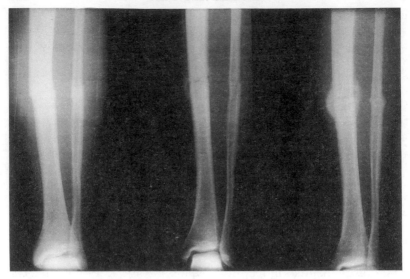

Figure 21.2. A midshaft fracture of the tibia and fibula. The X-rays were taken on the day of the injury (left), and at intervals of 4 weeks. An almost spherical blob of callus has formed.

stress to optimise the strength of the bone. Although the site of a freshly healed fracture is quite obvious on X-ray, the fusiform swelling in the bone steadily remodels so that an X-ray taken several years later may show no obvious abnormality at all.

There is no definite moment of fracture union. The strength of a healing fracture continues to increase to an arbitrary point at which the clinician feels that the risk of re-fracture is very low.

The ability to define a suitable end point is based on experience, using information such as the time from fracture, the X-ray appearance, the clinical feel of the limb and the presence or absence of pain. It is a quality judgement. Definitions of fracture healing based on stiffness measurements are already used in research and are beginning to be useful clinically. These techniques may eventually improve the informed clinical guess.

Primary bone healing

This process probably only occurs in artificial situations created by surgery and in undisplaced fractures.

Sir John Charnley discovered that a fresh osteotomy through cancellous bone can be made to heal very rapidly by compressing the cut surfaces together with a clamp. Unfortunately, this observation was erroneously extrapolated to support the practice of the plating of longbones. The AO (Arbeitsgemeinschaft fur Osteo-synthesenfragen) group, which was formed in Switzerland by Muller and his colleagues, set out to develop a properly engineered system for the internal fixation of fractures. The plates they designed have holes of a complex shape which allow compression of the fracture surfaces as the screws are tightened. These Dynamic Compression Plates (DCP) can produce very rigid internal fixation. So elegant was the system, and so persuasive the group's arguments, that it was quickly taken up throughout the world. There is no doubt that the perfect reduction of certain fractures, such as those involving joints, is beneficial. There is also no doubt that the rigid fixation of fractures allows for early movement of joints which reduces stiffness and swelling. Rigid fixation is a necessity to prevent metal fatigue and failure of the plate, but it abolishes the callus response.

The appearance of callus following plating is then taken to indicate movement due to inadequate surgical technique. To the Swiss, callus is anathema. The healing which occurs without callus in a rigidly plated longbone is called primary bone healing. It is probably the same mechanism as remodelling and only progresses slowly across the devitalised bone ends. The plate must therefore last as long as the callus which it prevented, and a plate failure may result in a non-union. Primary bone healing is therefore the second phase of physiological healing, artificially separated from the first phase (*Figure 21.3*).

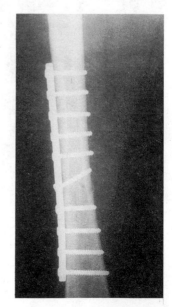

Figure 21.3. A rigidly plated fracture of the femur. After 4 months there is no callus. The plate must now survive for another year to allow healing by remodelling.

Fracture treatment

The aim of all orthopaedic treatment is to restore function and to minimise deformity. Immediately prior to their injury most patients have full function and no deformity. They have rightly come to expect complete recovery, and the demands of modern fracture treatment are therefore very exacting. The management of fractures consists of pain relief followed by painless reduction, and the maintenance of reduction in a way which does not interfere with bone healing or subsequent function (*Figure 21.4*).

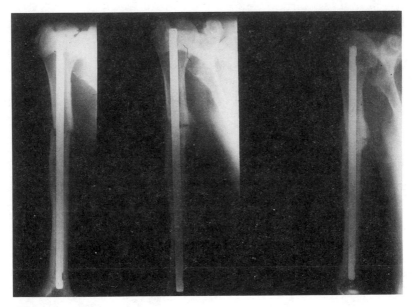

Figure 21.4. A humeral fracture treated with an intramedullary Küntscher nail. The X-rays were taken after 2 days (left), 4 weeks and 12 weeks (right) and show good callus production due to the limited movement permitted by the nail.

Reduction

Many fractures are minimally displaced and do not require reduction, but most displaced fractures must either be manipulated or reduced at operation.

Accurate manipulation is a subtle skill. Success depends on understanding the mechanism of injury and on taking advantage of the mechanical effect of undamaged soft-tissue structures.

Charnley emphasised the importance of the 'soft-tissue hinge' in reducing and holding fractures, and this is probably the most useful thing for the manipulator to bear in mind.

Open reduction

We know from experience that certain fractures cannot be reduced properly by closed manipulation. We also know that certain fractures will definitely require internal fixation, but some of these are still worth manipulating. If a fractured part is badly deformed, it will not only be extremely painful but also rapidly develop soft-tissue problems. If a badly displaced ankle fracture is left unreduced for a few hours, the skin stretched over the broken fragments may slough, but a timely manipulation will save the skin and will allow an open reduction to be performed later.

There is a wide spectrum of fracture reduction, from the Colles' fracture in an old person, which is almost invariably treated by closed manipulation, to the midshaft fracture of the radius and ulna, which is almost always internally fixed. Each fracture must be judged individually and in its relation to other injuries. Open reduction is almost always combined with some form of internal fixation (*Figures 21.5(a)* and *21.5(b)*).

Maintenance of reduction

The position may be maintained by plaster-of-Paris splintage, traction, external fixation, internal fixation, functional bracing or a combination of these.

Plaster of Paris

Plaster of Paris has good properties as a splinting material. It is easily applied, remains soft for a few minutes and suddenly sets hard. When set it is easily cut with a saw and withstands most patient abuse. It is radiolucent and may be repaired easily by adding extra layers. It also provides a perfect white surface for graffiti! There is danger in a plaster which completely encloses a freshly injured limb, as it will not expand to allow for swelling. The initial plaster is therefore applied as a slab or a cylinder which is split to allow expansion. This may be safely completed to a full plaster after about a week. The position of a fracture may be adjusted after a few weeks by plaster wedging, and windows may be cut out of the plaster for access to wounds. There are several synthetic casting materials, such as Scotchcast and Baycast. These tend to be lighter in weight, but are more difficult to apply and more expensive than plaster of Paris.

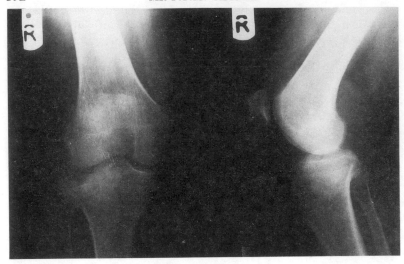

(a)

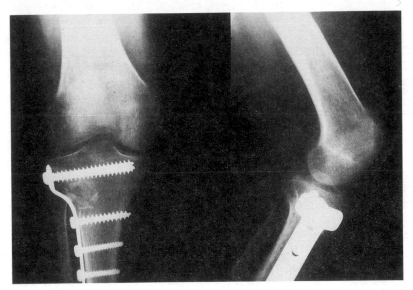

(b)

Figure 21.5. (a) A depressed lateral tibial plateau fracture in a pedestrian struck on the lateral side of the knee by a car bumper. (b) The plateau was elevated and held with cancellous bone graft from the iliac crest; a plate and screws hold the fracture and bone graft in place.

Conventional plaster treatment has the disadvantage of immobilising joints. Movement of joints has a beneficial effect on blood and lymph flow, reduces swelling, maintains muscle tone and bone strength, and circulates synovial fluid, which nourishes the articular cartilage. Prolonged plaster immobilisation tends therefore to maintain swelling and causes muscle wasting, stiff joints and ostopenia.

Traction

The unopposed pull of muscles tends to prevent reduction of longbone fractures. Traction counteracts this pull and straightens out the bone. It is used mostly in fractures of the femur, tibia and cervical spine, but may also be used in supracondylar humeral fractures (Dunlop traction). It allows for early movement of certain joints.

External fixation

Threaded pins are screwed into holes drilled into the bone via small incisions in the skin. The pins on each side of the fracture are then joined externally by a bar on which there are mechanisms to allow for adjustment. Once the fracture is reduced the mechanism is tightened to maintain the reduction (*Figure 21.6*).

External fixators have the great advantage of leaving the skin uncovered. This allows access to areas of tissue loss where further surgery or repeated dressings may be required. Because only the fractured bone is immobilised, the joints may be kept supple and the position of the fracture may be readjusted at any time. External fixation is useful in multiple injuries, as fractures may be immobilised relatively quickly to allow for soft-tissue surgery, such as vessel repair. It is easiest to use on subcutaneous bones, such as the tibia, but on deep bones (like the femur) the pins must pass through muscle, which therefore becomes tethered. This limits joint movement, causes pain and may result in infection passing down the pin tracks.

A higher rate of delayed or non-union is seen in fractured tibiae treated by external fixation than in those treated in plaster. This is partly because the fractures with more severe soft-tissue damage tend to be treated by external fixation and it is in these fractures that the blood supply to the bone is most disrupted. Rigid fixators tend to reduce the callus response but, in fact, most fixators allow some movement due to the elasticity of the pins. The Orthofix fixator allows axial movement when a screw on the telescope tube is released and this 'dynamisation' may help to induce callus if it is performed early enough.

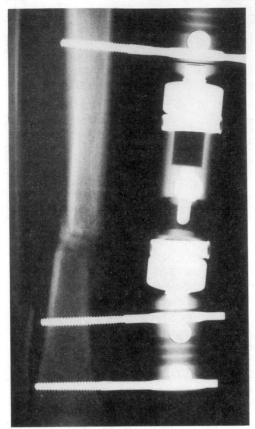

Figure 21.6. An 'Orthofix' external fixator maintains reduction in a fracture of the tibia and fibula.

Internal fixation

The great advantage of internal fixation is that even complex fractures may be anatomically reduced and held.

The great disadvantage is that periosteum and other tissues are damaged while gaining surgical access to the fracture. Healing is further compromised by rigid fixation and closed fractures are turned into compound ones.

Although these considerations must be carefully weighed before deciding to operate, there is no doubt that in expert hands, internal fixation has revolutionised the treatment of many types of fracture. Fractures of the radius and ulna, intertrochanteric fractures of the femur and femoral shaft fractures are now almost always treated by internal fixation, and the accurate reduction of intra-articular fractures cannot be achieved by any other means. Probably every type of fracture has been treated somewhere by internal fixation, but as with all surgery the ability to perform an

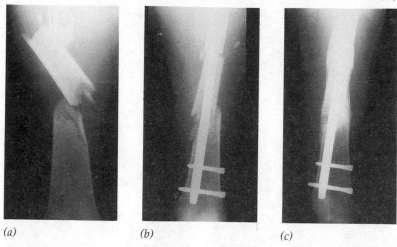

(a)   (b)   (c)

Figure 21.7. (a) A segmental fracture of the femur held with an interlocking intramedullary nail. (b) This second X-ray was taken immediately after the operation. (c) This X-ray, taken 18 months later, shows that the healed fracture has begun to remodel.

operation is not necessarily its indication (*Figures 21.8(a)* and *21.8(b)*).

Functional bracing

This is really just a conceptual shift in plaster-of-Paris treatment which allows for joint mobility. Sarmiento pointed out that most fractures will not displace any further than the initial displacement caused by the injury. In selected cases, therefore, it is possible to design a cast which allows joints to move, but prevents the fracture from displacing too much. Most functional braces employ hinges across joints and rely on the hydraulic effect of soft tissues confined in a cylinder or cone to control the fracture. Although considered a conservative option, they require constant vigilance. Like all new techniques, they were once applied to everything, but they have now found their place in tibial fractures and some femoral fractures. A femoral functional brace can be a useful adjunct to internal fixation around the knee, where some protection is required but movement is desirable.

Pain

Fractures are extremely painful and movement of a fresh fracture may be excruciating. There is hardly ever any reason to manipulate a fracture without proper regional or general anaesthesia. Once a

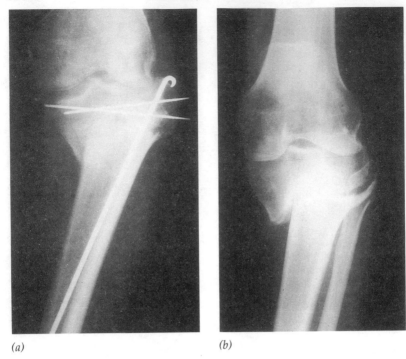

(a)   (b)

Figure 21.8. (a) A bizarre attempt at internal fixation leading to non-union of a fracture of the proximal end of the tibia (b).

fracture has been reduced and held, however, the severe pain will be relieved and replaced by a dull ache. Severe pain following reduction is a warning that something is wrong; it is usually caused by ischaemic muscle which has lost its blood supply because of arterial damage, compartment syndrome or a tight plaster. These problems are quite common and must be rectified quickly to prevent disaster. They are discussed in more detail later.

Some useful terms

Delayed union A fracture which has not united in the expected time.

Non-union A delayed union which appears likely to continue indefinitely.

Atrophic non-union A non-union in which the bone ends look inert and often tapered.

Hypertrophic non-union A non-union in which each bone end is surrounded by abundant callus, but the callus has not bridged the gap. It 'wants to unite', whereas the atrophic non-union does not.

Infected non-union Usually the end result of a compound fracture or unlucky internal fixation.

Union The moment when a healing fracture is thought to be strong enough not to refracture.

Malunion A fracture that has united in the wrong position. There may be rotational malunion, angulatory malunion, shortening, or a step in an articular surface.

Fibrous union A fracture will sometimes heal with fibrous scar tissue bridging the gap. It may be quite solid, but once it is established it will not proceed to bony union.

Pseudarthrosis Sometimes gross movement will continue at a fracture site producing a mobile non-union which is effectively a false joint.

Osteotomy A planned surgical fracture usually designed to correct a bony deformity.

Arthrodesis Bony union which occurs across a joint. It is usually the planned end result of surgery, but used to occur in untreated joint infections, particularly tuberculous. It is achieved by the same process as fracture healing.

Childhood fractures

Bones grow in childhood, which gives them some characteristics not found in mature bone. Although an immature bone may break cleanly, it may alternatively undergo a combination of cracking and bending, known as a 'green stick' fracture. Childhood fractures heal much faster than those in adults, and delayed union or non-union is very rare in children. Malunions, however, are more common. This is because, under certain circumstances, we are prepared to accept a poor reduction knowing that re-modelling will come to the rescue. It is safe to rely on remodelling only if its limitations are known. An angulated malunion near a growth plate will remodel better than one at the centre of a long bone, but rotational malunions hardly remodel at all. Remodelling will only tend to correct a malunion while the bone continues to grow and therefore has less effect in older children.

Fractures involving the growth plate may result in complete cessation of growth. More commonly, only part of the growth plate becomes fused while the rest continues to grow to produce a progressive deformity. This is a difficult situation to treat, but may be remedied by excising the bony tether, by fusing the rest of the growth plate, or by a corrective osteotomy when growth has ceased. The Salter–Harris classification which is used to describe these injuries is shown in *Figure 21.9.*

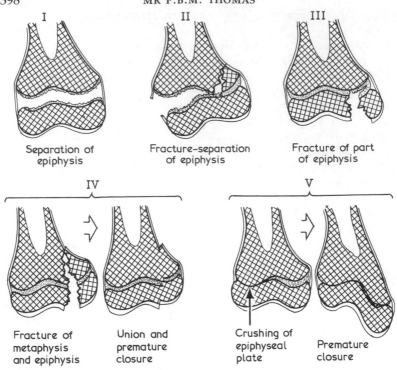

Figure 21.9. The Salter—Harris classification of epiphyseal injuries.

Dislocation

When a joint is disrupted in such a way that its articular surfaces are no longer in contact with one another, it is said to be dislocated. The abnormal position is then maintained by muscle spasm, which is extremely painful.

Reduction is usually achieved easily by a suitable manoeuvre once the patient is properly relaxed or anaesthetised, but sometimes it is prevented by the joint capsule or by the presence of a piece of bone or soft tissue jammed in the joint. In this situation, the joint is explored surgically and an open reduction is performed. A dislocation is not cured once it is reduced. The torn capsule and ligaments take several weeks to heal and must be protected by limiting movement during this period. If the patient with a dislocated shoulder is allowed free immediately after reduction, the capsule will heal lax and may allow recurrent dislocations to occur later. Dislocations are often associated with fractures and these combined injuries usually require open reduction and internal fixation.

Complications that affect the bone

Delayed union

This is usually due to damage to the blood supply of the bone caused by stripping of the soft tissues in the initial injury. It is therefore more common in high-velocity than in low-velocity injuries. It may happen if the callus is abolished by rigid fixation, and it is also more common in certain bones, such as the tibia, which have a precarious blood supply. Delayed union is treated by continuing splintage until the fracture eventually unites. The delayed union will be treated as a non-union if it shows no sign of healing after a reasonable length of time. This length of time is arbitrary and will vary from bone to bone and from surgeon to surgeon.

Non-union

The usual treatment for an established non-union is to open the fracture, clean out the fibrous scar and replace it with bone graft from the iliac crest. It is then held with a plate or an external fixator. This effectively creates a fresh fracture which usually unites. Compressing the fracture ends together with an external fixator may also cause a non-union to heal, even if the fracture itself is not grafted. The use of electrical stimulation and magnetic fields is still thought to be helpful by some and is based on the view that if mechanical stimulation produces electricity, which it does, then the application of electricity may stimulate bone to form. It is easier to achieve bone healing in a hypertrophic non-union than in an atrophic non-union. It is virtually impossible to achieve bone healing in an infected non-union until the infection has been eradicated (*Figures 21.10(a)* and *21.10(b)*).

Malunion

If the deformity compromises function or is cosmetically distressing, then the bone may be straightened by an osteotomy (*Figures 21.11(a)* and *21.11(b)*).

Infection

Pathogenic organisms may invade a fresh fracture if it is compound or if it is opened surgically. An acute infection may be successfully treated with antibiotics combined, if necessary, by the surgical removal of infected tissue and blood clot.

In acute osteomyelitis, the bone itself is colonised by organisms and, if some of the colonised bone is dead, then the infection will continue as chronic osteomyelitis. This is usually only cured by excision of all the dead bone, but as the dead bone is difficult to identify, infection may recur, sometimes years later.

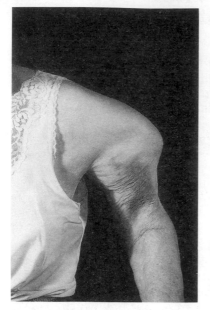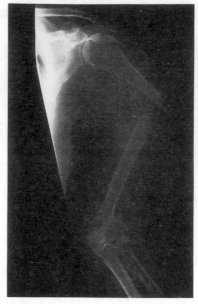

Figure 21.10. Established non-union of a midshaft fracture of the humerus, which had occurred 10 years before. Although there was more movement at the non-union than at the elbow, this patient's arm was comfortable and she declined further treatment.

Avascular necrosis

In certain bones, such as the scaphoid, the neck of the femur and the talus, a fracture can cause part of the bone to die. This is due to a peculiarity of the blood supply in these bones. The scaphoid, for instance, is supplied with blood only through its distal pole, so that a fracture through the waist will cut off nourishment to the proximal part. If the avascular bone is protected it will eventually be replaced by creeping substitution of new bone, but frequently the avascular part will simply collapse. Each site requires different treatment, some by bone graft in the early stages, and some by excision or prosthetic replacement later on (*Figure 21.12*).

Osteoarthrosis

If a fracture results in damage to the articular surface of a joint, then the distribution of load over the joint surfaces will change. This may cause pain and limitation of movement and may eventually lead to the changes of 'wear and tear' arthritis. For this

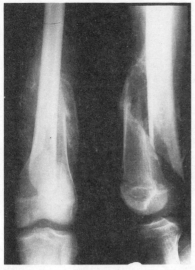
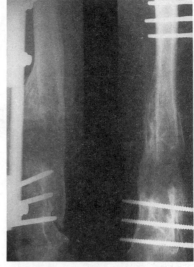

(a)   (b)

Figure 21.11. (a) Malunion of the distal end of the femur. This patient had a severe head injury and moved his leg a lot in traction which produced shortening and abundant callus. (b) The femur was lengthened again by callotasis using an external fixator. This technique would have helped Sir Astley Cooper's patient (see Figure 20.1).

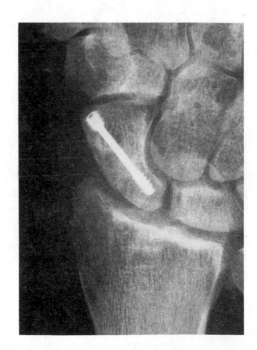

Figure 21.12. A fracture of the waist of the scaphoid was successfully treated with a Herbert screw, which has two threads of different pitches to produce compression. Avascular necrosis has not occurred.

reason, great care is taken to reduce intra-articular fractures as perfectly as possible.

Complications that affect the limb

Structures around a fracture are frequently damaged and each produces its own problems.

Blood supply

Arteries may be damaged in any part of a limb, but the commonest and most serious damage is to the popliteal artery in the supra-condylar femoral fracture and to the brachial artery in the supra-condylar humeral fracture. Sometimes reduction of a fracture will immediately improve the blood supply to a limb, but if there is any doubt then immediate surgical repair of the damaged vessel is mandatory. Dying muscle is extremely painful and severe pain following a good fracture reduction usually means a problem with the blood supply. If blood flow is not restored quickly, the muscle will die. Muscle which dies immediately will slough and may lead to amputation of the limb. Muscle which dies slowly will contract into a scar and cause clawing of the toes or the tragic Volkmann's contracture of the forearm and hand. These conditions should now be preventable, but sadly they still occur occasionally.

A tight plaster may also cause ischaemia and can be very dangerous, especially in children. Again, pain after adequate reduction means that something is wrong.

Compartment syndrome

Muscle groups are contained in inexpensile fascial sacks. If the muscle is damaged it swells, and the pressure in the compartment rises. This reduces the entry of blood, damaging the muscle further, and causing more swelling. When the compartment pressure exceeds the arterial supply pressure, the muscle will die. The process can be easily reversed by recognising the problem in time and surgically opening the compartments by fasciotomy.

Venous thrombosis

Damage to the wall of the vein, sluggish blood flow in an immobilised limb, and changes in clotting factor concentrations due to trauma may result in a deep venous thrombosis (DVT). This will cause swelling of the limb, which may become chronic, and a clot may travel in the venous circulation, causing a pulmonary embolus. The treatment is anticoagulation.

Peripheral nerve damage

Peripheral nerves may be contused (neurapraxia), more extensively damaged (axonotmesis) or divided (neurotmesis). A neurapraxia will recover in a few days, but an axonotmesis may take several months and it is important to maintain passive movement, especially in the hand, until recovery occurs. Divided nerves are usually repaired, and a continuing functional deficit may be treated by muscle transfer operations later on.

Joint stiffness

A normal knee may be immobilised for months in plaster and will not become stiff. If an injured knee is immobilised, however, it will become permanently stiff. The stiffness is due to inflamed structures around the joint becoming infiltrated with fibrous exudate and then stuck down by fibrous scar tissue. Ligaments and tendons are thus prevented from sliding normally, which reduces the range of motion of the joint. Immobilisation also reduces the nourishment of the articular cartilage by the synovial fluid. Early movement of joints is therefore a good thing and the modern treatment of fractures aims to allow this to occur as soon as possible.

Complications that affect the patient as a whole

Blood loss

Some fractures result in significant blood loss. A litre of blood will be lost in the thigh of a young adult with a fractured femur and many litres may be lost into a fractured pelvis. Hypovolaemic shock is treated by prompt intravenous fluid replacement and it is easy to underestimate the blood loss in a patient with multiple fractures.

Fat embolus

This curious condition is occasionally seen in a patient with at least one closed longbone fracture.

Mental confusion is followed by a slight rise in temperature and a petechial rash over the chest. The respiration rate increases and the patient may become drowsy. Arterial oxygen tension is found to be abnormally low and a chest X-ray shows fluffy opacities over the lung fields. There is still controversy about the true cause of the syndrome but it is probably a combination of embolising marrow fat (which is liquid at body temperature) and inadequately treated hypovolaemia. Complete recovery usually follows treatment with oxygen but, in the rare fulminating type, ventilation may be required and the patient may die from disseminated intravascular coagulopathy.

Metabolic changes

Any injury will produce general changes mediated by an increase in circulating catecholamines and corticosteroids. The patient with multiple fractures will enter a catabolic state for several days following injury and this often coincides with a period of low nutritional input. Management of this complex changing metabolic situation requires a good understanding of the physiology of trauma and patients with multiple injuries are often best treated in an intensive care unit for the first few days.

Psychological change

A fracture is a very alarming experience. A patient with a fresh fracture or dislocation is often terrified and will happily submit to any treatment which will relieve his pain and deformity. After surgery, he awakes in the alien environment of the ward and is immediately assailed by the horrors of injections and hospital food, as well as the indignities of bed pans and communal living. It is hardly surprising that he feels miserable and withdrawn as he tries to imagine his life reorganised around plasters and crutches. Function is our objective, and a cheerful patient will regain function much more quickly than a frightened one. Much of the problem is fear of the unknown and it is our job to explain treatment and predict outcome as accurately as we can. The better we predict each step in a patient's recovery the better we will be trusted. Once we have the patient's trust, then treatment becomes exciting and rewarding to everyone involved.

Bibliography

Introduction

DIAGNOSIS

Rogers, L.F. (1982). *Radiology of Skeletal Trauma*. Churchill Livingstone, Edinburgh.

PHYSIOLOGY OF BONE

Vaughan, J. (1981). *The Physiology of Bone*. Clarendon Press, Oxford.

Fracture healing

THE CALLUS RESPONSE

McKibbin, B. (1978). The biology of fracture healing in long bones. *Journal of Bone and Joint Surgery*, **60B**, 150–162.

REMODELLING
Currey, J. (1984). *The Mechanical Adaptations of Bone*. Princeton University Press, Surrey.
PRIMARY BONE HEALING
Charnley, J. (1953). *Compression Arthrodesis*. E. & S. Livingstone Limited, London.
Muller, M.E. *et al.* (1979). *Manual of Internal Fixation*, 2nd edition. Springer-Verlag, New York.

Fracture treatment

REDUCTION
Charnley, J. (1961). *The Closed Treatment of Common Fractures*, 3rd edition. Churchill Livingstone, Edinburgh.
OPEN REDUCTION
Crenshaw, A.H. (ed) (1987). *Campbell's Operative Orthopedics*, 7th edition, volume 3. The C.V. Mosby Company, Washington, D.C.

Maintenance of reduction

PLASTER OF PARIS
Watson-Jones, R. (1982). *Fractures and Joint Injuries*, 280–297. Churchill Livingstone, Edinburgh.
TRACTION
Galasko, S.C.B. (ed) (1984). *Principles of Fracture Management*, 46–63. Churchill Livingstone, Edinburgh.
EXTERNAL FIXATION
Mears, D.C. (1983). *External Skeletal Fixation*. Williams and Wilkins, London.
INTERNAL FIXATION
Uhthoff, H.K. (ed) (1980). *Current Concepts of Internal Fixation of Fractures*. Springer-Verlag, New York.
FUNCTIONAL BRACING·
Sarmiento, A. and Latta, L.L. (1981). *Closed Functional Treatment of Fractures*. Springer-Verlag, New York.
PAIN
Dodson, E.D. (1985). *The Management of Postoperative Pain*. Edward Arnold, London.
CHILDHOOD FRACTURES
Rang, M. (1974). *Children's Fractures*. J.B. Lippincott Company, Toronto.

Complications affecting bone

NON-UNION
Heppenstall, R.B. (1984). Bone graft surgery for non-union. *Orthopedic Clinics of North America*, **15**, 1, 113–123.
INFECTION
Galasko, C.S.B. (1989). The management of bone and joint infection. *British Journal of Hospital Medicine*, **42**, 32–44.

Complications affecting the limb

BLOOD SUPPLY
Cone, J.B. (1989). Vascular injury with fractures: *Clinical Orthopaedic and Related Research*, **243**, 30–35.

COMPARTMENT SYNDROME

Mubarak, S.J. *et al.* (1981). *Compartment Syndromes and Volkmann's Contracture.* Sanders.

VENOUS THROMBOSIS

Hull, R.D. *et al.* (1986). Prophylaxis of venous thromboembolic disease. *Journal of Bone and Joint Surgery,* **68A**, 146−150.

PERIPHERAL NERVE DAMAGE

Omer, G.E. (ed) (1982). Peripheral nerve injuries. *Clinical Orthopaedics and Related Research,* **163**, 1−106.

Complications affecting the patient as a whole

BLOOD LOSS

Baskett, P.J.F. (1990). Management of hypovocaemic shock. *British Journal of Medicine,* **300**, 1453−1457.

FAT EMBOLUS

Duis, H.J.T. *et al.* (1988). Fat embolism in patients with an isolated fracture of the femoral shaft. *Journal of Trauma,* **28**, 3, 383−390.

METABOLIC CHANGES

Jensen, J.E. *et al.* (1982). Nutrition in orthopaedic surgery. *Journal of Bone and Joint Surgery,* **64A**, 1263.

PSYCHOLOGICAL CHANGE

Bloor, R.N. (1990). Medicolegal reporting in orthopaedic trauma, in *Psychological Effect of Trauma,* Foy, M.A. *et al.* (eds), pp 457−468. Churchill Livingstone, Edinburgh.

22 Fractures – Physiotherapy and Charts of Fracture Management

C.E. Apperley and E.R.S. Ross

A fracture is a break in the continuity of a bone accompanied by soft tissue damage. Most bones do not break haphazardly, and the varieties of common fracture are limited. The clinical aspects are discussed in Chapter 21.

Treatment of a fracture begins immediately with first aid, relief of shock and clinical assessment. *Rehabilitation* begins when the fracture comes under definitive treatment. Adams (1983) states that rehabilitation is the most important of the three great principles of fracture treatment:

- Reduction is often unnecessary.
- Immobilisation is often unnecessary.
- Rehabilitation is always essential.

He also says that treatment of fractures without regard to rehabilitation could be worse than no treatment at all.

Fracture treatment aims at sound union of the bone ends in a good position, i.e. mechanically correct, the absence of stiff joints and atrophied muscles, and full restoration of function with the patient having confidence in using the part.

It is often a violent force that is required to break a normal bone. Therefore, there is also damage to other tissues; muscle fibres, fascia and other connective tissues may be torn, blood vessels are ruptured with resultant extravasation of blood, and nerves and skin may be damaged. Trauma may lead initially to bruising and oedema, with muscle atrophy, stiff joints, disturbed circulation and gross impairment of function following immobilisation.

The principles of physiotherapy aim to prevent this occurring by:

- The maintenance of normal movement and function of the uninjured structures.

- The restoration of normal movement and function of the fractured area as soon as possible.

New treatment methods, e.g. functional bracing, have increased patient mobility, which allows rehabilitation to be carried out as union proceeds.

The role of the physiotherapist

- To work as part of the multidisciplinary team.
- To assess the patient's condition and identify his needs.
- To explain any proposed physical treatment, and its aims, to the patient.
- To maintain respiratory function especially for those patients with respiratory disease, thoracic cage injury or spinal injury.
- To rehabilitate the patient back to independence.
- To be aware of likely complications and to report any untoward signs and symptoms to the nurse in charge of the ward (if relevant) and the doctor.

Assessment
Before beginning treatment the physiotherapist should make an assessment which should be repeated at intervals. This includes reading the medical notes and looking at the radiographs. The following should be noted:

- Diagnosis and date of injury.
- Cause of injury.
- Other injuries, illnesses or complications.
- Occupation.
- Home circumstances.
- *Symptoms*: ask about pain, stiffness and function
- *Signs at the fracture site*: local heat, redness, oedema, and tenderness.
- *Signs in the nearby joints*: effusion and range of movement.
- *Signs in the whole limb*: muscle power and/or wasting, and sensation.
- *General examination*: functional activity and respiratory function.

Fractures in splintage including functional bracing

The patient must continue to use the injured part as normally as he can. The degree of function related to the fracture area depends on the nature of the fracture, the risk of displacement and the extent of splintage.

Physiotherapy is usually possible from an early stage and will include:

- Elevation.
- Active exercises to mobilise all muscles and joints not included in the splintage. For example, a patient with a Colles' fracture must use the fingers, elbow and shoulder as normally as possible.
- Isometric exercises for the muscles enclosed in the splintage to preserve muscle function and prevent atrophy. These exercises help to pump away oedema, thereby avoiding the development of indurated and fibrosed tissues.
- Encouragement of normal patterns of movement; this will include gait if the lower limb is involved. If the patient is to be allowed non-weight-bearing or partial weight-bearing the use of crutches must be taught; this includes their use in rising from sitting, and from standing to sitting, a reciprocal gait (shadow walking if non-weight-bearing), steps and stairs.

On removal of the splintage a small amount of swelling in the fracture area is normal (being due to callus formation and a small amount of oedema); the physiotherapist must be aware of any signs of non-union or injection, i.e. swelling, heat, tenderness or reddening, which indicate an inflammatory state.

Following the removal of splintage the aims of treatment are to mobilise those joints which were immobilised, and improve the power of muscles and the condition of soft tissues. Even for patients with simple fractures which do not require physiotherapy, instruction on reducing pain and swelling with, for example, contrast bathing, mobilising and strengthening exercises can be beneficial.

In the case of more serious fractures or when a splint is temporarily, or totally, removed before consolidation, supervised physiotherapy is usually necessary. When there is sound union at the fracture site treatment can be increased with exercises being carried out against graduated resistance until normal power is regained.

Throughout treatment exercises should be given for the whole body together with functional activities. This stimulates co-ordination of one part with another and retrains independence. If the lower limb is affected, gait should be re-educated using the heel−toe pattern throughout, and the person rehabilitated until he has reached his normal level of fitness.

Fractures treated by early active motion

Physiotherapy now plays a greater role in the treatment of some fractures which, if immobilised, lead to joint stiffness and loss of function. For example, fractured metacarpals often have minimal displacement, but correct alignment is usually sacrificed for the return of good function — a beautiful radiograph but a stiff hand is useless!

Fractures which include cancellous bone, e.g. a crush fracture of the calcaneus, are often treated most effectively by physiotherapy. Ice therapy and elevation reduces pain and swelling, and movement of the ankle and subtalar joints must be early and repetitive. The activity moulds the fragments so that a useful range of movement is usually regained. Tibial condyle fractures also have improved reduction with movement, *but* this must be combined with continuous traction or cast bracing of the leg to prevent angulation at the knee.

Within this category is the elderly patient with an impacted fracture of the neck of the humerus (*Figure 22.1*). In this instance, physiotherapy should include techniques to aid relief of pain, active exercises, and graduated functional activities.

Fractures treated in traction

Prolonged traction as a treatment for some fractures is now being replaced, or supplemented, by other methods, especially functional bracing. For example, a patient with a fracture of the mid-shaft of the femur may be walking, partial weight-bearing in a cast brace, with a good range of hip, knee and ankle movement and muscle activity, possibly within 4—6 weeks of the injury. This is compared to the 12—16 weeks on traction alone, with subsequent stiff joints, especially the knee, and atrophied and fibrosed tissues.

Some fractures still require prolonged traction or internal fixation. These are fractures that are difficult to brace at the 'sticky stage', e.g. a fracture of the junction between the upper and middle thirds of the femur. Fixation of the proximal small segment is difficult, particularly when it is influenced by the strong flexor and abductor muscles of the hip.

Physiotherapy
Physiotherapy during traction includes:

• Maintenance of respiratory function.
• Circulatory exercises with ankle dorsiflexion, plantar flexion and deep-breathing exercises.

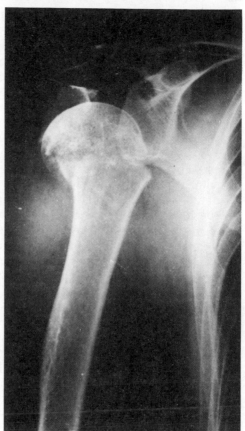

*Figure 22.1. Impacted
fracture of the neck of
the humerus.*

- Maintenance of the general tone of the body's muscles by:
  - (a) Strengthening exercises of the arms in preparation for crutch
    walking.
  - (b) Exercises for the unaffected leg. Care must be taken with
    resisted exercises in the first few weeks, because overflow
    of muscle activity to the affected leg may alter the position
    of the fracture and actually delay rehabilitation.
- Isometric contractions of muscles in the affected limb, especially
  the quadriceps group.
- Passive mobilisation of the patella of the fractured leg to prevent patello-femoral adhesions.
- At union of the fracture, knee flexion exercises may be permitted.

When traction is removed, treatment will be continued with
graduated exercise until acceptable function for the particular
patient's needs is regained.

Fractures treated by internal fixation

Internal fixation of a fracture is used when closed methods are *unsuitable*, e.g. holding a transverse fracture of the olecranon; or *inadequate*, e.g. a fractured neck of the femur. It is also indicated when precise reduction is required and is not possible by manipulation, e.g. intra-articular fractures, fractures of the medial malleolus, or the radius and ulna in the adult.

Internal fixation is not always adequate to hold a part, especially with stresses of weight-bearing, as the plate may break; it may be supplemented by external fixation, e.g. a plaster-of-Paris cast on cylinder. Plating the fracture allows active rehabilitation; the disadvantage of additional external fixation is that joint stiffness may be considerable, especially with the extra trauma of surgery. To avoid this stiffness, delayed splintage is often used. Postoperatively, the fracture area may be protected by a plaster-of-Paris back-slab. Treatment then consists of elevation of the limb and active movements to maintain the mobility of joints and muscles, as well as helping to pump away the inflammatory exudates. The patient is not allowed to weight-bear. After a few days, or when the stitches are removed, the patient should have a good range of movement in all joints. The plaster cast can then be completed, or splintage applied, and treatment continued as already described. There is little or no stiffness when the splintage is removed because the initial inflammation has been resolved, together with reabsorption of exudates.

Dislocations

Traumatic dislocation can occur at any joint, but those most commonly affected are the shoulder, elbow, interphalangeal and ankle joints. Dislocation may be associated with a fracture of adjacent bones, i.e. a fracture-dislocation. Dislocation cannot occur without damage to the joint capsule and ligaments – these are torn, which allows the articular surfaces to separate; or a ligament may be avulsed from its attachment.

Treatment is usually early closed reduction by manipulation, but sometimes surgical intervention is required, e.g. for an open reduction or ligamentous repair. When ligaments and the joint capsule are torn, the joint must be splinted in a position which will aid healing. The time of splintage depends on the part of the body which is affected, for example 6 weeks for a dislocated knee, 1 week for a finger, 3 weeks for the lateral ligament of the ankle.

The aims of physiotherapy are as those for fractures, but the affected joint will be stiff when the splintage is removed and may require intensive physiotherapy. During immobilisation, circulation of the limb should be stimulated, together with exercises to prevent muscle atrophy. When the plaster cast or bandage is removed, exercises are directed to gain range, strength and co-ordination of movement.

Physiotherapy when there are associated injuries or complications

If there are other injuries or complications the physiotherapy for the fracture must be adapted or, in some cases, completely withdrawn. Only complications that directly affect physiotherapy are considered here.

Joint complications

Joint injuries may include dislocation, subluxation, ligamentous rupture or strain, haemarthrosis, disruption by intra-articular fractures, or a penetrating wound into a joint with possible infection.

Joint stiffness is the most common complication of fractures and is predisposed by:

- *Peri-articular adhesion*: Injury to individual tissues, oedema and immobilisation cause adhesions between muscle, ligaments, capsule and bone. Some joints are more vulnerable than others, e.g. the knee, elbow and fingers stiffen easily with permanent impairment, while the hip and wrist usually regain movement more easily.
- *Intra-articular adhesions*: These occur when a fracture involves the articular surface, or is near to it. A haemarthrosis will result, which may be absorbed, or may organise forming adhesions. Physiotherapy is usually preventive, but if adhesions have occurred, then intensive treatment is necessary. Active and stretching exercises, ultrasound, local heat, and functional activities may be useful. If the physiotherapist is trying to mobilise a stiff joint before consolidation of the fracture, she must exercise caution, and be quite certain that the movement is at the joint and *not* at the fracture site. If a fracture is close to a joint, e.g. a supracondylar fracture of the femur, knee mobilisation may be delayed until consolidation has been achieved. If stiffness persists after consolidation and intensive physiotherapy, then manipulation under anaesthesia may be considered.

- *Infection*: This often causes stiffness of long duration.
- *Mal-union*: *see* Chapter 21.
- *Myositis ossificans*: This is post-traumatic ossification of haematoma around a joint. The cause is unknown. Passive movement may increase its production, and should be avoided with bone or joint injuries. The most usual site of myositis ossificans is at the elbow joint when, a few weeks after injury, the range of movement is noticed to be decreasing. Treatment is rest.
- *Sudeck's atrophy*: A painful osteoporosis occurring usually in the hand or the foot. Treatment is intensive physiotherapy, and occupational therapy, with active exercise, local heat, and elevation of the part. Interferential therapy has been found to be of value.
- *Osteoarthritis*: This is liable to follow malunion if the joint surfaces remain incongruous, or following avascular necrosis.
- *Unreduced dislocation*: If treatment is not progressing satisfactorily, then the therapist should check with the surgeon that it *was* reduced initially and has not re-dislocated.

Muscle complications

- *Torn muscle fibres* are common with fractures and may adhere to other structures during the healing process. If the affected muscles are treated while the fracture is healing, adhesions are reduced and the period of rehabilitation is shortened.
- *Disuse atrophy* can largely be prevented by repeated active exercises from the time of injury.

Tendon complications

- *Torn tendons*: These are rare, the most common example being a transverse fracture of the patella, which is usually associated with a tear of the extensor mechanism of the knee; repair is essential. This slows down rehabilitation, but unresisted active quadriceps exercises are usually permitted from the time of surgery. A protective back-slab is worn for walking until active knee extension, without a lag, is regained.
- *Avulsion fractures*: When the tendon pulls off a fragment of bone, e.g. the supraspinatus tendon at the shoulder, if the fragment is not severely displaced then gentle, graduated shoulder exercises can be started at once. Pendular exercises are especially useful in the first few weeks, as are elbow and hand exercises. If reduction was necessary, rehabilitation will be delayed and movement regained more slowly.

Nerve injury

This is not uncommon with fractures (see p. 403). It is usually in the form of a neurapraxia which recovers quickly. *Axonotmesis* occurs when the injury imposes a traction force on the nerve, and *neurotmesis* occurs with open fractures from penetrating injuries. Nerve injury should be diagnosed at the initial examination. Sensation and muscle power should be retested at subsequent assessments, because nerve damage may result from treatment or positioning, e.g. pressure of a below-knee plaster cast on the common peroneal nerve at the neck of the fibula. Physiotherapy will need to be adapted and treatment directed to maintain the mobility of those joints which are usually moved by the affected muscles. An example is an axillary nerve lesion associated with a fractured surgical neck of the humerus. Treatment should begin immediately in the form of gentle small-range pendular exercises of the shoulder, with the arm supported in a collar-and-cuff sling. At 3 weeks, post-injury union will have occurred; a greater range of movement can be achieved by careful active assisted movements. As previously mentioned, the physiotherapist must be sure that movement is at the shoulder joint and not at the fracture site. At 6 weeks the patient should be taught auto-assisted exercises, and the importance of maintaining mobility to prevent a 'frozen shoulder' should be explained to him. Throughout treatment, mobility and muscle power of the hand and elbow should be maintained. As the nerve lesion begins to recover, physiotherapy should include facilitatory and strengthening exercises.

If recovery of a nerve does not occur as expected, electromyography and exploration of the nerve may be indicated.

Other complications

- *Pressure sores*: If these should occur the physiotherapist may be asked to treat them by ice-cube massage, infra-red irradiation, ultraviolet irradiation or ozone therapy.
- *Infected wounds*: These are most likely to happen when the fracture site has been contaminated. Treatment may include extensive wound toilet and skin grafting. Physiotherapy is aimed at maintaining muscle power and, where possible, joint mobility.
- *Venous thrombosis*: If this occurs, physiotherapy will be in accordance with the wishes of the particular surgeon. Leg exercises and deep breathing exercises will have their place.
- *Adult respiratory distress syndrome (ARDS)*: The physiotherapist may well be the person who notices the first signs of this, particularly if it presents with typical chest symptoms which

call for 'chest physio'. The treatment is oxygen therapy and *not* conventional chest physiotherapy.

Not all fractures require physiotherapy and many patients only require to be taught simple exercises and to be advised to use their fractured limb in as normal a manner as possible. Every surgeon will have variations of treatment and the physiotherapist must always check what is required.

The following pages of charts give indications for the management and treatment of fractures in all parts of the body.

Abbreviations used in the following charts
IF   Internal fixation.
MUA Manipulation under anaesthesia.
OA   Osteoarthritis.
POP Plaster of Paris (cast, cylinder or black-slab).
RTA Road traffic accident.
THR Total hip replacement.

Charts of common fractures

When referring to this section, it is important to recall the previous detail which has been discussed. For example, soft-tissue damage will have occurred at the time of the fracture and may well influence the physiotherapy which is given, both in the early and late stages of rehabilitation.

Points to bear in mind when reading the charts
COLUMN 1   SITE
A broad anatomical classification is given. For greater detail see relevant texts.
COLUMN 2   USUAL AGE GROUP
This is, as it says, an indication of the age group which most frequently sustains this type of fracture. It must be remembered that almost any fracture can be sustained by a person of any age. Epiphyseal injuries are confined to the immature skeleton.
COLUMN 3   HOW INJURY OCCURS
This suggests the most usual, but by no means the only, way to sustain the fracture.
COLUMN 4   MOST USUAL METHOD OF TREATMENT
The surgeon will consider many factors before selecting his method of treatment. One or two more common methods have been listed here for the guidance of the physiotherapist.

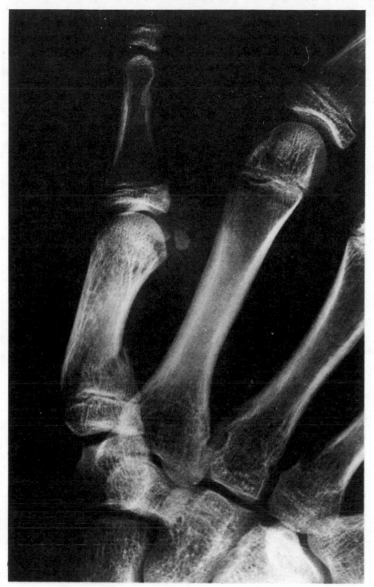

Figure 22.2 Salter II epiphyseal injury base of the first metacarpal.

COLUMN 5   MOVEMENT BEGUN

This is, of necessity, only a guide to timing. The surgeon will indicate his requirement, which will be based on local factors such as the general health of the patient, the degree of stability of

Chart 22.1. Fractures of the shoulder region.

Site	Age group	How injury occurs	Most usual method of treatment	Movement begun	Complications	Results and comments
CLAVICLE	All	Birth trauma Fall on outstretched hand Direct injury	Sling	As soon as pain permits	Neurovascular but uncommon	Excellent
SCAPULA • Glenoid • Neck • Acromion • Body	Adult	Direct blow	Sling	As soon as pain permits	—	Excellent
HUMERUS • Upper end • Neck (impacted; Figure 22.1)	All	Fall on outstretched hand	Sling	As soon as pain permits	Axillary nerve lesion	Good, especially in children
• 2/3/4* part fractures of upper end ± dislocation	Adult	Fall on outstretched hand	Sling Internal fixation Prosthetic replacement	Early	Stiffness Loss of function	Poor, but functional demand may be low
• Shaft	Adult	Direct, e.g. gunshot Fall on outstretched hand	U-slab or hanging cast Functional brace	2–3 weeks	Non-union	Good Considerable compensation possible if mal-union

* 2 part = neck (of humerus); 3 part = neck + greater tubercle; 4 part = neck + both tubercles.

Notes

The soft-tissue damage around a shoulder subjected to a fracture is considerable. The importance of early movement cannot be overstressed, but where early movement produces much pain it will be counter-productive. Better to allow the soft tissues to settle (2–3 weeks, and if pendular active movements can be begun, so much the better) and then start a vigorous programme.

COMPLICATIONS

Nerve lesions are associated more often than not with specific injuries, e.g. the axillary nerve in dislocation of the shoulder. Where such well-known associations exist, the nerve damage will be looked for automatically by examining: (a) the sensory component, i.e. loss of sensation to the skin; (b) the motor component, i.e. loss of muscle action. Pain may exclude adequate examination of both.

FRACTURED CLAVICLE

This can be treated with a 'figure-of-8' bandage but this does not support the fracture. It can cause great discomfort in the axillae. It is used less often now. This fracture, if combined with a 'flail' chest lesion, is serious.

FRACTURE-DISLOCATION OF SHOULDER

This is a common injury in the elderly. Range must be maintained. This can be done if great care is taken to support the weight of the limb when the patient is performing movements. Axillary nerve lesion is fairly common. It is not always easy to see whether deltoid muscle is working for several weeks, but the skin sensation of the C5 nerve will be altered. If the nerve is involved, the need for maintaining the range of movement is still of the greatest importance. In most instances there is spontaneous recovery from the nerve compression.

FRACTURED SHAFT OF HUMERUS

Blood vessel damage usually associated with open wounds, e.g. gunshot wounds. Usually picked up early in casualty. Radial nerve damage should always be sought and loss of wrist and/or finger extension is easily demonstrated.

Chart 22.2. Fractures of the elbow region.

Site	Age group	How injury occurs	Most usual method of treatment	Movement begun	Complications	Results and comments
Supracondylar	Child	Fall	• Collar and cuff • Dunlop traction • K-wire stabilisation	3 weeks	Myositis ossificans Malunion Volkmann's ischaemic contracture	Good
T- and Y-shaped fractures of lower humerus	Adult	Fall	• Early active movement • Internal fixation with screws and plates	As soft tissue recovery permits	Malunion Arthritis	Poor
Condylar	Child	Avulsion injuries	• Lateral usually fixed with K-wires or screws • Medial – may be left to form fibrous union	2 weeks	Non-union Malunion Late ulnar palsy	Good Good
Radial head	Any	Fall – usually an indication of severe medial soft-tissue damage to the elbow	• Collar and cuff • Excision (only in adult if badly comminuted) • Very rarely amenable to fixation	As pain permits	Stiffness Late OA	Good
Olecranon	Any	Avulsion or direct blow	Tension band wire Screw	Immediately	Stiff elbow	Excellent (usually some loss of

Notes

RANGE

Forearm rotation (pronation and supination): The functional usefulness of the hand after an elbow injury is proportional to the degree of rotation regained. It is re-educated in functional activity only.

Flexion: The hand must reach the mouth; beyond this, flexion is not essential.

Extension: While full-range movements are always the aim, an arm with no extension beyond 90° can be functional if the other movements are good.

Never attempt to increase the range by passive movements.

COMPLICATIONS

Volkmann's ischaemic contracture. This is rare in its full-blown form, resulting in muscle ischaemia and tissue necrosis with subsequent contracture. The flexor muscles of the forearm are specifically involved. The pulse is a poor indicator of forearm muscle ischaemia. It is much more important to heed a complaint of pain (a well-supported fracture will be relatively pain-free) in the forearm, especially if that pain is intense on passive finger extension. The capillary circulation to the fingers is also very important. The return of blood to the nail beds when blanched is a good indicator of this.

HAND SWELLING

It is important to avoid this since it may contribute to a poor functional result ultimately. Elevation and early finger exercises with careful attention to plaster or dressing tightness will avoid this.

SOFT-TISSUE DAMAGE

In elbow injuries this is often extensive, resulting in considerable swelling. In adults it tends to organise and give rise to permanent limitation of joint movements if it is not treated. Fortunately, few elbow injuries of adults need to be in plaster so ultrasound therapy can be given at once, even if movement is not permitted. In children, repeated manipulation must be avoided or myositis ossificans may result. Likewise passive exercising of elbow injuries is to be condemned.

FRACTURED OLECRANON

The triceps will displace a fracture of the olecranon when it acts. However, a tension band will convert the muscle force into an axial compression force on the fracture and, hence, early active rehabilitation should be the rule. Monteggia fractures represent a very severe injury to the whole elbow joint and, even if the ulnar fracture is well stabilised, it may not be possible to begin early movement.

Chart 22.3. Fractures of the radius and ulna.

Site	Age group	How injury occurs	Most usual method of treatment	Movement begun	Complications	Results and comments
ULNA SHAFT						
Isolated fracture	Any	Direct blow	Functional brace Long-arm cast	Immediately On cast removal	Non-union in adult	Excellent
Upper third with dislocation of radial head (Monteggia)	Any	Direct blow or forced pronation	*Child* – manipulate POP *Adult* – reduce radial head and plate ulna	On removal of POP at 3–6 weeks As soon as radial head thought to be stable	Radial nerve palsy rare	Excellent Poor
Ulnar and radial shafts	Any	Direct blow or fall	*Child* – MUA and long-arm cast *Adult* – plate	On removal of POP at 3–6 weeks Immediately	Malunion Non-union Cross-union	Good (some loss of rotation will always occur but may be unimportant functionally)
RADIUS						
Lower third with dislocation of lower radioulnar joint (Galeazzi)	Adult	Fall on outstretched hand	Internal fixation	Early	Loss of forearm rotation	Fair only
Lower quarter	Child	Fall	Plaster	On plaster removal	Malunion	Good Considerable moulding from growth can compensate for

	(Colles')			extensor pollicis longus Sudeck's atrophy Osteoarthrosis Malunion (common)	Good
		to fall	and shoulder straight away		Can be very poor where malunion occurs
Smith's	Adult	Fall	Plaster	As above	Stiffness of wrist
Barton's	Adult	Fall	Internal fixation	Immediately	

Notes

RANGE

Flexion and extension of the elbow and wrist are not affected unless the limb is put into a long plaster.

Forearm rotation: The alignment of the forearm bones is crucial to rotation. Also the upper and lower radioulnar joints must be correctly aligned. This, combined with uncertainty of union and late development of malunion, has led to wider acceptance of internal fixation in these fractures. In children, the exceptional recovery because of growth and the virtual certainty of union means non-operative treatment is advised. There are, however, cases which will require open reduction and internal fixation, e.g. as bone growth slows down in the late teens or where rotatory malalignment cannot be corrected by closed means.

Functional bracing in upper limb fractures: Sarmiento advocates bracing in certain fractures, e.g. humeral shaft, isolated ulna and Colles' fractures. There is little evidence as yet that such methods are widely applicable, but limited use suggests high union rates with good functional results.

POWER

This is quickly regained once firm union is established. The overall time for complete rehabilitation is often shortened if 'strengthening exercises' for the arm are delayed. The power of the hand in a 'gripping' action should be encouraged from the beginning.

COMPLICATIONS

Blood vessels and nerves are sometimes damaged at the same time since these fractures are usually the result of direct blows and often occur in road traffic accidents. However, they are not complications in the normal sense of the word, in that they do not occur as a result of the fracture.

Non-union is the most likely complication, particularly of the ulna, which is slow to unite. Heat, swelling or tenderness over the fracture area, or pain, or sudden loss of forearm rotation should be regarded as a possible indication of non-union or refracture.

PHYSIOTHERAPY

This must be directed towards encouraging use rather than attempting to 'hurry' recovery. These injuries are difficult to treat. Delaying movements may seem to be adding to joint stiffness, yet any attempt to force movements always meets with disaster.

Chart 22.4. Fractures of the carpus and hand.

Site	Age group	How injury occurs	Most usual method of treatment	Movement begun	Complications	Results and comments
Scaphoid	Young adult	Fall on outstretched hand or direct blow to back of wrist	Plaster immobilisation for 6–12 weeks	Immediate finger and elbow exercises	Non-union Avascular necrosis Late osteoarthritis	90% good results
Metacarpals	Young males	Classical 'punch' injury	None if isolated (may require fixation in severe and/or unstable injuries)	Immediately		Excellent – loss of knuckle contour may occur but functionally excellent
Bennett's (fracture-dislocation) (Figure 22.2)	Any	Direct blow	Bennett plaster K-wire or screw	On removal of plaster		Excellent provided the meta-carpophalangeal joint is reduced Even if fracture not reduced may give little trouble
Phalanges	Any	Direct blow Twisting injury	If stable, hold alignment by strapping to next healthy finger May require internal fixation with small screws or wires	Immediate use	Stiffness of fingers	Usually excellent, but if there are associated tendon or neurovascular injuries can result in a very stiff finger

Notes

FUNCTION

Power and pincer-type grips are the primary functions of the hand. In order to perform these actions effectively, normal kinaesthetic sensation, good joint range and controlled muscle power are needed.

RANGE

The joints of the wrist and hand are a complex structure designed to perform very strong and very delicate movements. The actual range of movement of each joint varies with the individual, and comparison with the uninjured hand is the only guide to its normal range.

Since function is the essential feature of the hand, it is this, rather than particular joint range, which should be the aim.

POWER

This is very important in the hand. All re-education should be designed towards power. Joint range is of no benefit if it is not controlled by strong muscle power.

COSMETIC APPEARANCE

This is often sacrificed in order to keep the functional range, e.g. fractured metacarpals usually result in the 'loss' of a knuckle because of a slight overlapping of the bone ends. To obtain a cosmetically perfect result would require an operative procedure which could result in a loss of metacarpophalangeal joint range.

SCAPHOID FRACTURES

It is now believed that a scaphoid fracture is only part of an injury to the wrist area. The bony injury may not indicate the severe damage which has occurred, especially to important volar ligaments. A condition of 'carpal instability' may exist which, if diagnosed early, requires the scaphoid fracture to be internally fixed to ensure its union and proper subsequent wrist function.

Chart 22.5. Fractures of the femur.

Site	Age group	How injury occurs	Most usual method of treatment	Movement begun	Complications	Results and comments
Sub-capital	60+	Fall, but some patients fracture, then fall	• Internal fixation • Prosthetic replacement, e.g. Moore, Hastings or THR	As soon as recovered from anaesthesia and all tubes and rains removed	• Non-union Avascular necrosis • Infection dislocation	Variable, but if case selection is good, very acceptable results from both forms of treatment
Intertrochanteric	Usually elderly	Fall	Internal fixation: • nail-plate • Ender-nail • compression screws	As soon as possible	Infection Failure of device	Good; results depend on type of fracture Compression screw devices appear to have some advantage
Subtrochanteric	Young adult	High velocity Direct violence Pathological*	Traction Internal fixation, e.g. Zickel nail	Will depend on treatment, but early	Malunion Non-union	Good
Shaft	All	Direct injury	• Traction 6/52 – cast brace • Internal fixation (IF) plates or intra-medullary	The ankle and knee should be exercised on traction from 10 days onwards With IF mobilisation can be begun on day after	Malunion Non-union Infection	Excellent results can be obtained by all methods

bearing may
be delayed for
12 weeks

children

Notes

* PATHOLOGICAL FRACTURES

A bone may be weakened by disease within the bone itself (e.g. Paget's disease), by disease which produces its effect on bone (e.g. osteomalacia), or by a disease process which only affects bone secondarily (e.g. a breast carcinoma which disseminates and produces skeletal deposits' secondaries). All such processes may precipitate a fracture in bone by an injury which otherwise would not result in a fracture. All fractures in almost any bone in an elderly patient must be regarded suspiciously, but spinal fractures, upper femoral fractures and rib fractures especially.

UPPER FEMORAL FRACTURES

The hazards of traction for the elderly are bronchopneumonia, pressure sores and DVT. Selected cases can do very well but, in the main, operative treatment offers early mobility and is therefore widely practised.

Range

Usually these patients want only to be able to enjoy 'quiet' living, i.e. the ability to sit (90% of hip flexion), stand and walk (some extension of hip if possible), toileting (30% abduction). A much greater range is desirable, but not essential.

Power

Personal independence is only possible if the muscle power is sufficient to perform the action. Encouragement to keep practising sitting, standing or walking is very important. The quadriceps, hamstring and glutei muscle groups are the most important ones to maintain.

FEMORAL SHAFT FRACTURES

Range

The quadriceps muscle must clearly be working normally to allow full knee flexion. In shaft fractures the muscle may be damaged, be trapped in the fracture, be involved in callus, be adherent to the femoral shaft or be grossly atrophied by prolonged disuse. Some loss of flexion almost always occurs, but severe loss of flexion fortunately occurs only rarely. When this happens it may be possible to free the quadriceps (quadricepsplasty) and regain flexion. The importance of maintaining quadriceps bulk cannot be too strongly emphasised since it contributes to knee stability, which is perhaps even more important than range.

Power

The quadriceps muscle atrophies very quickly. It is important to encourage its use as quickly as possible after injury.

Complications

Overdistraction on traction (if used) is to be avoided. Non-union should not result from treatment, but may still occur in compound fractures as a result of the initial severe damage.

Chart 22.6. Fractures around the knee.

Site	Age group	How injury occurs	Most usual method of treatment	Movement begun	Complications	Results and comments
Supracondylar	Any	Direct in young High violence May be due to twisting injury in elderly	• Traction to reduce fracture • Internal fixation (especially if intra-articular component)	Quadriceps exercises early for all Knee mobilisation early, i.e. 10 days following internal fixation, but weight-bearing deferred for 9 weeks and full weight-bearing for 12 weeks	Neurovascular to popliteal vessels and nerve	Overall fair If simple non-comminuted fracture, fixation or bracing can give excellent results
Patella	Any	Direct blow Avulsion if quadriceps act strongly, but knee unable to extend	Internal fixation Plaster cylinder Excision	Straight away On removal of cast 6 weeks	Retro-patellar arthritis	Excellent
Upper tibia	Adults	Valgus or varus stress drives femoral condyle into upper tibia	• Perkins method • Internal fixation	In the first few days	Superficial peroneal nerve palsy Malunion Instability Osteoarthritis	Generally excellent or good
Tibia shaft	Any	Direct or indirect	Longleg plaster Functional brace Internal fixation	Removal of POP 3 weeks	Non-union Malunion Compartment	The result must be viewed in terms of the initial

the calf

and the available
techniques; no
generalisation
can be made

Notes

FRACTURES OF THE FEMORAL CONDYLES OR TIBIAL PLATEAUX

Unless the bone architecture is restored after these fractures, the normal joint is deranged. Instability results in pain and loss of normal joint range. The type of trauma which gives rise to these injuries will usually have caused some degree of dislocation of the joint, often damaging the soft tissue very considerably.

Range

Full extension is the primary aim; without this the quadriceps muscles cannot act efficiently. A patient can learn 'to live with' a stiff straight knee, but a loss of 10°, or more, of extension creates a weak, painful joint and a poor gait. It is seldom possible to regain full-range movements after these fractures in the middle or older age groups, so that full extension is the most important movement.

Power

Controlled movements of the knee joint are essential in walking, sitting and standing. Whatever movements are restored to the joint, these are only as useful as the degree of muscle power controlling them. Every effort to maintain the power of the quadriceps muscle must be made, even if the knee joint cannot be moved because of fixation.

FRACTURE OF THE PATELLA

The patella is a sesamoid bone in the tendon of the quadriceps. When fracture occurs, it may do so leaving the overlying periosteum and ligaments intact, e.g. stellate fracture in the elderly. These simply require removal of the haemarthrosis, a few days' rest, then active exercise. Where, however, the fracture is pulled apart and loss of extension of the knee occurs the fracture must be held together till union occurs or, if too comminuted, removed and the quadriceps mechanism repaired. The patella lends itself to a technique similar to the olecranon, i.e. tension-band wiring. A figure-of-eight wire passed through the upper and lower poles of the patella over its anterior aspect is all that is required, unless several fragments are present in which case it is excised. As soon as wound healing has occurred, quadriceps exercises and knee flexion are started. If the patella has been excised, 6 weeks in a plaster-of-Paris cylinder is necessary to allow the quadriceps mechanism to heal.

It is important to keep the quadriceps muscle as strong as possible. A 'lag' occurs if the patella is removed because of the change in the angle of pull of the muscle. This lag, or loss of full extension, is a feature of most fractures of the patella in the early stages of rehabilitation and must be overcome if the knee is to regain full stability.

FRACTURES OF THE SHAFT OF THE TIBIA

Simple transverse fractures of the tibia occur, but road traffic accidents result in high velocity injuries many of which are compound, many comminuted. The problem can be divided into: (a) care of the soft tissues and (b) care of the bone.

Treatment will depend on the degree of damage to each. In severe injuries which might have resulted in an amputation in the past external, fixation has allowed stabilisation of the skeleton, thus permitting soft-tissue repair.

Chart 22.7. Ankle fractures.

Site	Age group	How injury occurs	Most usual method of treatment	Movement begun	Complications	Results and comments
Malleoli	Any	By talus rotating in the ankle mortice	1. Plaster – long leg 2. Internal fixation	1. On removal of POP 2. Day 2	Stiffness of the joint Infection Osteoarthritis may occur in either treatment	Results can be excellent but again are dependent on the type of fracture
Talus neck	Young adult	Severe dorsiflexion injury	Internal fixation	Early if well stabilised	Avascular necrosis	Bad; the blood supply is cut off to the body which then dies Revascularisation can occur but damage to the ankle and subtalar joints leads to OA
Calcaneus	Adult	Falls from a height, landing on heels	• Early movement, non-weight-bearing } Straightaway • Internal fixation		Poor function in the subtalar joint	Bad; the involvement of the subtalar joint leads to loss of function, i.e. inversion and eversion; if, in addition, such movement as persists is painful arthodesis may be necessary

| Metatarsals (5th) | Adult | Avulsion injury as foot inverts | Below-knee walking plaster for 3/52 | As soon as plaster removed | Non-union very occasionally | Excellent |

Notes

FRACTURES OF THE ANKLE AND HINDFOOT

The function of the foot on the lower leg is to perform the actions required for propulsion of the body over uneven surfaces at varying speeds. The injuries that can be sustained vary from a simple strain to complex fracture-dislocations involving one or more joints. Unless the bone and joint architecture can be restored to normal, the function of the foot is restricted and usually painful.

Range

Inversion and eversion are the most important movements to restore. Without them, walking on uneven surfaces is painful or even impossible.

Loss of dorsiflexion is a serious problem and leads to back kneeing.

Complications

Avascular necrosis of the talus is evident within a week or two on bone scanning. Fortunately, this is a rare injury.

Chart 22.8. Fractures of the pelvis and acetabulum.

Site	Age group	How injury occurs	Most usual method of treatment	Movement begun	Complications	Results and comments
Stable, e.g. iliac wing; pubic ramus	Adult	Direct blow or fall	Bed rest	As soon as initial pain settles encourage free movement in bed and walk as soon as possible, i.e. 3–4 days	Haematoma	Excellent Sometimes mistaken for a fractured upper femur in the elderly
Unstable, e.g. both rami on one side with dislocation of the ipsilateral sacro-iliac joint	Adult	Crush injury	Internal or external fixation Pelvic sling at bed rest for up to 6 weeks	Can sometimes sit out after 3–4 days On removal of traction	Haemorrhage Ruptured urethra Ruptured bowel Ruptured spleen Ruptured diaphragm	Variable Long-term back pain, short leg; pelvic disproportion may become a very real problem
±Dislocation of the hip	Adult	Dashboard injury, i.e. blows on flexed knee and hip Direct blow to greater trochanter	Traction 4–6 weeks Increasingly internal fixation	Gentle assisted movement while on traction as soon as pain permits Internal fixation can be followed by immediate movement, but not weight-bearing	Sciatic nerve palsy Avascular necrosis Myositis ossificans Osteoarthritis	50% good and excellent results claimed for non-operative management 75–80% good results claimed for operative management

Notes

PELVIC GIRDLE

A single fracture of the pelvic girdle (i.e. one ramus or the wing of the ilium) does not significantly alter the stability of the pelvis. Early walking should be encouraged.

Multiple fractures which break the ring in two places, e.g. two rami on the same side plus a disrupted sacro-iliac joint render the pelvic girdle unstable. If non-operative management is used, weight transmission through the pelvis must await union of bone. Some exercises may be permitted for the remainder of the limb and the rest of the body. External fixator systems may be strong enough to allow the patient to get up, weight-bearing as early as 1 week.

Complications

The force which fractures the pelvis may either directly injure abdominal organs (e.g., liver, spleen, bowel) or bone may damage the bladder and urethra, or the increased abdominal pressure may rupture the diaphragm. Such severe injuries may require, e.g. temporary diversion of the urine or faeces by suprapubic cystostomy and colostomy. These other injuries will determine whether operative intervention for the fractures is possible and will alter possible physiotherapy measures.

Chart 22.9. *Fractures of the spine.*

Site	Age group	How injury occurs	Most usual method of treatment	Movement begun	Complications	Results and comments
Flexion unjuries	Any	Fall or something falling on patient	Bed rest Cervical collar Traction Fusion	Depends on severity and level of lesion	Neurological	Excellent
Extension injury	Adults	Car accident, especially rear-end collisions	Collar	6 weeks+	—	Bad; usually so-called 'whiplash' injury which has no fracture at all Good if only a fracture of a spinous process
Crush injury	Adults	Force exerted from above or below, e.g. fall from a height	Bed rest Spinal support	Move as pain decreases	Neurological	Good if not associated with severe deformity
Flexion-rotation Fracture-dislocation	All	Direct forces, e.g. RTA	Bed rest 6–8 weeks Fixation with distraction rods	Early passive movements of all joints	Neurological (*see Cash's Textbook of Neurology for Physiotherapists*, Chapters 5–9)	Usually neurological involvement which produces greater or lesser permanent disability

the fracture, etc. The terms *weight-bearing* and *non-weight-bearing in plaster* indicate the time at which some weight can be expected to be taken on the limb.

Broad outlines only of treatment are given, and the reasons for them. It must be remembered that all injuries are different, as are the people who sustain them. The treatment must be given to meet the needs of the particular patient, *not* as they appear in any book.

Reference

Adams, J.C. (1983). *Outline of Fractures, Including Joint Injuries*, 8th edition. Churchill Livingstone, Edinburgh.

Acknowledgements

The charts on management of fractures have been adapted and enlarged from those first used by Miss M.K. Patrick, OBE, MCSP, in *Cash's Textbook of Some Surgical Conditions for Physiotherapists*, 6th edition. The authors of the chapter are grateful to her for their use. Similarly *Figures 22.1* and *22.2* are reproduced by permission of Miss Patrick.

23 *Advanced Rehabilitation Following Trauma*

S.H. McLaren

This chapter on rehabilitation concerns therapy of people by people and not by machine. There is obviously a place for treatments from highly sophisticated electromedical equipment and, possibly, a niche for computerised statistics on patient numbers and types of remedial procedures available, but *not* in this chapter! Here is considered 'person to person' therapy — where the *method of approach* to the injured human being and the *tone of voice* used are of paramount importance in the treatment regime.

In a more leisurely past (the so-called 'good old days') the individual with a problem could find a sympathetic listener and confidant in his home doctor or parish priest but now, sadly, pressure of work (frequently of the 'paper' variety) tends to close the door on this source of 'face-to-face' communication. The therapist should be able to fill this role in part — *time* should be allowed during the rehabilitation programme for conversation. Often a vital glimpse of the patient's innermost soul may be gained and a reason elicited for his apparent excessive pain or a reluctance to return to his work situation or even to his family.

The previous chapters have dealt with the patient's regime both pre- and post-operatively and the charts on pages 418–434 provide an excellent guide to the type of fracture the therapist may be expected to encounter. Also included are the various methods of treatment employed (both surgical and non-surgical) and the length of time required before each case is likely to be ambulant. With all this information to hand and the surgeon's permission to act it's 'all stations go' for the Advanced Rehabilitation stage!

The end of the beginning

Rehabilitation of the patient begins at the moment of accident. For example, a middle-aged man takes his dog for a customary walk along the usual route. Uppermost in his mind is a personal problem with which he is wholly preoccupied so that he crosses a familiar road without due care and attention into the path of an oncoming vehicle.

The first person on the scene should speak the truth to the injured man — 'You have broken your right leg but we will soon have you in St Blogg's Hospital and on the road to recovery. We will contact your wife and/or mother with the news of your mishap as soon as possible and, don't worry, your little dog is quite safe and is in good hands.' The dazed, frightened victim now knows:

- *What* has happened to his limb and *why* he is experiencing pain.
- *Where* he is going.
- That his dependants are aware of his plight.
- That his much-loved dog is perfectly safe.

With all these immediate problems 'solved' his mind is then more receptive to the replanning of his temporarily altered life-pattern and, out of recent chaos, organised rehabilitation for his future has begun.

Causes of accidents
Many people have accidents because they are:

- Physically exhausted.
- Mentally depressed.
- Suffering intense feelings of anger.
- In a temporary state of euphoria.

All these conditions render the human body more prone to traumatic incident. The careless pedestrian, the bored machine operator, the frustrated car driver and the love-sick adolescent are all high on the list of homo sapiens most likely to 'meet with an accident going somewhere to happen'.

Advanced rehabilitation is not just a restoration of the patient to his or her pre-accident state — but to a much healthier, more *vital* life altogether (*Figure 23.1*).

'Category' of patient
It is the therapist's job to 'rehabilitate', but the methods and approach may vary with each type of patient.

Examples
- The amputee needs extra *time* to make the required psychological adjustment to an altered physical state.

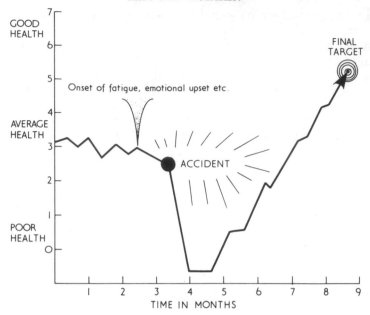

Figure 23.1. Diagrammatic representation of restoration to a better degree of health following an accident.

- The patient who has undergone surgery to arthrodese an ankle or knee joint must master a new techique of propulsion.
- The patient who has had a joint replacement must also master a new technique of walking. Usually these patients have suffered a painful circulatory or arthritic condition for some considerable period of time before the surgical intervention and the type of rehabilitation required would be a continuation of the pre-operative treatment programme with progression as feasible.
- Pre- and post-natal rehabilitation require a somewhat different technique from the therapist – assuming that the condition in which the patient finds herself is an anticipated event imposed upon her voluntarily.

These example patients have all experienced a doctor's surgery or a hospital department and are acclimatised. Not so the normally healthy victim of a road traffic accident (RTA) who, in a state of surprised shock, finds himself compulsorily detained in a hospital bed with his leg residing in a warm damp plaster cast.

Treatment regime

'A man is not fully rehabilitated until he is again paying income tax.' There is therefore a great deal of work to be completed by both the victim of trauma *and* the therapist before the former is able to resume a normal, fully active life.

'The dictionary is the only place where success comes before work.' It is therefore vital that the patient understands that *active participation* in his own treatment programme is essential.

Patient involvement

Rehabilitation is one continual process and must involve the complete person as a whole being. In many instances too much emphasis is laid on the injured part and the patient then becomes morosely absorbed by the presence of the fractured limb. It is the therapist's job to restore the patient's confidence in the affected part and *not* allow it to become the focal point of morbid fascination to that patient.

The success or failure of advanced rehabilitation depends almost entirely on the *atmosphere* in which it is conducted:

ENTHUSIASM IS CAUGHT AND NOT TAUGHT!

The ingredients for the making of a good rehabilitationist might well be:

- An extrovert personality.
- A sense of humour.
- A delight in taking classes of patients for group exercise.
- A commanding voice which will carry conviction.

Sense of humour − or lack of it   Frequently, the patient's sense of humour has wilted or even disappeared by the time his plaster cast has dried out, and restoration of the ability to laugh at tribulation − *and* at himself − is *vital*. A good therapist will be able to thread humour back into the treatment pattern.

> LAUGHTER IS A GOOD ABDOMINAL EXERCISE
>
> and
>
> HE WHO LAUGHS − LASTS!

To advance is to 'encourage the progress of . . .' and, from the outset, the patient should be involved in a forward-thinking regime. This pattern of activity should be designed not only to prime him for his 'bread-and-butter' work, but also to consider his free time expenditure of energy.

Social needs The patient may push a pen in an office from 09.00h to 17.00h Monday to Friday, but lead an energetic golf-playing, sailing, cycling, footballing, dancing or gardening life in the evenings or at the weekend. Any one of these activities requires a very high standard of stamina, co-ordination and general physical fitness. Into the majority of these extra-mural exertions creeps an element of competition. This is important and can be utilised with success when injected into the patient's treatment programme:

- Patient *versus* therapist.
- Patient *versus* patient in a one-to-one capacity.
- Patient *versus* several other patients in a group situation.

Rehabilitation centres

'A rehabilitation centre is for a man who is run down to go to be wound up.' Throughout the United Kingdom there are specialised units where traumatic cases are admitted for concentrated treatment. Some centres are for patients requiring 24-hours-a-day, 7-days-a-week attention, a number accommodate both residential and day patients from Monday to Friday, and others are day centres only.

In these centres the patient learns to be a 'little fish in a big pond' instead of being the 'only pebble on the beach'. In his own home he may be surrounded by a doting family, waited on hand and foot, except when the ambulance transports him two or three times a week to a hospital outpatient department. The conscientious, non-compensationitis fellow will practise his basic home exercises between hospital visits, but the awareness of his injured limb is heightened when there is no other traumatised person present. He has no one with whom to share the experience of trauma, nobody similarly afflicted with whom to discuss the subsequent pain or discomfort and the obvious limitation of movement in normal activity. He may well become introspective. **'The man who gets wrapped up in himself makes a very small parcel.'** A rehabilitation centre or unit provides a varied daily programme which covers most activities over a full working week.

Treatment variations   There are given in *Table 23.1*. The rehabilitation centre provides many advantages, whether residential or not. The patient may see the medical staff *in situ* instead of making a tedious journey to a hospital to wait in a frustratingly long queue. He may contact the administration staff concerning sick notes or

Table 23.1. Treatment variations.

Group exercise classes	
• Competitive	
• Non-competitive	
Individual treatment sessions (as required)	
Hydrotherapy:	A. Passive − aeration baths:
	1. One limb
	2. Whole body immersed
	B. Active:
	1. Organised group exercise (in treatment pool excluding swimming)
	2. Swimming and diving in standard-size swimming pool
Circuit training:	(a) Non-weight-bearing
	(b) Weight-bearing
	(c) For general activity
	(d) To work-specific area only, competing against other members of the group
	(e) Working to improve an individual score
Weight lifting:	(a) For correction of lifting techniques *only*
	(b) To develop strength and endurance − brick-layers, etc.
Weight and pulley work:	(a) To encourage joint mobility
	(b) To increase muscle power
Functional tests:	1. In a specially devised area, e.g scaffold climbing, rough ground walking and crawling − pushing and pulling (a) 'free' (wheelbarrow loaded or empty), (b) vehicle on rails containing variable weights.
	2. In a workshop situation (a) woodwork, (b) car maintenance
Outdoor work:	1. Walks − various
	2. Gardening
	3. Logging
	4. Leaf sweeping, snow clearing, etc.
Games*:	1. Indoor ⎫ in teams, with a partner or
	2. Outdoor ⎭ individually against an opponent (see Chapter 24).

* The rules for 99% of all games can be adjusted to suit a specific need. The patient with normal intelligence is usually able to adapt his thought processes rapidly and easily to the altered situation and gain added enjoyment from the 'new' approach to an 'old' game.

benefits without travelling to some distant ministerial building there to wait in another long queue, at the end of which is an unfamiliar face.

The unit administrator is available to discuss alternative employment using the patient's existing skills or to arrange retraining for more suitable work developing some latent or new dexterity. All these points assist the patient to regain his equilibrium mentally as well as physically, especially if his injury is likely to render him permanently disabled to some degree. There are at least two sides to everything and conflict between one therapist and another as to the correct approach to rehabilitation is inevitable. Provided the ultimate aim of 'restoring the patient' is achieved, then 'let variety be the spice of life'.

Debatable points

The following 'debatable points' are designed deliberately to provoke controversy. As well as a standard comment, the author's own point of view is expressed and openly invites criticism.

STANDARD COMMENT	AUTHOR'S VIEWPOINT
A1 The same exercises should be repeated at each session so that the patient achieves a high standard of performance in one particular movement before progressing to another.	A2 Different exercises should be given at each session so that boredom is avoided (for both the patient *and* the therapist) and, with a wider range of general activities, a greater variety of joint movement is obtainable.
B1 The patient should have individual gait-training to prevent a limp-pattern forming and no attempt should be made to progress to a trot until a limp-free walk is established. This prevents the formation of bad postural habits.	B2 The patient should be encouraged to trot, run and jump, swerve and possibly fall over, laugh, get up off the floor, and try again regardless of a limp or any other irregular pattern of movement. By this means he will prove to himself that he is ambulant once more and only *then* should formal correction of gait be introduced into this treatment programme.
C1 The patient's clothing should be reduced to the minimum to allow for freedom of movement and so enable the therapist to observe the precise working of muscles and joints.	C2 The patient should be allowed considerable freedom in the choice of clothing worn during treatment sessions. This prevents embarrassment or other mental discomfort which

D1   All exercises and activities in group therapy should be non-competitive thus preventing overstrain of the injured limb. This ensures that the less competent patient never feels inferior to his fellow patients.

could inhibit natural movement. Muscle groups contract and relax whether or not they are visible to the therapist.

D2   A high proportion of exercises and activities in group therapy should be competitive so that the patient exerts himself to the fullest extent as soon as possible. This aim of competition prepares him for a return to the outside world and the inevitable rat race. Learning to laugh at himself when he fails dismally in some minor game or contest will stand him in good stead once he leaves the sheltered hospital environment behind.

E1   When patients are required to work in pairs during a treatment session always ensure that (a) the injuries of each are at the same stage of recovery; (b) the two patients are of the same sex and within the same age group; and (c) that both are of similar build.

E2   Make sure that everyone partners everyone else, regardless of injury, sex, age or size. Life in the world outside the hospital walls is not designed to accommodate people in neat pigeon-holes. 'The wind blows as hard on the weak as it does on the strong.'

F1   The patient should be treated two or three times each week in a hospital outpatient department. This enables him to continue a normal life at home with his family and friends, thus aiding his recovery in a familiar environment. Good training in basic home exercises is sufficient to guarantee development of mobility and muscle power both in the affected limb and in the body generally.

F2   The patient gains most benefit when he is outside his home environment and may learn to become independent more rapidly when he is living and working with others similarly disabled. Very few patients work their muscles and joints to full capacity when performing formal exercises solo at home!

G1   A man's hobby is his own concern and no time should be allotted to this during a treatment session. His ability to perform leisure-time activities

G2   The average man works one-third of a 24-hour span in order to play for the second eight-hour period, and sleep; to recover from both types of will return naturally with time. All effort should be concentrated on the work situation.

exertion commandeers the remaining one-third. To promote full rehabilitation, time should be allowed for the patient to discover whether or not his leisure activities – be they boisterous football, peaceful fishing or relatively strenuous gardening – are again possible.

Dos and don'ts

The following 'dos' and 'don'ts' are not laws so much as comments. They are designed to stimulate discussion and provoke argument out of which may arise a new approach or a treatment scheme ideal for the particular unit or department.

Dos

1. DO believe in what you are doing.
2. DO keep the final aim in view, i.e. to rehabilitate the patient to a 24-hours-a-day life.
3. DO remember rehabilitation is a team effort with the patient as the focal point.
4. DO work to restore confidence, stamina and co-ordination, a sense of community living and, above all, a sense of humour.
5. DO use 'contact exercises' wherever possible. So many jobs these days are computerised, mechanised and conveyor-belted and person-to-person contact is often absent. Advanced rehabilitation can help to restore this deficiency.
6. DO remember that 'the injured man is stronger than the average woman' and female therapists should not underestimate the ability of patients – severely injured or not. So much time is wasted by giving 'feeble' exercises.
7. DO remember full and correct use of the voice is vital if success is to be maximal. '**Enthusiasm and laughter are like the measles – infectious**.' Let the patient laugh at you so that you are then entitled to laugh at him too. Develop the power of repartee, which can be used to great advantage in class work.
8. DO use the patient's name. This is a personal touch and reduces his feeling of being merely a number on a filing card. Introduce yourself to your class whenever a new patient is injected into it.

9. DO offer the patient a challenge and the latent *caveman instinct* will rise to the occasion:

(a) Let them cheat a little — but catch them at it.

(b) Let them make a noise whenever it is feasible to do so — a cathedral atmosphere is not conducive to merriment — but make sure there is silence when you wish to give a command or correction.

(c) Always remember to announce the winners of a race or competition — a little praise goes a long way.

(d) Devise a 'penalty or prize plan' — a press-up is an excellent exercise in itself and may be utilised as a 'penalty' for anything from being late for class to 'cheating' in a game. Most male patients *delight* in the opportunity to display their prowess in this direction. The therapist also must be prepared to pay the same penalty for a misdemeanour. It is not 'one rule for them and another one for us'. The 'prize' need not be an enormous one. Sometimes a mere reduction in the number of penalty press-ups which may have accrued is sufficient reward. (Some rehabilitation units provide a *Personalised Prize* in the shape of a keyring, a coaster or a bookmark with suitable words inscribed, and the effort expended by the majority of patients in the attempt to win these 'favours' is well worth any initial financial outlay involved. A simple inexpensive item stamped *Super Star of the Year Award* becomes tantamount to the World Cup in value. Try it.)

10. DO 'trick' the patient into using his injured limb during group therapy. During individual treatments it is more advantageous to allow the patient to demonstrate a movement with his unaffected limb which will then 'teach' the injured limb what is required of it.

11. DO remember to have enough apparatus for everyone in the class to work simultaneously:

(a) This equipment should be basic, inexpensive and easily obtainable for use in the home, so that activity can be continued outside the hospital or centre. Many children would delight in the opportunity to 'play' with Daddy or Grandpa when he returns from hospital and teaches the family the exercises and activities he has been doing.

(b) Use a piece of apparatus if it either makes the exercise more interesting (*Figure 23.2*) or distracts the patient's attention from the injured area (*Figure 23.3*).

12. DO try to keep the number of patients down to a maximum of 12 for class work. This allows for a greater use of available space and reduces the risk of collision, etc., and, with a small number, there is a better chance that the individual patient

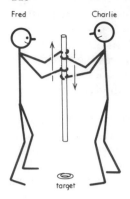

Fred   Charlie

target

Figure 23.2. Challenge for patients with painful hands, arms or shoulders. Charlie attempts to pull the pole downwards towards the target while Fred prevents him. The challenge offered to both men is sufficient to overcome a 'normal' pain; at any point either man can concede victory to his opponent by merely 'giving in' to the superior opposition and so prevent overstrain of a joint or muscle group.

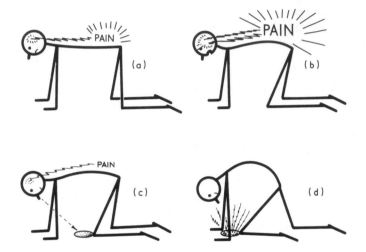

PAIN (a)

PAIN (b)

PAIN (c)

(d)

Figure 23.3. (a) Patient in prone kneeling in preparation for a hip and spine flexion exercise (to mobilise joints following removal of plaster jacket or the equivalent). (b) Increase in awareness of pain on movement of one hip.
(c) Add a piece of apparatus, e.g. a rubber quoit or bean bag (not a ball). The 'awareness' is now divided between pain and the piece of apparatus.
(d) Flexion of same hip pushing the bean bag with knee towards the thumb.
Target: *To propel the bean bag beyond the thumb and double the range of movement is achieved. 'Pain' is now in the bean bag as the thought processes concentrate on knee and thumb regions.*

can be seen and praised – or corrected – and the personal level is maintained.

13. DO remember to keep the patient on the move, especially if an outpatient where time is limited. 'Waiting for one's turn' in a game or activity is a time-waster.

14. DO teach lifting techniques as part of any class activity regardless of injury. 'Prevention is better than cure.' It is hoped that the correct lifting of stools, forms or medicine balls will become automatic eventually.

Don'ts

1. DON'T give 'lethal' exercises:
   (a) where one patient is 'fixed' to another and, therefore, unable to free himself when he wishes. *Examples*: (i) arms linked (*Figure 23.4*) and (ii) 'wheelbarrows' (*Figure 23.5*).
   (b) (i) leapfrog over a partner's back (*Figure 23.6*), (ii) somersaults (*Figure 23.7*), and even (iii) double leg raising (*Figure 23.8*). These are all potential 'hazard exercises'. **Avoid them.**
2. DON'T stop the class following a minor incident, e.g. a grazed knee or a 'jumped' finger or a nose bleed. Send the patient to the nearest first aid department, in company with a volunteer from the same class, and carry on as before. School children, sportsmen and housewives are prone to minor accidents and are used to 'just getting on with it'.
3. DON'T demonstrate an exercise badly or half-heartedly. If you can *do* the exercise − do it well; if not − don't do it all. Instead, declare your inability to do a press-up or touch your toes, or whatever, to your class and the patients will gleefully attempt to succeed where you have failed.

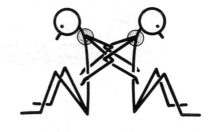

Figure 23.4. Two patients sitting back to back with both arms linked and pulling in opposite directions.
○ = *area likely to be overstrained with no chance of escape from an opponent's grip.*

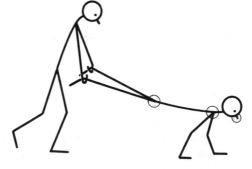

Figure 23.5. Two patients acting as wheelbarrows.
○ = *areas likely to suffer injury if the wheelbarrow 'pusher' is overenthusiastic.*

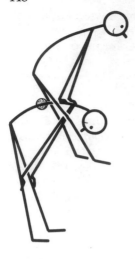

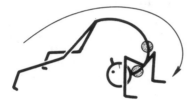

Figure 23.6. Leapfrog. ○ = area which could succumb to forced flexion, especially in the patient who is not expecting his partner to 'land' on his back.

Figure 23.7. Somersaults. ○ = areas most vulnerable to damage when the weight of the body, travelling at speed, hits the ground.

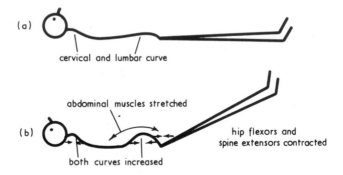

(a)

cervical and lumbar curve

abdominal muscles stretched

(b)

hip flexors and spine extensors contracted

both curves increased

Figure 23.8. Double leg raising. (a) Body in normal black-lying position. (b) Double leg raising. The patient usually holds his breath, thereby increasing his abdominal pressure to abnormal heights.

4. DON'T sit down or lean against the wallbars with arms folded or hands resting on the hips (teapot!) when taking a class. The *voice* gives the command and the hands and arms should be

used to emphasise the order 'Make a circle right round the room' or 'Jump up'.

5. DON'T join in as a fully participating member of the group activity. You will see more of the work your class is doing if you are an active spectator, involved without being embroiled.

After all these DON'TS, the final declaration is a DO:

Make your patient work *so* hard that it is easier for him to return to his work than it is to continue on an advanced rehabilitation programme. He will have proved to himself that he is able to cope with the unexpected as well as with routine requirements in his daily life and the therapist will have the satisfaction of knowing that it has been human endeavour and not a machine-wrought treatment that has brought the patient to 'the end of the beginning'.

Acknowledgement

The author acknowledges the co-operation, inspiration and toil of all the patients, staff and students at The Hermitage Rehabilitation Centre, County Durham; without it this chapter would not have been written.

24 'Maxercises'

S.H. McLaren

Illustrated by M. Rutter

A **Maxercise** = maximum physical and mental exercise combined with an element of fun in a competitive atmosphere within the group. A Maxercise is not a formal exercise, nor is it purely a game. Patients are placed in a one-to-one situation, working either against an opponent or together with a partner versus other competing pairs within the group.

These particular Maxercises each utilise one or two pieces of basic apparatus:

- A pole.
- A pole and a quoit.
- A strong blanket.
- A plastic football.
- A large medicine ball.

After many years of experimentation at The Hermitage Rehabilitation Centre the idea of using the same equipment for a 30–40-minute group treatment session has been found to be more advantageous than exchanging one piece of apparatus for another at the end of each exercise. A different piece of equipment may be used the following day (see *A2*, p. 442). The introductory cartoon figures (*Figure 24.1*) – burly, affable Alf and thin, aesthetic, humourless Ernest – typify two patients, one at each end of the 'brawn *versus* brain' range. Variety in the choice of Maxercises should ensure that both Alf and Ernest each win one or more events so that the honours are equally divided. Success and achievement count for a great deal in total rehabilitation.

The key to the amount of difficulty each Maxercise offers is shown in the facial expression (*Figure 24.2*). A *smile* indicates the easier situation, e.g. where Alf is sitting passively on the blanket waiting to be pulled across the floor by the lighter-weight Ernest, who is (understandably) *frowning* at the daunting prospect (see *Figure 24.19*, p. 000). In *Figure 24.17* (p. 464) Ernest is able to shake the quoits over Alf's wrists more easily because he is the taller of the two men and has the advantage that extra height gives him,

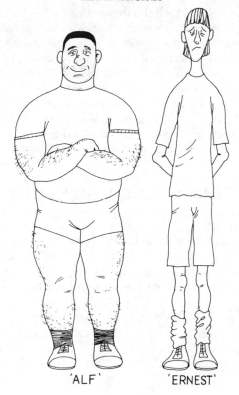

'ALF' 'ERNEST'

Figure 24 1.

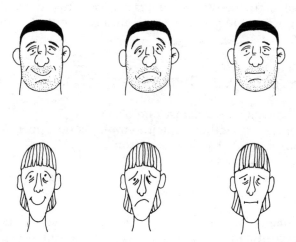

Figure 24.2.

so *he* wears the *smile* and Alf the *frown*. Where the facial expressions are *neutral* the effort is shared equally between Alf and Ernest who are partners and not opponents in this instance (see *Figure 24.29*, p. 478). The amount of co-ordination and physical stamina required to bounce and catch a ball from the surface of a second ball is no greater for one than for the other.

You have now made the acquaintance of Alf and Ernest: let them introduce you to some simple Maxercises which are suitable for the rehabilitation of many different injuries and conditions in male and female patients from teenage upwards.

Group 1 Maxercises using poles

Apparatus required
Industrial weight broom-shanks 30–36in long. These are reasonable in price and will last for many years if linseed oil is applied liberally some days before the initial use. A full length new shank makes two adequate pieces of equipment for this type of activity.

Space required
Sufficient to prevent accidents when moving poles are involved, particularly at head level (see *Figure 24.17*, p. 464), preferably an area large enough to move at least 3m from one side of the room to the other.

Floor surface
For exercises shown in *Figures 24.12–24.16* inclusive, there should be no carpets or rugs and the floor should be scratchproof. A good polyurethane-type coating is sufficient to prevent permanent marking when the poles are used in direct contact with the floor surface.

Maxercise No. 1 *(Figures 24.3–24.6)*

Type: Competitive – against one opponent.
Use: General strengthening with emphasis on upper limbs.
Apparatus required: 1 pole per person.
Space required: Minimal.

Aims

Alf	Ernest
To maintain the poles in the starting position.	To pull one or both poles downward until the ends touch the floor.

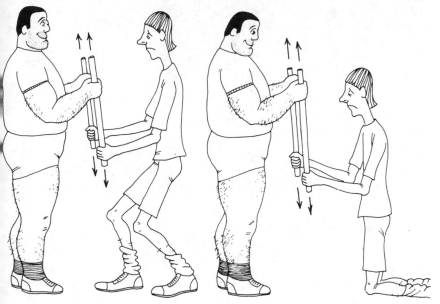

Figure 24.3.

Figure 24.4.

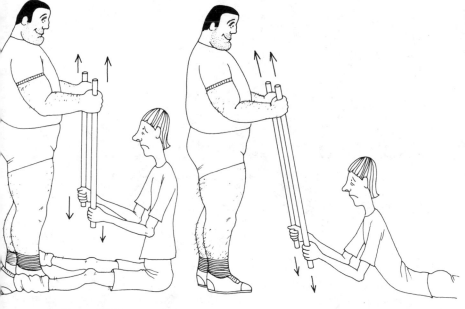

Figure 24.5.

Figure 24.6.

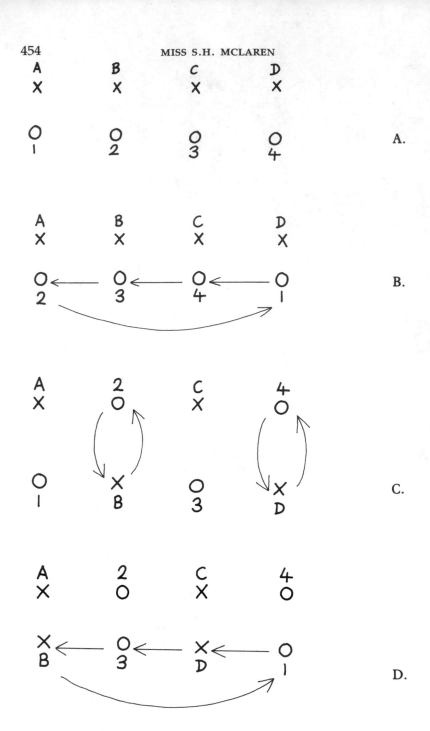

A.

B.

C.

D.

Figure 24.7.

Teaching points

1. Check that Alf and Ernest are holding the poles correctly — Alf near the top and Ernest at the bottom.
2. Give a clear command to Ernest 'Ready — Pull!' — slowly and steadily without jerking towards the floor. Alf stands still. If Ernest reaches floor level with the pole ends he is the winner.
3. Give a clear, decisive 'stop' after 15–20 seconds — resting briefly before Ernest holds the poles at the top and Alf pulls downwards.
4. Congratulate the winner by *name* — for all to hear (see Chapter 23, p. 445, 9c).
5. Remember to change partners frequently (see E2, p. 443). *Figure 24.7* shows quick methods of partner changing.

This Maxercise may be performed in a variety of starting positions. Some examples are shown in *Figures 24.4–24.6.*

If both partners are non- or partial-weight-bearing or wheel-chair-bound this Maxercise may be performed in long sitting on the floor or sitting on a chair. Remember to apply the brakes firmly if the patient is in a wheelchair. The advantage is nearly always with the partner who is keeping the poles stationary. The flexor muscles are much more powerful than the extensors in the region of the shoulder girdle. The exception will be Alf, who will probably unfurl Ernest without undue strain.

Maxercise No. 2 (*Figures 24.8* and *24.9*)

Type: Competitive — against one opponent.
Use: Co-ordination and reflex training.
Apparatus required: 1 pole per pair of patients.
Space required: Minimal. (If Alf and Ernest both stand on a mat the sound of a dropped pole is reduced.)

Figure 24.7. Changing partners: (a) A, B, C and D each have a partner 1, 2, 3 and 4. (b) A, B, C and D stand still while 1 moves to the other end of the line to partner D. Next time 2 moves up to partner D. Continue in that manner until 1 is back to the starting position (a). (c) The next move is for B and D to change with 2 and 4 respectively, before in (d) 1 moves once again to the other end of the line followed by B; then 3, and so on, until A and 1 are back together again. In order to give everyone a chance to partner everyone else the final move is a diagonal one. A changes with D and 2 changes with 1 and again the 'top' line of people remains stationary. B moves to partner 4, followed by 3, A and 2.

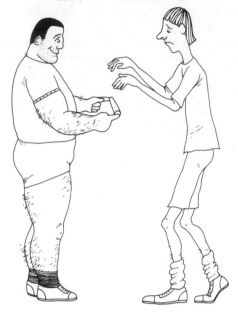

Figure 24.8.

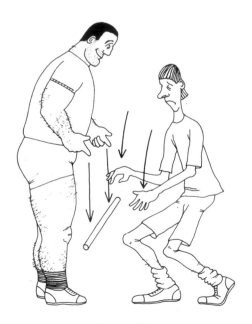

Figure 24.9.

Aims

Alf	Ernest
To open his arms, unobtrusively allowing the pole to drop from between his fingertips down toward the floor without prior warning to Ernest of his intention.	To catch the pole from above before it hits the floor, which requires speed of action in conjunction with a good eye for movement.

Teaching points

1. Make sure that Alf is balancing the pole between his index fingers only and is staring Ernest in the eyes before he drops it.
2. Check that Ernest's hands are above the pole and that he does not turn them palm upwards in order to catch it.
3. Ensure that Ernest drops the pole next time regardless of winning or losing on Alf's drop. This way each will have an equal opportunity to score. Allow time for both partners to try three or four times each before stopping the activity and enquiring who caught how many.
4. Change partners as before.

Variation: Other apparatus (rubber quoits, bean bags) may be used in place of the heavy and noisy poles, especially by teams of chairbound participants.

Maxercise No. 3 *(Figures 24.10 and 24.11)*

Type: Competitive − working with a partner against other pairs in the group.
Use: General body movement at speed: (a) elevation of shoulder girdle; (b) knee and spine flexion; and (c) training in running and fast turning (if space permits).
Apparatus required: 1 pole per pair of patients.
Space required: Minimal if standing still. (If space allows, Alf runs across the room to the stationary Ernest and back to the starting point between each pole action.)

Aims

Alf	Ernest
To grip the pole tightly at each end and pass it over Ernest's head, down behind his knees	To step over the pole at the appropriate moment without endangering Alf's front teeth with

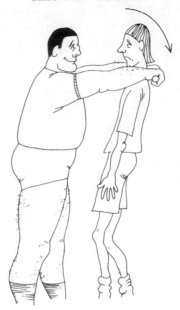

Figure 24.10.

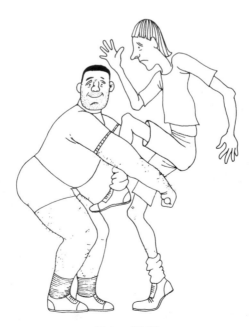

Figure 24.11.

and under his feet three times as quickly as possible without leaving hold of the pole at either end.

an overenthusiastic knee and hip flexion movement.

Teaching points

1. Emphasise the necessity for *control* of movement to Alf's team wielding the pole and Ernest's team high-stepping to avoid it.
2. Watch out for cheating by Alf's line of pole-holders who will probably learn at an early stage that taking one hand off the pole makes life simpler. The press-up makes an excellent penalty — if not a deterrent — to dishonest folk!
3. Alter the race by reversing the direction of the movement, i.e. starting at Ernest's feet and finishing over his head.
4. Note and congratulate the winners and change partners as before.

Variations: This Maxercise allows for umpteen variations on the same theme. The following may all be used to perform this activity:

- A skipping rope folded in half or, indeed, several times.
- Team bands; a metre of carpet binding stitched to form a circle.
- A twisted blanket (*see Figure 24.24a*, p. 472).

With these pliable materials it is possible to alter the starting positions so that Alf is kneeling while threading the skipping rope (or equivalent) over the head (or feet) of a *sitting* or *back lying* Ernest.

Maxercise No. 4 *(Figures 24.12–24.16)*

Type: 'Skiing' with variations — working with a partner — non-competitively to begin with and then, when skilled enough, as a race against other pairs.
Use: Development of balance, co-ordination and rhythm with essential physical support from partner. Very strong arm work required by Ernest, while Alf develops his ankle muscles.
Apparatus required: Two poles per partnership.
Space required: Large clear area to move across from one side to the other while balancing on 'skis'.

Aims

To re-establish a sense of team-work — through physical contact. It requires considerable confidence in one's own muscle power (if

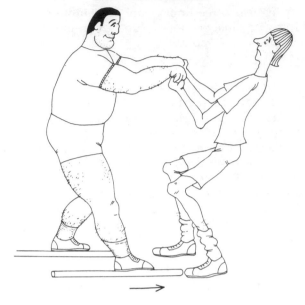

Figure 24.12.

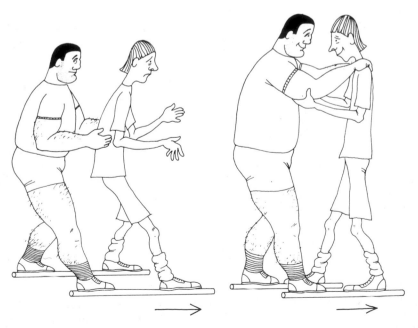

Figure 24.13.

Figure 24.14.

you are Ernest's weight) to maintain Alf's bulk upright on a pair of cylindrical poles.

Teaching points

1. Clarify the hand and finger grip. Alf's fingers are curled over Ernest's with his hands in a prone position, while Ernest's palms are facing upwards.
2. Alf slides his feet one by one — Ernest does *not* tow him across the floor.
3. Allow a generous time for practice.
4. Specify any rules regarding falling off the poles, e.g. (a) return to starting line and begin again, or (b) stand still until remounted on poles, or (c) invent a house rule of your own.
5. Give a clear command 'Ready — Go!' and, if the winners achieve a first-class performance, give them an opportunity to make a demonstration run for the benefit of the others. This is extra exercise and a morale booster.
6. Change partners as before, but allow a short rehearsal time as each individual has a different rhythm and method of propulsion.

Variations: The illustrations are self-explanatory. Alf and Ernest are working in harness on the same 'skis' — first travelling forward and then Ernest faces Alf and moves backward.

Although this is an excellent activity for regaining control of foot and ankle movements for rough ground work and scaffold climbing, it is often too painful for a bare foot to tolerate. Do *not* insist on the removal of shoes.

Maxercise No. 5 *(Figures 24.15 and 24.16)*

Type: Non-competitive activity working closely with partner, who is essential for maintenance of starting position.
Use: For developing or maintaining balance, co-ordination and concentration, with particular emphasis on ankle stabilisation.
Apparatus required: Two strong poles, one laid across the other.
Space required: Minimal.

Aims

Alf	*Ernest*
To balance on the top pole while performing weight transference from his left foot to his right foot and back again.	As supporting partner, works twice as hard to prevent Alf from being dislodged. A press-up penalty could be imposed if the support permits the balancer to topple off his perch.

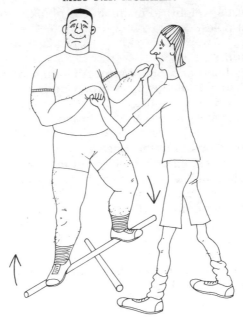

Figure 24.15.

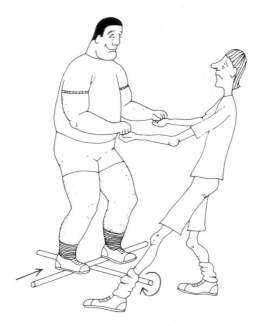

Figure 24.16.

Teaching points

1. Once again, note the finger grip and position of the hands. Ernest needs to assume a wide base for maximum balance and stability, while Alf rocks from one foot to the other tilting the pole until it makes audible contact with the floor.
2. Once the participants have learnt to rock adequately let them choose a well-known tune − e.g. 'For he's a jolly good fellow' − and each note is then tapped out in the correct rhythm by the movement of alternate feet. Once again, the champion 'musician' and his partner might enjoy giving a command performance for the benefit of the others.

The Maxercise shown in *Figure 24.16* is difficult, but not impossible. By lungeing from one leg to the other, Ernest assists Alf to 'roll' himself from side-to-side across the revolving lower pole. Alf's feet remain stationary while Ernest and the supporting pole act as the moving parts.

This is *not* a suitable exercise for use as a race. It requires concentration and control to be a safe activity and both these qualities vanish in the face of competition at speed.

Maxercise No. 6 *(Figure 24.17)*

Type: Another competitive activity in which Alf and Ernest are antagonists instead of buddies.
Use: To gain full elevation of the shoulder girdle and a spontaneous spring action out of the feet and legs.
Apparatus required: Two poles and two rubber quoits for each pair.
Space required: A moderate amount.

Aims

To encourage spring at full stretch in both combatants by attempting to hook the two quoits over the opponent's wrists before he can do the same to you. Height is an advantage, though the shorter person with an ability to jump upwards from a standing start may often be successful. In *Figure 24.17*, Ernest is applying his extra height to good advantage although the small quoit may not slip over Alf's chunky fists too easily.

Teaching points

1. Space the pairs wisely with adequate distance between neighbouring couples so that there is room to jump about and 'stab' with the poles without endangering others in the group.
2. Note grip position in *Figure 24.17*: for safety reasons the hands never move from the ends of the poles.

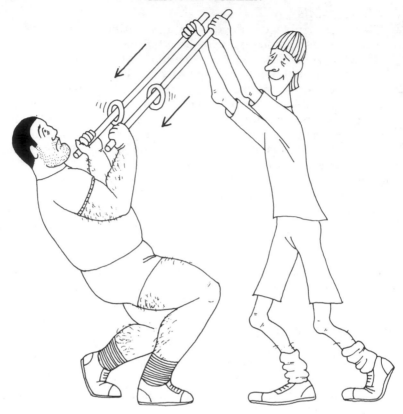

Figure 24.17.

3. Remind both partners to stop immediately, again for safety reasons, should one of them leave go of either or both poles.
4. Make sure that the command – 'Ready – Go!' is heard by all participants and that nobody jumps the gun. Speed of reaction to the challenge has its reward in both this Maxercise and Maxercise No. 7.

Maxercise No. 7 *(Figure 24.18)*

Type: A competitive activity ideally suited as a follow-on to Maxercise No. 6 as the body movements are downward in a flexed or crouch position, as opposed to an upward, stretching-in-extension attitude.

Use: Development or maintenance of a good reflex action combined with general flexion of knees and ankles.

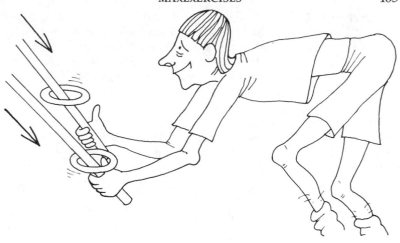

Figure 24.18.

Apparatus required: As for Maxercise No. 6.
Space required: Minimal.

Aim

To gain gravity's aid before one's partner does so, in order to hook the quoits over one's own thumbs. Quick reflexes (and a cunning streak) are guaranteed to bring victory.

Teaching points

1. Dissuade Ernest and others like him from assuming the stance shown in *Figure 24.18*. The command 'Knees bend-Back straight' was intended as an *upright* position to prevent strain on the spine.
2. Watch out for the cheat who slides his hand along a pole, grabs a quoit and scuttles back to the starting position with his trophy. This is decidedly 'not cricket'.
3. Change partners frequently.

Group 2   Maxercises using blankets

Apparatus required

Blankets: Army-type grey blankets — single-bed size — are designed to withstand stress and strain and are virtually indestructible. Even the voracious moth appears to avoid them. Any energy expended in obtaining such blankets is amply rewarded by the amount of useful life they provide.

Space required

A large hazard-free area, such as a gymnasium or an assembly hall. Plenty of ventilation is advisable as fluff and dust can accumulate and cause distress to people with chest problems.

For safety reasons the number of participants in this Maxercise should *not* exceed 12 regardless of floor space available.

Floor surface

As for the pole Maxercises, i.e. a smooth, ideally wooden, floor with a good quality polyurethane coating. No carpets or rugs.

Maxercise No. 8 *(Figure 24.19)*

Type: Competitive − working in conjunction with a partner not against him.

Use: To provide strong back extension work and powerful finger-grip action for people returning to heavy labouring jobs.

Apparatus required: One strong blanket per partnership.

Space required: A large area.

Aim

Alf	Ernest
To remain balanced at the end of the blanket without holding on with hands or feet.	To tow Alf's passive weight smoothly across the room until he can touch the wall − at which point the roles are reversed and Alf pulls Ernest back to the starting point.

Teaching points

1. *It is essential that a trial run in slow motion precedes this competition at speed.* Ernest must be reminded throughout the activity to lean forward. Should he tilt backward and suddenly lose his grip or should Alf roll off the end of the blanket, then Ernest is liable to fall heavily.

2. On the return journey, when Alf is towing Ernest's comparatively negligible weight, emphasise that *control* is the keyword. If Ernest rolls off because Alf is careless and jerks the blanket thoughtlessly then the press-up penalty comes into its own.

Variation: Instead of remaining passive, the passenger can sit holding on with hands and feet and a greater yet safe towing speed can be achieved.

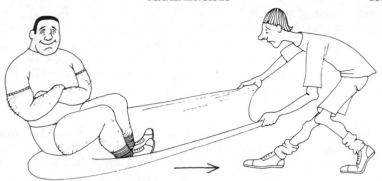

Figure 24.19.

Maxercise No. 9 *(Figure 24.20)*

Type: Co-operating partners in a competitive situation.
Use: For strengthening of shoulder girdle muscles, hip abductors
and evertors of feet.

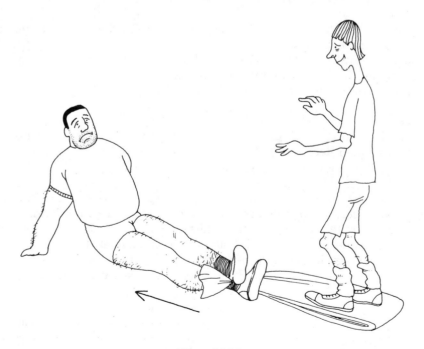

Figure 24.20.

Apparatus required: One blanket.
Space required: As for Maxercise No. 8.

Aim

Alf tows the balancing Ernest using only his crossed feet to hold the blanket and his hands to 'grip' the floor.

Teaching points

1. Alf draws his feet slowly towards his hands so that Ernest is not jerked off the blanket. Ernest bends his knees slightly and uses his arms outstretched to act as a counter-balance.
2. The winners are the two who arrive across the floor first, *without* having lost the passenger off the blanket. This encourages more control of movement and is therefore less likely to lead to a dangerous situation being created by an unthinking enthusiast.
3. Remember to change roles and partners frequently and do *not* leave the Maxercise asymmetrical, e.g. pull the blanket with the *opposite* foot on top during the second run.

Maxercise No. 10 *(Figure 24.21)*

Type: Alf and Ernest in harness working for the good of the partnership.
Use: Teamwork with emphasis on knee and ankle work.
Apparatus required: One blanket (folded).
Space required: As for Maxercise No. 8.

Aim

To develop a rhythm of movement so that, by jumping and sliding their feet, both Alf and Ernest (*and* the blanket) travel across the floor simultaneously.

Teaching points

1. Note position of Ernest's feet − gripping folds of the blanket between them using his adductors strongly. Alf's stance should be a wide one with knees slightly bent and feet flat.
2. Allow practice time for a rhythm to be established.
3. Change places so that Ernest has a fair share of the easier position.
4. Encourage 'more haste less speed'. Congratulate the pair who travel the greatest distance without losing contact with the blanket.

Variation: This is an energetic 'fun' activity if attempted in lines of four each holding on to the body in front. The leader grips the

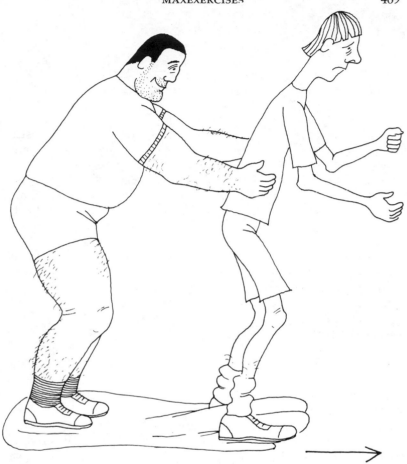

Figure 24.21.

blanket with his feet and the back marker calls 'mush, mush'. The team moves forward as one unit on each 'mush'. Practice time is essential. It is very difficult to stay on the front end of the blanket when three stalwarts are pushing with enthusiasm from behind! The winning team is the one which arrives intact.

Maxercise No. 11 *(Figure 24.22)*

Type: Competitive – against an opponent.
Use: The offer of a challenge of this ilk awakens the most dormant of creatures.
Apparatus required: One blanket per pair.
Space required: Moderate.

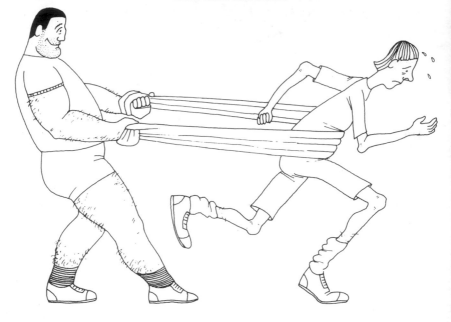

Figure 24.22.

Aim

Alf
To prevent Ernest reaching the far side of the room by standing still and restraining him with a blanket 'rein'.

Ernest
To summon up enough strength to pull himself *and* Alf across the room.

Teaching points

1. Note Alf's grip on the blanket. There is only a loop around his hands, which he is gripping with his fingers, *not* a rigid knot. This is important, for Alf must be able to leave go should he feel the strain is too great on an injured area.
2. The position of the loop of blanket around Ernest's abdomen. His thorax is not encased so there is little or no restriction on his breathing apparatus. Any ground he gains he can keep: Alf must *not* pull him backward to the starting line, for this is both dangerous and demoralising for Ernest.
3. Change over so that the horse becomes the driver after 15–20 seconds – and change partners so that Ernest has a glimmer of a chance against some lesser Samson.

Maxercise No. 12 *(Figures 24.23 and 24.24)*

Type: Brain teaser which gives both Alf and Ernest an equal
chance to get their breath back from the previous Maxercise.
Use: An activity which develops brain rather than brawn.
Apparatus required: One blanket.
Space required: Minimal.

Aim

Alf
To assist Ernest where possible
without leaving go of his end
of the blanket 'rope'.

Ernest
To make a complete knot in the
blanket without loosening his
grip on the blanket end (*Figure
24.24B*). To do so disqualifies
the partnership.

Teaching points

1. Make a good 'rope' by holding the diagonal corners of the
   blanket and swirling it round (*Figure 24.24A*).

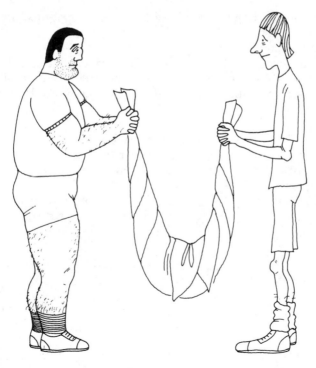

Figure 24.23.

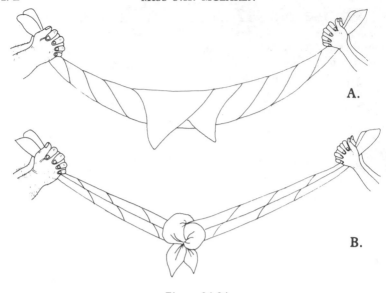

Figure 24.24.

2. Insist that the fingers are entwined in a 'wasps' nest' position (*Figure 24.24A*).
3. Allow 'thinking' time.
This Maxercise does not make a good race as it encourages cheating from the not-so-bright participants, who find it impossible to reason along scientific lines! Ernest should shine brightly in this activity.

Variations: (i) Alf makes the first knot while the blanket 'rope' is at its longest. Ernest, being the thinner of the partners, ties the second knot on top of the first. It is not impossible to tie three knots in some blankets.
(ii) Untie knots with feet only — either standing up or sitting down. The winners are the two who have all their knots untied without being tempted to use their hands or teeth.

Maxercise No. 13 *(Figure 24.25)*

Type: Non-competitive *or* a competitive activity depending on the degree of fitness of the patient. Performed in pairs.
Use: Co-ordination, rhythm and teamwork development.
Apparatus required: One blanket, one wallbar fitment or fellow patient to act as an anchor for one end of the 'rope'.
Space required: Large area.

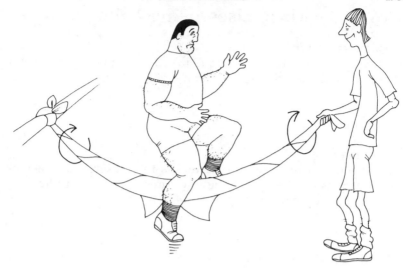

Figure 24.25.

Aim

Alf	Ernest
To step or jump over the blanket 'rope' a given number of times.	To turn the 'rope' over Alf's head and under his feet smoothly and rhythmically.

Teaching points

1. Make certain that (a) the end of the blanket is securely tethered to the wallbar or equivalent; and (b) the 'rope' continues to twist in a tightening direction once Ernest begins to turn it. An unravelling blanket can become a hazard.
2. Insist that the 'rope' hits the floor on each downward movement. It can be dangerous to the skipping partner if an airborne blanket catches him at knee height. Someone of Alf's weight falls very heavily when tripped up.

Variations: (i) In teams of four: Nos 1 and 2 hold the 'rope' while Nos 3 and then 4 each complete three skips in turn. Nos 3 and 4 then hold and turn the 'rope' while Nos 1 and 2 take their turn to skip three times each. This encourages team-work and timing.

(ii) Instead of skipping over it, Alf runs *under* the turning 'rope' without making contact with it, turns and jumps over it at ground level as it comes towards him.

(iii) Alf and Ernest each hold one end of the 'rope' and, standing side by side, skip three times while turning the 'rope' together. This develops partnership rhythm – making each man aware of the natural speed of the other.

Group 3 Maxercises using balls

Apparatus required
Lightweight plastic footballs (standard size) (*Figures 24.26–24.29*)
or 6, 7 or 10lb medicine balls (*Figures 24.30–24.32*).

Space required
Moderate.

Floor covering
The presence of mats or carpets makes the Maxercises easier in
some respects. Certainly, it is more comfortable for Alf to lie on a
carpet than on a bare floor (*Figure 24.27*).

Maxercise No. 14 *(Figure 24.26)*

Type: Competitive against partner.
Use: To test the ability of the patient to withstand jarring actions.
Apparatus required: One plastic football each.
Space required: Moderate in size, and without hanging light fit-
    ments and uncovered windows.

Aim

Alf	Ernest
To knock Ernest's ball down- ward in order to make Ernest drop his ball without letting go of his own ball.	To grip the ball tightly so that Alf cannot dislodge it with his ball.

Teaching points

1. Note position of Alf's hands, which are slightly curved over
   the top surface of his ball, while Ernest cradles the ball from
   underneath.
2. The feet remain more or less stationary while Alf taps Ernest's
   ball lightly several times before increasing the amount of power
   behind the blows. Should Alf lose his grip while hitting Ernest's
   ball, Ernest becomes the winner through default.
3. Noses, front teeth and spectacles may all be in danger if this
   Maxercise is not taught correctly. Do *not* allow hitting from
   below the ball unless each participant is fully aware of the
   danger of behaving in an uncontrolled manner.
4. Change the ball over as well as the partners. A football with
   less air in it is easier to hold between the palms and so
   becomes an unfair advantage if not circulated round the group!

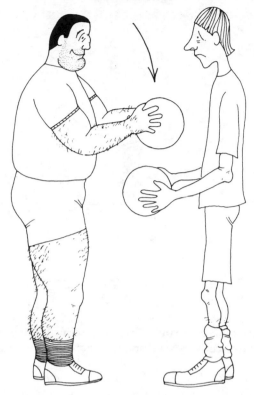

Figure 24.26.

Maxercise No. 15 *(Figure 24.27)*

Type: Competitive – working in conjunction with a partner.
Use: Development of co-ordination in eye, hand and foot.
Apparatus required: One plastic football per pair.
Space required: Moderate.

Aim

Alf

To kick back the ball rhythmically using the soles of both feet simultaneously.

Ernest

To throw (and catch) the ball accurately so that Alf can kick it back speedily and directly a given number of times.

Teaching points

1. Emphasise that the kick is to come from both feet at once.

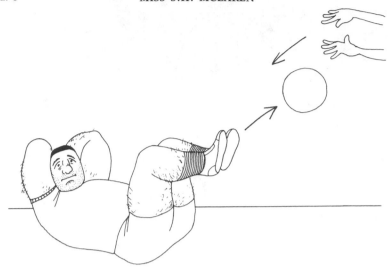

Figure 24.27.

2. A dropped ball by Ernest does not count towards the final score. This encourages effort to reach for the more difficult catch.
3. Change places after a short time and change partners frequently. Some unathletic types find the eye—foot co-ordination required for this Maxercise almost impossible.
4. Do encourage the kicker to maintain a bent-knee position to prevent strain on the spine. With good timing, the ball can be returned with sufficient force to reach its target without the knee extensors being used in the middle to inner range.

Maxercise No. 16 *(Figure 24.28)*

Type: Competitive — working in a one-to-one situation.
Use: Balance — particularly Ernest on his one leg.
Apparatus required: One plastic football per pair.
Space required: Minimal.

Aim

Alf	Ernest
To retain the ball firmly between his inverted feet while maintaining his balance on adducted legs.	To balance on one foot and pull the ball away from Alf's feet using the heel of the other foot.

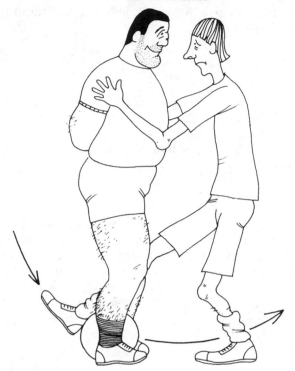

Figure 24.28.

Teaching points

1. Allow Ernest to support himself lightly against Alf's frame. This is a 'trick' Maxercise particulary useful for recalcitrant leg and ankle injuries – so remember to change from one leg to the other when Ernest and his line are battling for the ball. To begin with, allow Ernest to choose which leg he wishes to use to pull the ball away from Alf's feet. The second one works doubly hard to support his weight while he is concentrating his effort on the 'active' limb. Use the other leg on the second attempt to win the ball.
2. Coach Alf by suggesting he should bend his knees and turn his toes inward after Ernest's leg has passed through the space above the ball.
3. Instruct Ernest to 'pull' rather than 'kick' the ball out – this is less traumatic for the stationary Alf.
4. Change over after 15–20 seconds so that Ernest has a chance to grip and keep the ball.

5. Change partners to give those with less weight behind them a chance to succeed.

Maxercise No. 17 *(Figure 24.29)*

Type: Competitive — working in conjunction with a partner against the remainder of the couples.
Use: Co-ordination of hand and eye.
Apparatus required: One plastic football each.
Space required: Moderate.

Aim

Alf

To hold one ball tightly between both palms while using it as a 'bat' to return the ball thrown by Ernest three times.

Ernest

To throw accurately and catch quickly as his missile bounces off the curved surface of Alf's 'bat'. This requires co-ordination and quick reflex action by both men.

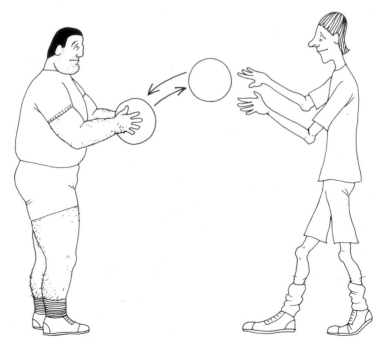

Figure 24.29.

Teaching points

1. Stand close together for the short practice session, then gradually space Alf and Ernest wider and wider apart.
2. Give praise where due, for three catches without a drop in between.
3. Change the ball as well as the partners. Well-inflated ones make better 'bats' than the softer kind.

Variations: Only possible on hard surface without carpets:
(i) Ernest *bounces* the ball diagonally down to the floor towards Alf who sends back a catch from his 'bat'.
(ii) Ernest *throws* the ball and Alf *bounces* it back.
(iii) Ernest *bounces* the ball to Alf who *bounces* it back off the 'bat'.
(iv) Alf throws the ball high into the air and 2 seconds later Ernest attempts to knock it out of the sky by throwing his ball as if it were a missile. This is *not* suitable for highly excitable people in a room with unprotected windows on all sides or hung with chandeliers. Be sensible in the use of it as a Maxercise.

Maxercise No. 18 *(Figure 24.30)*

Type: Co-ordination and balance using partner as a support.
Use: Knee and ankle work to increase stability.
Apparatus required: One large medicine ball each.
Space required: Minimal.

Aim

To support each other while balancing on a large ball and 'see-sawing' alternately into a squat position.

Teaching points

1. See that both men know what they are expected to do. Practise on the floor beside the ball to establish a see-saw rhythm before climbing aboard.
2. Vary the speed of ascent and descent. The slower the timing the more difficult the Maxercise.
3. Progress to using only one hand for support.
4. Congratulate the smooth performers who remain aloft.

Variations (Figures 24.31 and 24.32):
(i) Ernest remains on the ball and, helped by Alf, rolls it under his feet alternately so that he (and it) move forward slowly and steadily.

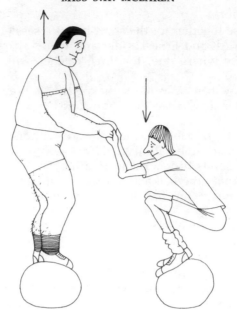

Figure 24.30.

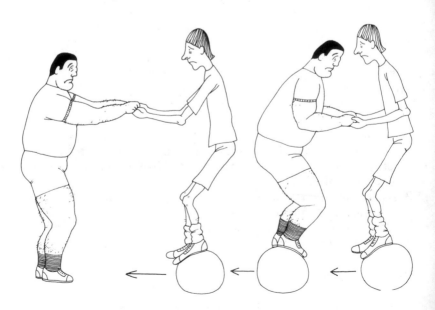

Figure 24.31.   *Figure 24.32.*

(ii) Both Alf and Ernest are mounted on medicine balls and, working as a team, propel themselves across the room without falling off. The speed of progress depends on the skill of the one travelling backward — he has the most difficult task. Reverse direction after a short period so that each partner experiences the sensation.

Conclusion

A Maxercise is a self-propagating animal. New ideas, developments and variations on old, well-tried Maxercises are born during advanced group work. Watch out for them, and record them.

It is almost impossible to perform any one of these Maxercises without using every joint and muscle group in the body at some stage — albeit reluctantly. Surely, this is a good test for a patient who intends to return to a full working situation?

Therapists who are purists dislike Maxercises because (a) they are not specific for the treatment of any one injury or joint; and (b) when taught in an inadequate or careless manner could constitute a risk to the therapist, the patient or the department décor. *Patients* who want to get better enjoy them because they offer a challenge to which they can respond and, in so doing, tend to forget or disregard the injured limb.

25 'School for Bravery' – An Approach to the Management of Chronic Pain

C.M. Ellingworth

Introduction

Some of the basic concepts expressed in this chapter will seem familiar to most physiotherapists. Many of today's practitioners would agree that interdependence of the body and the mind cannot be ignored. Physiotherapists soon realise that during the assessment of a patient, non-verbal messages may be far more informative than the actual words expressed by the patient. Some physiotherapists, however, still have difficulty in interpreting and responding to psychological factors.

There is today a wide acceptance that health and illness are the result of a mutual interaction with and influence of the psychological, physical and social factors in a person's life. The relationship between psyche and soma has been the centre of attention and research for several decades. The 'School for Bravery' is an approach that has been developed over the past few years; the techniques involved are aimed particularly at that group of patients with chronic pain and associated illness behaviour.

The management of chronic disabling pain has generally been neglected in the undergraduate curriculum and, until recently, has hardly been touched on in postgraduate education. This is understandable since, traditionally, education of student physiotherapists has been based on the acquisition of assessment, diagnostic and technical skills. We are taught to establish a physiotherapy diagnosis based on the assessment of the patient and, subsequently, select and implement appropriate physiotherapy. With the patient who presents with chronic pain problems, however, routine physical assessment is very often inhibited due to his innappropriate behaviour. Consequently, treatment is limited to the attempted relief of his symptoms, because no specific underlying physical problem can be identified.

Apart from a very few individuals who have a congenital inability to feel pain, each of us structures his own idea of pain from the data of personal experience. Our reaction to pain is largely learned from childhood. Hannington-Kiff (1981) discusses the different interpretations of pain according the point of view taken. If you are a physiologist, intense stimulation as registered in terms of action potentials is pain; to a pharmacologist, pain is something to be relieved by drugs; to a neurologist, a vocal complaint or the withdrawal of a limb after a pinprick demonstrates the ability of a person to feel pain. Thus, for the clinical physiotherapist who has to deal with chronic or recurrent pain, a definition of pain has to be multifaceted. It has to explain the clinical vagaries of pain; why there is no one-to-one relationship between the intensity or apparent intensity of stimulation, as judged by visible pathology, and the complaint of pain. Undoubtedly, some patients make use of the subjective nature of pain for secondary gain, especially in a welfare state, because they know that there is no way a doctor can categorically dismiss their claim that they are suffering.

The various textbook definitions of pain express the view that pain is a sensation with specific nerve endings, nervous pathways and higher centres in the brain. Continuing research substantiates that there are nervous pathways largely devoted to the neural traffic associated with pain, and that the higher centres associated with the perception and interpretation of pain are located mainly in the areas of the brain which subserve emotion. The latter relationship is very important, because it helps to justify why chronic pain can provoke deep behavioural changes in some patients. It is a mistake, therefore, to look upon the patient with chronic pain as the relatively passive recipient of an overwhelming input of sensory stimulation. Many of these patients have only a niggling background of low-key pain, but they take a negative attitude toward it, deciding that they cannot live with their perceived handicap. Such a decision may be made at either a conscious or subconscious level, during which pain, emotion and personality are closely interwoven. Hannington-Kiff (1981) defined pain as a stack of chips, with each chip representing a clinical feature of pain.

This definition of pain as a 'set' illustrates that the contribution of one or more subsets or the addition of new sets can alter the nature of pain (*Figure 25.1*).

Clinically, therefore, attempts can be made to modify those factors which seem to be most evident. For example, a strong stimulus might be interrupted by a nerve block; abnormal nervous input might be modified by transcutaneous nerve stimulation; mood change might be controlled by an antidepressant drug;

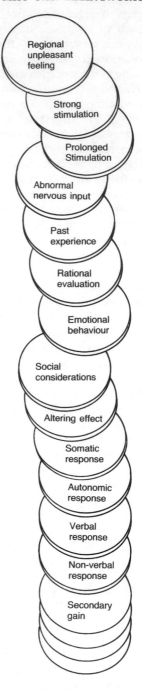

Figure 25.1. The many possibilities in the 'pain game'.

and secondary gain might be satisfied by payment of financial compensation.

Chronic pain, like any other chronic illness, often has a profound impact on a patient's functional capacity. A patient with chronic pain may frequently display marked disability that pervades all aspects of his life, such that he is often unable to engage in gainful employment. A patient with chronic pain may also develop a syndrome characterised by marked functional impairment, chemical dependence, emotional distress, marital and family disruption and vocational difficulties, in addition to the subjective experience of intractable pain (Bergquist-Ullman and Larsson, 1977). The scope and complexity of this syndrome is such that these patients often fail to improve with the conventional management of pain, and repeated efforts to find a successful intervention lead to excessive demands on health-care facilities.

The 'School for Bravery' approach

Many patients with chronic pain link their pain with impairment of function and disability, believing that they are unable to live normal lives as long as they have pain. The extent to which they are able to function is inversely proportional to the level of their pain. Indeed, these patients typically regard relief of pain as a prerequisite to resuming a normal, active lifestyle, and they are often seen to engage in a relentless search for the 'magic cure'. In the absence of such a panacea, these patients remain disabled, stretch health-care resources and often become progressively more disenchanted, frustrated and hostile in their interactions with health care providers.

Catastrophe theory

The many definitions and complexities of pain, and in particular chronic pain, are of our own making. There is not a scientific model which adequately describes and predicts events in the field of pain. Catastrophe theory, as described by the French mathematician Professor Thom, demonstrates that there is a stable situation in which the patient who continuously complains of pain can suddenly have relief of that pain, either long-term or even permanently, by brief and simple procedures, such as transcutaneous nerve stimulation or acupuncture. The application of his theory to chronic pain is argued as follows. The diffuse lasting background element of pain involves the emotional centres in the brain, the limbic lobe. The discriminative element of pain involves the discrete mapping on to the neothalamus and post-central cortex. The specific function of this system is to evaluate the noxious stimuli in terms of time and space. It is recognised, in our language of emotional decisions, that a continuous behavioural situation can suddenly change, e.g. something becomes 'the last straw'. A small or trivial upset can swing our whole emotional behaviour to the extreme opposite.

Professor Thom's catastrophe theory provides a theoretical framework to account for these two-way changes. Catastrophe theory describes, using mathematical formula and graphic representation, a situation in which there are two opposing stable states and, between them, an overlapping period where instability exists. *Figure 25.2* illustrates how it is possible to move rapidly from one stable state to another.

The upper stable state Z–B is equivalent to the feeling of wellness, and the lower stable state A–X to the feeling of illness. Therefore, the period of time X–Z is equivalent to the rapid change from one state to the other. It must be emphasised that this change describes feelings and emotional states, and not physical conditions.

The patient identified as appropriate for the 'School for Bravery' can be described as being at point A on the graph. He is in a

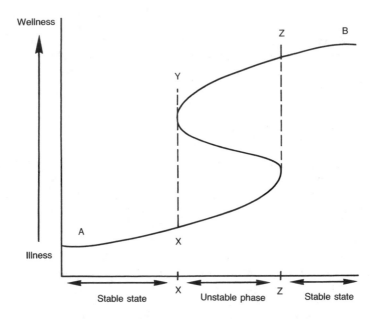

Figure 25.2. Graph to illustrate catastrophe theory.

stable state of long-term illness behaviour. As he commences on the programme, this state eases during the first few days − X. As normal activity is positively rewarded and wellness behaviour is reinforced, he changes rapidly and moves to point Y. With continuing positive rewards and reinforcement of his wellness behaviour, he steadily climbs the slope Y−Z, until he reaches the stable state of wellness once more, Z−B. It is at this stage that the patient will appear to recognise the uphill climb that he has made and will spontaneously say 'I'll never let myself get like that again.'

The physical or sensory aspect of chronic pain has two controls, rational (discriminative) and emotional (affective), as shown in *Figure 25.3*. The pain which a patient complains about is represented by the intersection of all three components.

A patient with chronic back pain is far more likely to decide that the pain is tolerable if he can come to terms with the rational significance of the pain. Whereas, if he is frightened and reacts emotionally, the pain will be more likely to become intolerable and he will become a pain-invalid. In chronic pain, the evolution of the associated mood with time is important and catastrophe theory enables the prediction that any such system which has a divergent tendency (i.e. rational − tolerable pain; emotional − intolerable pain) will assume one or other extreme of behaviour.

The principal aim of the 'School for Bravery' approach is designed to modify perceived intolerable chronic pain to a level

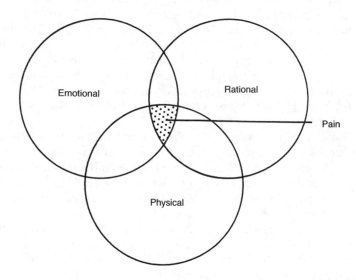

Figure 25.3. The three attributes of pain.

which is accepted as tolerable. The complete relief of pain must not be expected, either by the patient or the physiotherapist. An empathetic physiotherapist who provides an explanation for a patient's pain can positively contribute to the conversion of an intolerable pain into a tolerable one. As pain becomes chronic, behavioural changes occur and so any situational improvement may provide a large improvement in mood and have a beneficial effect on the pain. The emotional centres of the brain, which are deeply involved in chronic pain perception, characteristically swing from one extreme of activity to another.

The 'thick file' syndrome

Pain and illness behaviour is present to some extent in almost every patient that physiotherapists see, so changing patients from an illness state to a wellness state is fundamental to their work. Some patients demonstrate illness behaviour more than others, but the majority recover from it and return to confident adult behaviour in a normal way. In a proportion of chronic pain patients, however, this exaggerated pain and illness behaviour appears to linger, and very quickly a vicious cycle is demonstrated. The patient often has an initial minor problem, but if this coincides with a period of personal stress or worry the problem becomes magnified. The patient then turns to the caring professions for help in a childlike way, expressing his fears by exaggerated pain and illness symptoms. The usual advice given is to rest, be careful, stop if it hurts and not to overdo it. At every appointment he is asked solicitously how his pain is and listened to as he describes it at length. The more pain he describes, the more attention and care he receives. His friends and family protect him, the feeling of concern about being ill deepens and is confirmed by everything around him. Hidden fears set in and he listens to his pain as it rules his life.

In despair, the professions try various interventions and, at each expressed twinge of pain, the patient's anxiety levels increase, panic sets in and the pain becomes worse. The patient's whole life becomes a seeking of care and attention to the carers' apparent distress. The professionals, too, become trapped because, as experts, they must find an answer. The medical file of tests, admissions and re-referrals grows. The patient soon becomes discouraged as the medical profession can do no more and, in fact, he is told that he will have to live with his problem.

Sympathy very quickly evaporates and, in desperation to regain care and attention, the patient takes to stumbling, staggering, collapsing, using a wheelchair and adopting an invalid lifestyle. In these final stages, he loses all interest in his hobbies, and disability pensions, mobility and attendance allowances begin. The development of this syndrome is diagrammatically represented in *Table 25.1*. There is a growing need for physiotherapists to be able to identify the development of this syndrome in its early stages in order to change the way the patient with chronic pain is being handled; preferably, identification should be early enough to prevent its happening at all.

Table 25.1. Diagrammatic repesentation of the 'Thick File' Syndrome.

PAIN INCIDENT + LIFE TENSIONS >>> Fear >> Anciety >>>
   SEEKS HELP > Bed rest/concern/care
      I MUST BE ILL >>>> Fear >>> Increasing pain >> Anxiety
         WORRY >>>>> SEEK 2nd OPINION
         FURTHER INVESTIGATIONS >> Treatment > Advice >
         Warnings
            I MUST BE REALLY ILL >>>>> Fear >> Increasing pain
  6 PANIC SETS IN >>>> What about the future?
  7 DEPRESSION
  8 PAIN BEHAVIOUR >>>> Signals for help
  9 Told 'YOU WILL HAVE TO LIVE WITH THE PAIN'
10 ADOPTS AN INVALID ROLE
11 >>>>> HELP >>>>>

Identifying the problem

Patients who have pain engage in certain behaviours that communicate the fact to others. These behaviours, termed pain behaviours, are increasingly viewed as important targets for chronic pain assessment and intervention. Pain behaviours include activities that can be recorded by means of daily diaries, such as the time spent in bed during the day, visits to health-care professionals, or taking medications. They also include discrete motor behaviours, such as guarded movement, pain avoidant postures, or pain-related facial expressions. Psychological research on the determinants of chronic low back pain behaviour generally falls into two categories. The first is that chronic low back pain behaviour can be seen as a function of the environment and, secondly, as a function of a defect in the 'milieu interieur', such as nociception, pain perception or personality (Schmidt *et al.*, 1989).

Physiotherapists have valuable expertise in analysing movement, a skill that can be utilised to the full when observing illness behaviour. It is necessary to define the observable symptoms of pain and illness behaviour in terms of the patterns of posture, gait and movement used by patients who wish to signal that they are in pain or are ill. Once these symptoms are described, they can be contrasted with the normal movement patterns of other adults who have a similar physical problem, but who are well adjusted and coping with it. The ability to recognise these illness and pain behaviour symptoms is an essential and valuable diagnostic tool when assessing the somewhat uncertain case. *Table 25.2* lists the observable chronic pain with illness behaviour signs and symptoms. Patients who exhibit six or more of the listed behaviours should raise the suspicion of an illness behaviour syndrome.

Table 25.2. Observable chronic pain and illness behaviours.

- Lack of eye contact
- Expressionless, unsmiling face, sad and anxious
- Stooping, depressed posture
- Look much older than their years
- Often neglected, dirty appearance
- Have overt badges of invalidism − collar, stick, wheelchair
- Excessively slow movements when asked to show something
- Inappropriate co-contraction and eccentric muscle work
- Apparent excessive effort and unnecessary difficulty in performing ordinary activities
- Auto-assisted movements
- Use of pain gestures to indicate suffering − clutching or rubbing affected area, wiping brow, puffing
- Abnormal gait and movement patterns
  Absence of head/trunk/body rotation
  Arms held to side
  No arm swing
  'Waddling' gait.
- Abnormal balance reactions
- Attention-seeking, by saying that they feel faint or dizzy
- Exaggerated sway or stagger, *but* never actually falling
- Apparent neurological tremors or spasms
- Lack of spontaneous social gestures

Patient category

A patient suitable for selection for the 'School for Bravery' approach is one who demonstrates at least four of the following criteria:

- A thick medical file.
- A long-standing history of pain for which no treatment has been effective.

- Inappropriate, observable pain behaviour.
- Exaggerated movements or abnormal posture.
- Has been told by a doctor that nothing more can be done for his problem.

A patient with at least four of the above, if treated in a lively physiotherapy gymnasium using a behavioural modification programme, where pain and the pain areas are ignored and activity and wellness are rewarded, will show significant improvement in function in 1 week. He will describe himself as 'feeling fit' and 'living again' within 4 weeks. He will abandon all invalid props, return to a normal lifestyle, sustain and maintain his improvement and, in 50% of cases, will continue to describe the pain as 'copeable'.

Principles of the approach

The principles of the 'School for Bravery' approach are based on catastrophe theory and behaviour modification techniques that modify overt behaviour, combined with the traditional rehabilitation skills of physiotherapists.

The approach must be positive at all times and structured to precise behavioural goals to achieve the normal recovery pattern of this syndrome. The medium is exercise and functional activity in a lively physiotherapy gymnasium.

The principles can be summarised as follows:

1. Reduction of fear by the translation of pain from dangerous to 'it only hurts' or 'it's OK'.
2. Rebuilding of confidence and self-esteem by constant praise and rewarded achievements, structured in small goals, combined with empathy and laughter.
3. Extinguishing overt pain and illness behaviour by ignoring it.
4. Encouraging regrowth of normal activity by positive feedback on every occasion that normal activity is attempted.
5. Changing from illness to wellness behaviour.
6. A deliberate movement by the physiotherapist away from the traditional professional caring expert in charge to a relationship where the patient is seen as an equal adult who has a problem which he is teaching himself to tackle and cope with.
7. Provision of the opportunity for the patient to be recognised in public to have earned a legitimate recovery by hard work and his own efforts. This is essential to the patient's self-esteem and future social well-being, especially if it had been suggested to his family and friends that 'it was all in his mind'.

Basic treatment techniques

The 'School for Bravery' approach is a carefully progressed programme of gymnasium activities designed to build confidence
and fitness, combined with a behaviour modification programme.

The patient is given the choice of the frequency and duration
of attendance, provided that the goals agreed between him and
the physiotherapist are being met. Most patients choose to attend
daily, beginning with a duration of an hour and increasing to a
whole morning. The first 2 days are usually individual sessions
and, from the third day, the patient progresses to more general
gymnasium activities and circuits. The exercise programme is *not*
in any way directed at his area of complaint. In fact, it is deliberately planned to keep attention away from it. The main techniques
are:

- To reduce fear.
- To build confidence.
- To reduce pain and illness behaviours and increase wellness
  behaviour.
- To achieve adult behaviour.

Reduce fear
This is the most important part of the programme in the first few
days. A patient who exhibits normal pain behaviour has his fear
easily reduced with simple explanations over a model spine. For
a patient with abnormal pain behaviour, however, a simple explanation is not always helpful. Indeed, it can have an adverse
effect, increasing the patient's fear and anxiety because he tends
to concentrate again on his problem.

The technique is to reassure the patient indirectly by the way
we react to pain. It is necessary to convince him that pain is not a
dangerous sign and, therefore, unimportant. An authority figure
is needed to tell the patient that pain is 'OK', that 'it only hurts'
and 'yes, it should hurt when you start using your muscles
again'. The physiotherapist must translate the patient's pain for
him, so that overcoming it becomes a challenge, like an athlete
overcoming the pain barrier, rather than something for the patient
to fear.

Build confidence
Confidence is rebuilt by the structuring of small progressive
goals to follow a recovery sequence. The goals are presented in
the guise of exercises or movements which serve to provide the
opportunity to praise the effort and achievement. Constant com-

pliments and positive feedback rebuild the patients' personal pride and help to enhance their self-image.

Reduce pain and illness behaviours and increase wellness behaviours

A patient with abnormal pain and illness behaviour consistently dwells on his problem. Therefore, the physiotherapist must cheerfully attempt to ignore his complaints of pain, and reward him with maximum interest, attention and praise for whatever activity he has been able to do in spite of the pain. Noticing and praising each and every *positive* attempt the patient makes is the crux. There needs to be a conscious practice of this to prevent physiotherapists from falling accidentally into the concern for pain that is the normal habit.

After 2 weeks, the majority of patients will no longer exhibit pain and illness behaviour. Movements are no longer exaggerated or abnormal. The patient has ceased from signalling continual pain and is moving normally and showing adult wellness behaviour, including enjoying social games. However, he will still describe himself as having pain, although he can cope and live with it. He begins to behave and react like most mature adults who have problems they live with. He learns to grin and bear it and not let pain affect his life. The patient's positive experience of being treated as normal and well will help him to become so. A patient who does not show the beginnings of this transition to normal wellness behaviour by the end of the second week, however, is likely to fail to respond to the 'School for Bravery' approach.

Change to adult behaviour

The best results are achieved when the physiotherapist accepts the problem as the patient describes it and this is not challenged or discussed. The patient seems to be able to do his own thinking once he has re-established his physical confidence. He soon regains control of his life and stops crying for help from the professionals. The pride of adulthood returns and the patient begins to tackle his own personal problems without assistance. Throughout the programme, the patient is given the choice and control of what he does. The physiotherapist might make recommendations, but the patient always makes the decision. The patient who meets the criteria for selection for the 'School for Bravery' has to relearn to take charge of his own life and to make his own decisions once again.

For successful rehabilitation of the patient, the physiotherapist must enter into a contract with him prior to his commencing the programme. There should be agreement on what may or may not be achieved, and that the patient can continue the programme only if he shows signs of improvement.

Any patient accepted for the 'School for Bravery' is expected to take responsibility for his own share of the effort. The more usual patient—therapist role changes to an adult-to-adult discussion and agreement. Contracting is essential to specify the patient's own responsibility in his rehabilitation, and to prevent the physiotherapist from falling into what has become known as 'the parent trap'. This term developed because frequently the patient turns to the physiotherapist, as if to a parent, for sympathy, understanding, comfort and wisdom, with the expectation that he will sort out his problem for him. The patient—physiotherapist role will very quickly become a parent—child role, especially if the physiotherapist is willing to take responsibility for the patient, his problems and the pain. Like catching falling patients, however, it is not easy to stop speaking to patients as a wise or caring parent. It is something that all physiotherapists do automatically.

The assessment

This is an initial exploration in which the patient is brought to admit to the reality of his lifestyle and that no one can offer any foreseeable hope of change. This assessment forces the patient into a position of having to recognise and face up to the consequences of his abnormal behaviour problem, as an adult.

The assessment procedure is done gently and non-accusingly, using very practical, factual questions that are couched in non-emotional terms. Empathy and concern should be evident, but the patient is firmly led to see the effect on his life and lifestyle, e.g. the loss of any hobbies, loss of status, loss of friends, the effect on his family life and social pleasures. The person the patient used to be is explored and contrasted with the current version and the prospects for the future are investigated. The assessment is drawn to a conclusion, having reached the point where all appears lost and hopeless. The patient is offered the opportunity and challenge of at least becoming physically more fit, if he has the courage. It is the patient's choice. The physiotherapist must never insist, cajole or persuade the patient to accept the challenge. It is essential that the physiotherapist pursues the following procedures when assessing a patient for the 'School for Bravery':

1. Thoroughly read through all the patient's past and present medical notes.

2. Perform a quick physical assessment of the patient, without concentrating on his problem area.
3. Observe and listen throughout for:
   (i) Abnormal pain behaviours, especially those defined as
      (a) *Guarding* − this is an abnormally stiff, interrupted or rigid movement while moving from one position to another.
      (b) *Bracing* − this is a stationary position in which a fully extended limb supports and maintains an abnormal distribution of weight.
      (c) *Rubbing* − this is touching, rubbing or holding the affected area of pain for a minimum of 3 seconds.
      (d) *Grimacing* − this is an obvious facial expression of pain, which may include furrowed brow, narrowed eyes, tightened lips, corners of mouth pulled back, clenched teeth.
      (e) *Sighing* − this is an obvious exaggerated exhalation of breath, usually accompanied by shoulders first rising and then falling; the cheeks may be expanded.
   (ii) Tension, anxiety, worries, fears.
   (iii) Patient's appearance, lack of eye contact, posture.
   (iv) Descriptions of pain.
   (v) Actual movements and how they are performed.
4. Interview the patient to establish how he perceives the problem in terms of:
   (i) What the doctor has told him.
   (ii) When and why it began.
   (iii) His current lifestyle and role within the family unit.
   (iv) What he has lost.
   (v) How he describes his confidence levels − in self, in the future.
   (vi) What he has to gain, i.e. financial, emotional.
5. Test the patient's reaction to the programme:
   (i) Challenge him as an adult.
   (ii) Has he any courage?
   (iii) Is he willing to pay the cost of pain?

The recovery sequence

Five hundred patients with the previously described observable and abnormal behaviour patterns have been successfully treated by the 'School for Bravery' approach; they have all been observed to have followed a well-defined sequence of recovery and to the time-scale that is indicated below.

Day 1

- Eye contact made — approx. 4 minutes.
- Smile — approx. 5 minutes.
- Relaxation of tension, head erect — approx. 12 minutes.
- Attempts first movements, stands without help — approx. 30 minutes
- Takes a few steps without props — within 1 hour.

Day 2

- Arrives wearing 'fitness' clothes.
- Improved general appearance, looks brighter.
- Works hard and will attempt previously impossible movements.
- Pain gestures and staggering behaviour are virtually extinguished.

Days 3—4

- Spontaneous social gestures reappear.
- Erect posture and obvious pride in appearance and achievements.
- Rotation of trunk and unlocking of body segments.
- Arm swing returns.
- Voluntarily joins in games and laughter.
- Abandons invalid props.

Day 5

- Stride lengthens and weight-bears equally.
- Normal postural and balance reactions reappear.
- Seeks to attempt more advanced activities and to progress on to circuits within the gymnasium.

Week 2

- Attention-seeking behaviour reduces as patient discovers self-rewards.
- Complaints of pain and aching decrease and become extinguished.
- Patient will attempt previously painful activities.
- Seeks to join in and compete with others.
- Increased confidence levels are demonstrated.
- Independent adult behaviour is restored.

Week 3

- Returns to previous hobbies and lifestyle.
- Dawning recognition of previous state and expression of determination never to slide backward.
- Sets up own fitness programme for home.
- Can safely be weaned off the programme.

These recovery stages are illustrated by Mrs X, a 32-year-old who had spent 2 months in a neurological unit because of apparent loss of lower-limb motor function. She was eventually discharged home with a diagnosis of 'functional parapareisis'.

On *Day 1* she came to the gymnasium in a wheelchair and wearing her nightdress. She repeatedly collapsed, made gestures of pain and generally had a depressed air about her. She spent an hour in the gymnasium working individually to improve her standing balance and weight-transferance.

On *Day 2* she came in trousers and sweater, looked brighter and was chatting. Within the hour she had progressed to walking alone. The collapsing, staggering and overt pain gestures had ceased, but her gait still remained rigid and unnatural.

On *Day 3* began with the same gait pattern but as she was put into a wellness setting of a badminton game, with her stick being replaced by a racket, her trunk rotation suddenly reappeared. This was quickly followed by a series of spontaneous social gestures and normal balance reactions. Within 10 minutes of entering the gymnasium, she could walk on a 4in wide balance beam with confidence.

At *Week 3* she was a happy, confident, attractive young woman with a fun-loving stride and totally unrecognisable as the patient who arrived on Day 1.

Conclusion

The majority of patients, after 2 weeks on the 'School for Bravery' programme, will have almost extinguished their abnormal pain and illness behaviours. Their movements are no longer exaggerated or abnormal. They have ceased demonstrating continual pain signals and are moving and functioning normally. However, 70% of them will still describe themselves as having pain, but say they can cope and live with it. At this 2-week stage, these patients are still vulnerable and if they are given conventional physiotherapy or seen or reviewed by a doctor, they will immediately return to an illness state. The third week is therefore vital if they are to complete the course satisfactorily and make the transition to a wellness state and maintain it.

When patients have been interviewed following completion of their programme, it is quite evident that very few of them have any idea of the nature of their problem. Almost all of them believe it to have been physical and continue to do so. All of them admit to having been deeply depressed.

The 'School for Bravery' approach demonstrates that if patients are treated as if they are well and normal, and they are conscious of this as a positive experience, they will become so. Good health is a mind and body phenomenon and physiotherapists need expertise and skills in both areas. The 'School for Bravery' allows physiotherapists to combine behavioural assessment techniques with their traditional skills to produce an exciting and powerful tool for rehabilitation and ongoing good health.

References

Bergquist-Ullman and Larsson (1977). Acute low back pain in industry – a controlled prospective study with special reference to therapy and confounding factors. *ACTA. Orthop. Scand.*, **170**, 1–117.

Hannington-Kiff (1981) *Pain*, Update Books, London.

Bibliography

Ahles, T., Cassens, H.L. and Stalling, R.B. (1987). Private body consciousness, anxiety and the perception of pain. *Journal of Behavioural Therapy and Experimental Psychiatry*, **18**, 215–222.

Barsky, A.J. and Klerman, G.L. (1983). Hypochondriasis, bodily complaints and somatic styles. *American Journal of Psychiatry*, **140**, 273–283.

Beers, T.M. and Karoly, P. (1979). Cognitive strategies, expectancy and coping style in the control of pain. *Journal of Consultative Clinical Psychology*, **47**, 179–180.

Brands, A.M.E.F. and Schmidt, A.J.M. (1987). Learning processes in the persistence behaviour of chronic low back pain patients with repeated acute pain stimulation. *Pain*, **30**, 329–337.

Broadbent, D.E. (1958). *Perception and Communication*. Pergamon Press, London.

Ciccone, D.S. and Grzesiak, R.C. (1984). Cognitive dimensions of chronic pain. *Social Science Medicine*, **19**, 1339–1345.

Fernandez, E. (1986). A classification system of cognitive coping strategies for pain. *Pain*, **26**, 141–151.

Fernandez, E. and Turk, D.C. (1989). The utility of cognitive coping strategies for altering pain perception: a meta-analysis. *Pain*, **38**, 123–135.

Feuerstein, M., Papciak, A.S. and Hoon, P.E. (1987). Biobehavioural mechanisms of chronic low back pain. *Clinical Psychiatric Reviews*, 7, 243–273.

Fordyce, W.E. (ed) (1976). *Behavioural Methods for Chronic Pain and Illness*, Mosby, St Louis, MO.

Fordyce, W.E., Roberts, A.H. and Sternbach, R.A. (1985). The behavioural management of chronic pain: a response to critics. *Pain*, 22, 113–125.

Gill, K.M., Keefe, F.J., Crisson, J.E. and Van Dalfsen, P.J. (1987). Social support and pain behaviour. *Pain*, 29, 209–217.

Kanfer, F.H. and Philips, J.S. (1970). *Learning Foundations of Behaviour Therapy*. Wiley, New York.

Keefe, F.J., Wilkins, R.H. and Cook, W.A. (1984). Direct observation of pain behaviour in low back pain patients during physical examination. *Pain*, 20, 49–54.

Keefe, F.J. and Gil, K.M. (1985). Recent advances in the behavioural assessment and treatment of chronic pain. *Annals of Behavioural Medicine*, 7, 11–16.

Keefe, F.J., Wilkins, R.H., Cook, W.A., Crisson, J.E. and Muhlbaier, L.H. (1986). Depression, pain and pain behaviour. *Consultative Clinical Psychology*, 54, 665–669.

Keefe, F.J., Bradley, L.A. and Crisson, J.E. (1989). Behavioural assessment of low back pain: identification of pain behaviour subgroups. *Pain*, 40, 153–160.

McGill, J.C., Lawlis, G.F. *et al.* (1983). The relationship of Minnesota Multiphasic Personality Inventory (MMPI) profile clusters to pain behaviours. *Journal of Behavioural Medicine*, 6, 77–92.

Porter, R.W., Ellingworth, C.M., Hughes, T. and Trailescu, F. (1989). *Assessment of a 'School for Bravery'*, *Back Pain*. Manchester University Press.

Schmidt, A.J.M. (1987). The behavioural management of pain: a criticism of a response. *Pain*, 30, 285–291.

Schmidt, A.J.M. and Brands, A.M.E.F. (1986). Persistence behaviour of chronic low back pain patients in an acute pain situation. *Journal of Psychosomatic Research*, 30, 339–346.

Schmidt, A.J.M., Gierlings, R.E.H. and Peters, M.L. (1989). Environmental and interoceptive influences on chronic low back pain behaviour. *Pain*, 38, 137–143.

Sternbach, R.A. (1974). *Pain Patients, Traits and Treatment*. Academic Press, New York.

Williams, J.I. (1989). Illness behaviour to wellness behaviour: the School for Bravery Approach. *Physiotherapy*, 75, no 1.

Acknowledgement

The author expresses her thanks to Mrs J.I. Williams, BA, FCSP, DIP TP, for her help and advice throughout the years involved with the establishment of the 'School for Bravery' and also for granting permission to use material from her article published in 1989.

Index